HANDBOOK OF CANINE AND FELINE EMERGENCY PROTOCOLS

Handbook of Canine and Feline Emergency Protocols

Editor:

Stephen Rego, Ph.D.

Delve Publishing
www.delvepublishing.com

Handbook of Canine and Feline Emergency Protocols
Editor: **Stephen Rego, Ph.D.**

708 3rd Avenue, 6th Floor
New York, NY 10017
United States of America
www.delvepublishing.com

ISBN: 978-1-68095-866-9

Library of Congress Control Number: 2016951619

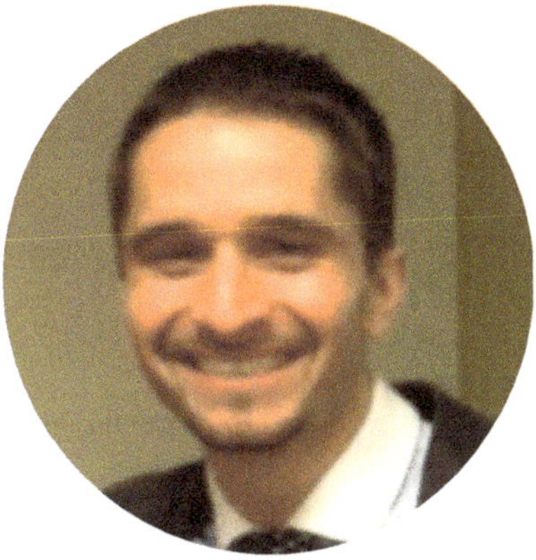

About the Editor

Stephen Rego, Ph.D.

Stephen obtained his PhD from the University of North Carolina at Charlotte in 2013 where his graduate research focused on cancer immunology and the tumor microenvironment. He received postdoctoral training in regenerative and translational medicine, specifically gastrointestinal tissue engineering, at the Wake Forest Institute of Regenerative Medicine. Currently, Stephen is an instructor for anatomy and physiology and biology at Forsyth Technical Community College.

Contents

List of Contributors

Alice Critti
Departamento de Ciências Veterinárias, Universidade Lusófona de Humanidades e Tecnologia, HVA - Hospital Veterinário da Arrábida, Portugal

João Requicha
Departamento de Ciências Veterinárias, Universidade Lusófona de Humanidades e Tecnologia, HVA - Hospital Veterinário da Arrábida, Portugal

Ângela Martins
Departamento de Ciências Veterinárias, Universidade Lusófona de Humanidades e Tecnologia, HVA - Hospital Veterinário da Arrábida, Portugal

Marcela da Costa Gomes
School of Veterinary Medicine and Animal Science, Universidade Estadual Paulista "Júlio de Mesquita Filho", Botucatu, SP, Brazil

Noeme Sousa Rocha
Universidade Estadual Paulista "Júlio de Mesquita Filho", School of Veterinary Medicine and Animal Science, department of Veterinary Clinic, Botucatu, SP, Brazil

Adriana Tomoko Nishiya
Department of Pathology, School of Veterinary Medicine and Animal Science, University of São Paulo, Av. Prof. Dr. Orlando Marques de Paiva, 87, CEP 05508-270, São Paulo, Brazil

Cristina Oliveira Massoco
Department of Pathology, School of Veterinary Medicine and Animal Science, University of São Paulo, Av. Prof. Dr. Orlando Marques de Paiva, 87, CEP 05508-270, São Paulo, Brazil

Claudia Ronca Felizzola
Department of Pathology, School of Veterinary Medicine and Animal Science, University of São Paulo, Av. Prof. Dr. Orlando Marques de Paiva, 87, CEP 05508-270, São Paulo, Brazil
Surgical Oncology Rua Antônio Alves Magan, 124, CEP 01251-150, São Paulo, Brazil

Eduardo Perlmann
Department of Surgery, School of Veterinary Medicine and Animal Science, University of São Paulo, CEP 05508-270, São Paulo, Brazil

Karen Batschinski
Department of Pathology, School of Veterinary Medicine and Animal Science, University of São Paulo, Av. Prof. Dr. Orlando Marques de Paiva, 87, CEP 05508-270, São Paulo, Brazil

Marcello Vannucci Tedardi
Department of Pathology, School of Veterinary Medicine and Animal Science, University of São Paulo, Av. Prof. Dr. Orlando Marques de Paiva, 87, CEP 05508-270, São Paulo, Brazil

Jéssica Soares Garcia
Department of Pathology, School of Veterinary Medicine and Animal Science, University of São Paulo, Av. Prof. Dr. Orlando Marques de Paiva, 87, CEP 05508-270, São Paulo, Brazil

Priscila Pedra Mendonça
Department of Surgery, School of Veterinary Medicine and Animal Science, University of São Paulo, CEP 05508-270, São Paulo, Brazil

Tarso Felipe Teixeira
Pathology Veterinary Medicine, FEPI Itajubá University Center, Dr. Antonio Braga Filho Street, 687, Itajubá, 37.501-002 Minas Gerais, Brazil

Maria Lucia Zaidan Dagli
Department of Pathology, School of Veterinary Medicine and Animal Science, University of São Paulo, Av. Prof. Dr. Orlando Marques de Paiva, 87, CEP 05508-270, São Paulo, Brazil

Nikolaos Dervisis
Virginia Maryland College of Veterinary Medicine, 245 Duck Pond Dr., Blacksburg, VA 24061, USA

Shawna Klahn
Virginia Maryland College of Veterinary Medicine, 245 Duck Pond Dr., Blacksburg, VA 24061, USA

Sparkes AH
The Feline Centre, School of Veterinary Sciences, University of Bristol, Langford House, Langford, Bristol BS40 SDU, UK
Veterinary Director, International Cat Care and International Society of Feline Medicine, Tisbury, UK

Tasker S
The Feline Centre, School of Veterinary Sciences, University of Bristol, Langford House, Langford, Bristol BS40 SDU, UK

Thibault JC
Merial, Lyon Gerland Laboratory, 254 rue Marcel Merieux, 69007 Lyon, France

Poulet H
Merial, Lyon Gerland Laboratory, 254 rue Marcel Merieux, 69007 Lyon, France

Jyotika Varshney
Masonic Cancer Center, University of Minnesota, Minneapolis, MN 55455, USA
Department of Surgery, University of Minnesota Medical School, Moos Tower, 11-212420 Delaware Street, S.E.; MMC 195, Minneapolis, MN 55455, USA

Milcah C. Scott
Masonic Cancer Center, University of Minnesota, Minneapolis, MN 55455, USA
Animal Cancer Care and Research Program, University of Minnesota, St. Paul, MN 55455, USA

Department of Veterinary Clinical Sciences, College of Veterinary Medicine, University of Minnesota, St. Paul, MN 55108, USA

David A. Largaespada
Masonic Cancer Center, University of Minnesota, Minneapolis, MN 55455, USA
Department of Pediatrics, University of Minnesota, Minneapolis, MN 55455, USA

Subbaya Subramanian
Masonic Cancer Center, University of Minnesota, Minneapolis, MN 55455, USA
Department of Surgery, University of Minnesota Medical School, Moos Tower, 11-212420 Delaware Street, S.E.; MMC 195, Minneapolis, MN 55455, USA

Shiho Usui
School of Agriculture, Meiji University, Kawasaki, Japan

Hidemi Yasuda
Spectrum Lab Japan, Midorigaoka, Meguro-ku, Tokyo, Japan

Yuzo Koketsu
School of Agriculture, Meiji University, Kawasaki, Japan

Marina Mickael
Marshall University School of Pharmacy, West Virginia, USA

Eric Morris
Marshall University School of Pharmacy, West Virginia, USA

Mollie M Roush
Marshall University School of Pharmacy, West Virginia, USA

Inder Sehgal
Marshall University School of Pharmacy, West Virginia, USA

August S. Bassani
Professional Compounding Centers of America (PCCA), Houston, Texas, USA

Daniel Banov
Professional Compounding Centers of America (PCCA), Houston, Texas, USA

Chris Simmons
Professional Compounding Centers of America (PCCA), Houston, Texas, USA

Ha Phan
Professional Compounding Centers of America (PCCA), Houston, Texas, USA

Miyu Mercier
VCA Aurora Animal Hospital, 2600 West Galena Blvd, Aurora, Illinois, 60506, USA

Heidi L. Barnes Heller
VCA Aurora Animal Hospital, 2600 West Galena Blvd, Aurora, Illinois, 60506, USA

Mickael Weber
Royal Canin Research Center, Aimargues, France

Laura Sams
Royal Canin Research Center, Aimargues, France

Alexandre Feugier
Royal Canin Research Center, Aimargues, France

Sandrine Michel
Royal Canin Research Center, Aimargues, France

Vincent Biourge
Royal Canin Research Center, Aimargues, France

Kristin Kirkby Shaw
Animal Surgical Clinic of Seattle, Seattle, Washington, USA

Lesley C. Rausch-Derra
Aratana Therapeutics, Inc., Kansas City, Kansas, USA

Linda Rhodes
Aratana Therapeutics, Inc., Kansas City, Kansas, USA

Rachael Thomas
Department of Molecular Biomedical Sciences, College of Veterinary Medicine & Center for Comparative Medicine and Translational Research, North Carolina State University, Raleigh NC 27607, USA

Domenico Santoro
Department of Small Animal Clinical Sciences, College of Veterinary Medicine, University of Florida, Gainesville, FL 32610, USA

Rosanna Marsella
Department of Small Animal Clinical Sciences, College of Veterinary Medicine, University of Florida, Gainesville, FL 32610, USA

Micaela Cipolla
Department of Veterinary Science and Public Health (DIVET), Università degli Studi di Milano, via Celoria 10, 20133 Milano, Italy

Luigi Bonizzi
Department of Veterinary Science and Public Health (DIVET), Università degli Studi di Milano, via Celoria 10, 20133 Milano, Italy

Alfonso Zecconi
Department of Veterinary Science and Public Health (DIVET), Università degli Studi di Milano, via Celoria 10, 20133 Milano, Italy

Alan Wells
University of Pittsburgh, USA

Mariely Lima
Superior School of Education Paula Frassinetti, Portugal

Karine Silva
University of Porto, Portugal

Preface

Canine and feline emergency protocols are important topics in veterinary medicine and will be commonly utilized by anyone entering the field. With the broad scope of topics associated with canine and feline emergency protocols this book provides an array of articles covering various topics including, trauma, cancer, diabetes, thyroid disease, skin disease, meningoencephalomyelitis, pain and inflammation and allergies. This book may interest both lay and professional individuals interested in furthering their understanding of a wide array of emergency veterinary topics. The final section of this book discusses innovative strategies that may one day be widely used in the field of emergency veterinary medicine, namely stem cells. Additionally, the utilization of animals in primary human care facilities is introduced as a way to connect pets to human health. The text is comprised of seventeen chapters. First chapter presents an overview on the application of cold intermittent pneumatic compression in the rehabilitation of multiple trauma dogs and cats or after surgery. Second chapter aimed at verifying the morphologic expression of parameters used in the cytopathological diagnosis of spontaneous OSAs in dogs of several breeds, including mixed-breeds. It also aimed at analyzing the possible concordance between cytopathological and histopathological parameters of these bone neoplasms. The aim of third chapter is to report a comparative approach of the etiological, epidemiological, pathological, and molecular aspects of melanomas in dogs. Chapter four and chapter five highlights therapeutic innovations, and the efficacy of a non-adjuvanted canarypox virus vectored vaccine and a sub-unit vaccine individually. Sixth chapter attempts to address many of the unanswered questions pertaining to osteosarcoma by focusing on recently acquired knowledge from a multi-species approach. Furthermore, the objective of the seventh chapter was to characterize DM in dogs by using a mixed-effects modelling approach to identify characteristic factors and estimate their effects. Chapter eight covers the most common endocrine diseases of dogs and cats and in vitro characterization of the percutaneous absorption of tramadol into inner ear domestic feline skin using the franz skin finite dose model has been presented in ninth chapter. A prospective study on the efficacy of glucocorticoid monotherapy for treatment of canine meningoencephalomyelitis of unknown etiology is presented in chapter ten. The aim of eleventh chapter was to assess the impact of psyllium husk and the influence of different levels of total dietary fibre on faecal hair excretion in short and LH cats by directly measuring hair in their faeces. Twelfth chapter reviews the mechanism of action of anti-inflammatory drugs for use in animals and introduce the first-in-class drug for managing pain and inflammation associated with osteoarthritis (OA) in veterinary patients: grapiprant, an EP4 prostaglandin receptor antagonist (PRA). Thirteenth chapter provides an overview on advances and opportunities of cytogenomics of feline cancers, and fourteenth chapter discusses the various models by focusing on the primary manifestation of allergy. Fifteenth chapter examines the role of health communication and sixteenth chapter represents a new approach to cellular support for dysrepair. Last chapter shows that owning a pet dog can have prophylactic and therapeutic value, but that incorporating these animals into clinical practice, can have a number of benefits for different types of patients. Dogs can also fill the role of assistants for people with disabilities, bringing important physical, psychological and social positive effects for their handlers, and even be trained to alert to seizures in epileptic patients and to changes in blood sugar levels in diabetics. In light of this, a significant "push" is currently being made by a number of researchers to integrate dogs into mainstream healthcare, notably through family medicine.

Editor

Stephen Rego, Ph.D.

INTRODUCTION

There are two canines in each jaw, each situated between the second incisor and the first premolar. In some animals (e.g. herbivores, such as giraffes and rabbits) canine teeth are absent. "canine tooth." A Dictionary of Biology. . "canine tooth."

Canidae

The biological family Canidae is a lineage of carnivorans that includes domestic dogs, wolves, foxes, jackals, dingoes, and many other extant and extinct dog-like mammals. A member of this family is called a canid.

The cat-like feliforms and dog-like caniforms emerged within the Carnivoramorpha 43 million years before present. The caniforms included the fox-like Leptocyon genus whose various species existed from 34 million years before present before branching 11.9 million YBP into Vulpini (foxes) and Canini (canines).

Canids are found on all continents except Antarctica, having arrived independently or accompanied human beings over extended periods of time. Canids vary in size from the 2-m-long (6 ft 7 in) gray wolf to the 24-cm-long (9.4 in) fennec fox. The body forms of canids are similar, typically having long muzzles, upright ears, teeth adapted for cracking bones and slicing flesh, long legs, and bushy tails. They are mostly social animals, living together in family units or small groups and behaving cooperatively. Typically, only the dominant pair in a group breeds, and a litter of young is reared annually in an underground den. Canids communicate by scent signals and by vocalizations. They are very intelligent. One canid, the domestic dog (including the dingo), long ago entered into a partnership with humans and today remains one of the most widely kept domestic animals.

Taxonomy

All living canids as a group form a monophyletic relationship with the extinct borophagines through both groups having a bicuspid (two points) on the lower carnassial talonid, which gives this tooth an additional ability in mastication. This together with the development of a distinct entoconid cusp and the broadening of the talonid of the first lower molar, and the corresponding enlargement of the talon of the upper first molar and reduction of its parastyle distinguish these late Cenozoic canids and are the essential differences that identify their clade.

Phylogenetic relationships

Skulls of various Canid genera; Vulpes (corsac fox), Nyctereutes (raccoon dog), Cuon (dhole) and Canis (golden jackal)

Within the Canidae, the results of allozyme and chromosome analyses have suggested several phylogenetic divisions:

The wolf-like canids, (genus Canis, Cuon and Lycaon) including the dog (Canis lupus familiaris), gray wolf (Canis lupus), red wolf (Canis rufus), eastern wolf (Canis lycaon), coyote (Canis latrans), golden jackal (Canis aureus), Ethiopian wolf (Canis simensis), black-backed jackal (Canis mesomelas), side-striped jackal (Canis adustus), dhole (Cuon alpinus), and African wild dog (Lycaon pictus).

The fox-like canids, which include the kit fox (Vulpes aelox), red fox (Vulpes vulpes), Cape fox (Vulpes chama), Arctic fox (Vulpes lagopus), and fennec fox (Vulpes zerda).

The South American canids, including the bush dog (Speothos venaticus), hoary fox (Lycalopex uetulus), crab-eating fox (Cerdocyon thous) and maned wolf.

Various monotypic taxa, including the bat-eared fox (Otocyon megalotis), gray fox (Urocyon cinereoargenteus), and raccoon dog (Nycteruetes procyonoides)

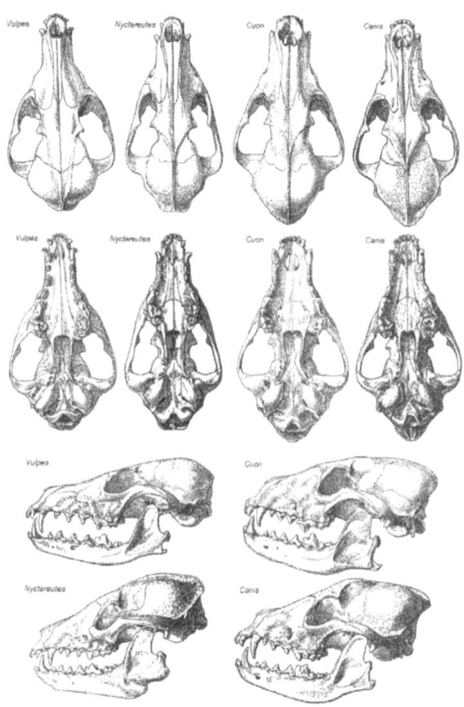

DNA analysis shows that the first three form monophyletic clades. The wolf-like canids and the fox-like canids together form the tribe Canini. Molecular data imply a North American origin of living Canidae some ten million years ago and an African origin of wolf-like canines (Canis, Cuon, and Lycaon), with the jackals being the most basal of this group. The South American clade is rooted by the maned wolf and bush dog, and the fox-like canids by the fennec fox and Blanford's fox. The grey fox and island fox are basal to the other clades, however this topological difference is not strongly supported.

Evolution

The Canidae today includes a diverse group of some 34 species ranging in size from the maned wolf with its long limbs to the short-legged bush dog. Modern canids inhabit forests, tundra, savannahs and deserts throughout tropical and temperate parts of the world. The evolutionary relationships between the species have been studied in the past using morphological approaches but more recently, molecular studies have enabled the investigation of phylogenetic relationships. In some species, genetic divergence has been suppressed by the high level of gene flow between different populations and where the species have hybridized, large hybrid zones exist

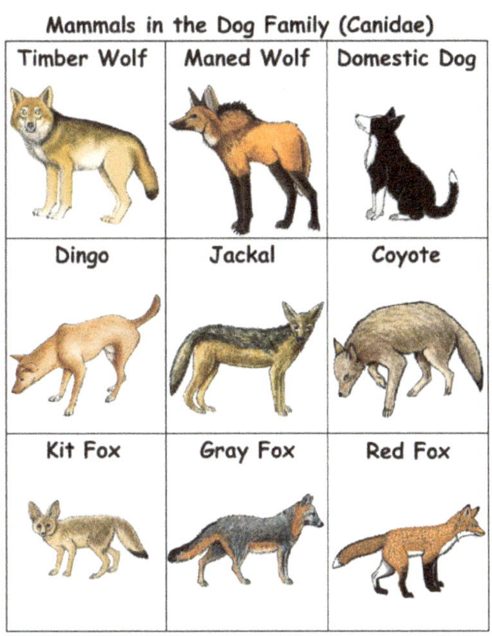

Characteristics

Wild canids are found on every continent except Antarctica, and inhabit a wide range of different habitats, including deserts, mountains, forests, and grasslands. They vary in size from the fennec fox, which may be as little as 24 cm (9.4 in) in length and weigh 0.6 kg (1.3 lb), to the gray wolf, which may be up to 160 cm (5.2 ft) long, and can weigh up to 79 kg (174 lb). Only a few species are arboreal – the North American gray fox, the closely related Channel Island fox,[24] and the raccoon dog habitually climb trees.

All canids have a similar basic form, as exemplified by the grey wolf, although the relative length of muzzle, limbs, ears and tail vary considerably between species. With the exceptions of the bush dog, raccoon dog, and some domestic breeds of Canis lupus, canids have relatively long legs and lithe bodies, adapted for chasing prey. The tails are bushy and the length and quality of the pelage varies with the season. The muzzle portion of the skull is much more elongated than that of the cat family. The zygomatic arches are wide, there is a transverse lambdoidal ridge at the rear of the cranium and in some species, a sagittal crest running from front to back. The bony orbits around the eye never form a complete ring and the auditory bullae are smooth and rounded.

All canids are digitigrade, meaning they walk on their toes. The tip of the nose is always naked, as are the cushioned pads on the soles of the feet. These latter consist of a single pad behind the tip of each toe and a more-or-less three-lobed central pad under the roots of the digits. Hairs grow between the pads and in the Arctic fox, the sole of the foot is densely covered with hair at some times of year. With the exception of the four-toed African hunting dog (Lycaon pictus), there are five toes on the forefeet but the pollex (thumb) is reduced and does not reach the ground. On the hind feet, there are four toes, but in some domestic dogs, a fifth vestigial toe, known as a dewclaw, is sometimes present but has no anatomical connection to the rest of the foot. The slightly curved nails are non-retractile and more or less blunt.

The penis in male canids is supported by a bone called the baculum. It also contains a structure at the base called the bulbus glandis which helps to create a copulatory tie during mating, locking the animals together for up to an hour. Young canids are born blind, with their eyes opening a few weeks after birth. All living canids (Caninae) have a ligament analogous to the nuchal ligament of ungulates used to maintain the posture of the head and neck with little active muscle exertion; this ligament allows them to conserve energy while running long distances following scent trails with their nose to the ground. However, based on skeletal details of the neck, at least some Borophaginae (such as Aelurodon) are believed to have lacked this ligament.

Social behavior

Almost all canids are social animals and live together in groups. In general, they are territorial or have a home range and sleep in the open, using their dens only for breeding and sometimes in bad weather. In most foxes, and in many of the true dogs, a male and female pair work together to hunt and to raise their young. Gray wolves and some of the other larger canids live in larger groups called packs. African wild dogs have packs which may consist of twenty to forty animals, and packs of fewer than about seven individuals may be incapable of successful reproduction. Hunting in packs has the advantage that larger prey items can be tackled. Some species form packs or live in small family groups depending on the circumstances, including the type of available food. In most species, some individuals live on their own. Within a canid pack, there is a system of dominance so that the strongest, most experienced animals lead the pack. In most cases, the dominant male and female are the only pack members to breed.

Canids communicate with each other by scent signals, by visual clues and gestures, and by vocalizations such as growls, barks, and howls. In most cases, groups have a home territory from which they drive out other conspecifics. The territory is marked by leaving urine scent marks, which warn trespassing individuals. Social behaviour is also mediated by secretions from glands on the upper surface of the tail near its root and from the anal glands.

Reproduction

Canids as a group exhibit several reproductive traits that are uncommon among mammals as a whole. They are typically monogamous, provide paternal care to their offspring, have reproductive cycles with lengthy proestral and dioestral phases and have a copulatory tie during mating. They also retain adult offspring in the social group, suppressing the ability of these to breed while making use of the alloparental care they can provide to help raise the next generation of offspring.

During the proestral period, increased levels of oestradiol make the female attractive to the male. There is a rise in progesterone during the oestral phase and the female is now receptive. Following this, the level of oestradiol fluctuates and there is a lengthy dioestrous phase during which the female is pregnant. Pseudo-pregnancy frequently occurs in canids that have ovulated but failed to conceive. A period of anoestrus follows pregnancy or pseudo-pregnancy, there being only one oestral period during each breeding season. Small and medium-sized canids mostly have a gestation period of fifty to sixty days while larger species average sixty to sixty-five days. The time of year in which the breeding season occurs is related to the length of day, as has been demonstrated in the case of several species that have been translocated across the equator to the other hemisphere and experiences a six-month shift of phase. Domestic dogs and certain small canids in captivity may come into oestrus more frequently, perhaps because the photoperiod stimulus breaks down under conditions of artificial lighting. The size of a litter varies, with from one to sixteen or more pups being born. The young are born small, blind and helpless and require a long period of parental care. They are kept in a den, most often dug into the ground, for warmth and protection. When the young begin eating solid food, both parents, and often other pack members, bring food back for them from the hunt. This is most often vomited up from the adult's stomach. Where such pack involvement in the feeding of the litter occurs, the breeding success rate is higher than is the case where females split from the group and rear their pups in isolation. Young canids may take a year to mature and learn the skills they need to survive. In some species, such as the African wild dog, male offspring usually remain in the natal pack, while females disperse as a group, and join another small group of the opposite sex to form a new pack.

Feline

Feline (family Felidae), any of 37 cat species that among others include the cheetah, puma, jaguar, leopard, lion, lynx, tiger, and domestic cat. Cats are native to almost every region on Earth, with the exception of Australia and Antarctica. They are carnivorous mammals that live in a wide variety of habitats, but they are typically woodland animals.

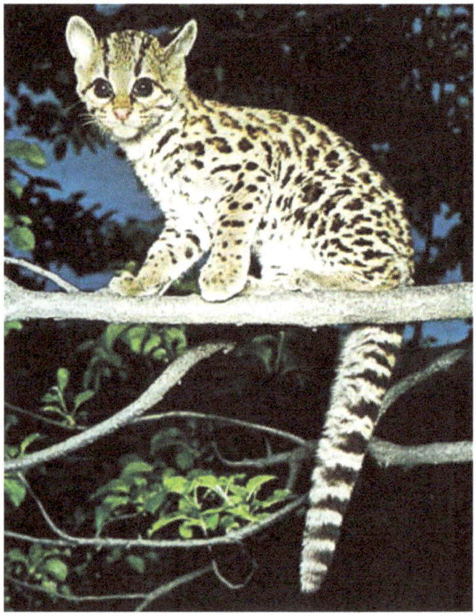

Most cats are patterned with spots, stripes, or rosettes, but some, such as the puma (Puma concolor), jaguarundi (Herpailurus yaguarondi), and lion (Panthera leo), are uniform in colour. Black or nearly black coats occur in individuals of several species. Although lynx (genus Lynx) have a stubby tail, most cats have a long tail that makes up about a third of the animal's total length. The head is characterized by a short nose and round face, usually with short ears. The only cat with a well-developed mane is the male African lion. Cat feet have sharp claws that are retractile except in the cheetah. In most felids the male is larger than the female.

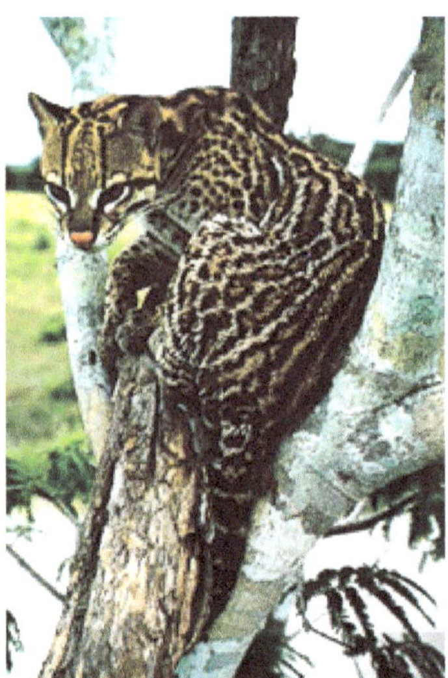

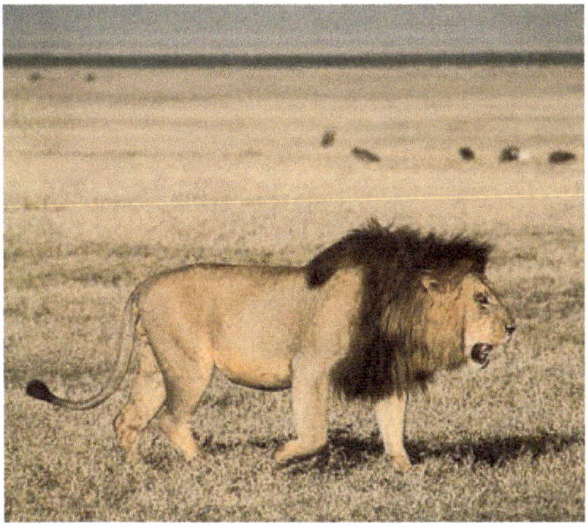

Cats are noted for purring when content and for snarling, howling, or spitting when in conflict with another of their kind. The so-called "big cats" (genus Panthera), especially the lion, often roar, growl, or shriek. Usually, however, cats are silent. Many cats use "clawing trees," upon which they leave the marks of their claws as they stand and drag their front feet downward with the claws extended. Whether such behavior is for the purpose of cleaning or sharpening the claws or simply to stretch is debatable, but the behavior is innate; kittens raised in isolation soon begin to claw objects.

The larger cats are strong, fierce, and extremely dangerous when hungry. Because of their large size, they occasionally attack humans. Although tigers and leopards are most noted as man-eaters, lions and jaguars can also be dangerous. In North America the puma, also known as the cougar or mountain lion, tends to avoid contact with humans, but a few attacks occur annually, especially in areas where development encroaches on areas of high puma density, such as the western United States. Similarly, attacks on livestock often necessitate removal of problem animals.

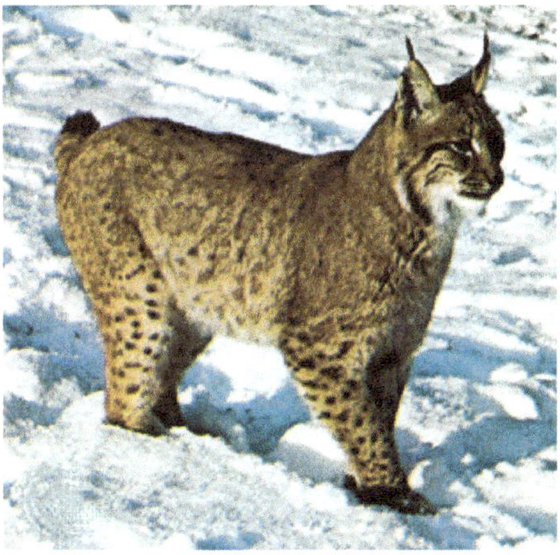

The fur of some cats is sometimes in great demand, especially fur with contrasting colours and patterns such as spots or stripes. The demand is such that some rare cats are hunted and trapped illegally and are in danger of becoming extinct. In North America none of the cats used by the fur trade is endangered. Strict regulations allow a sustainable take of animals from healthy populations of Canada lynx (Lynx canadensis), bobcat (Lynx rufus), and puma.

Form and Function

The agility of a cat is evident in its anatomy. The clavicle, or collarbone, is much reduced in size. It does not connect with other bones but is buried in the muscles of the shoulder region. This allows the animal to spring on its prey without danger of breaking the bone. The hind legs are well developed, with powerful muscles that propel the cat in its spring toward or onto prey. In addition to the power of the hind legs, the animal uses strong back muscles to straighten the spinal column and provide extra force in springing and running.

Cats are generally nocturnal in habit. Their large eyes are especially adapted for seeing at night. The retina has a layer of guanine called the tapetum lucidum, which reflects light and causes the eyes to shine at night when illuminated. Cats have good senses of sight and hearing, but their sense of smell is not as developed as that of the canids, a fact suggested by the cat's short snout.

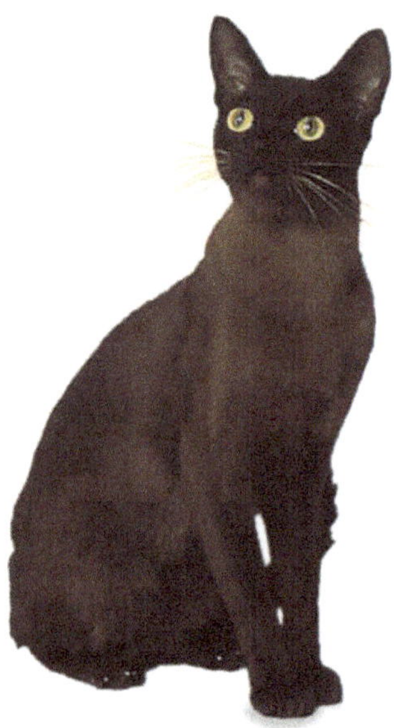

A predisposition to cleanliness is well established among cats. They groom themselves with their rasping tongue, preening at length after a meal. Feces and urine are covered as a matter of habit. Cats differ in their reaction to water; most species are reluctant to enter it but will swim readily when necessary. Nervous tail wagging is common to all cats, from the lion to the house cat. Kittens learn it from the mother; the behavior is associated with play, which is a prelude to predation as an adult. Cats are the most highly specialized of the terrestrial flesh-eating mammals. They are powerfully built, with a large brain and strong teeth. The teeth are adapted to three functions: stabbing (canines), anchoring (canines), and cutting (carnassial molars). Cats have no flat-crowned crushing teeth and thus do not chew or grind their food but instead cut it. All cats are adapted to be strict flesh eaters, an assumption made primarily on the basis of their digestive tract and dentition. In keeping with a carnivorous habit, the cat has a simple gut; the small intestine is only about three times the length of the body. The tongue in all cats has a patch of sharp, backward-directed spines near the tip, which has the appearance and feel of a coarse file; these spines help the cat lap up liquids and groom itself. There are five padded toes on the front foot and four on the rear. The first toe and its pad on the front foot are raised so that only four toes register in a track.

Cats have a reduced number of premolar and molar teeth; the typical dental formula includes only 30 teeth. The incisors are small and chisel-like, the canines long and pointed. The premolars are sharp, and occasionally an upper premolar may be lacking. The lower molar is elongate and sharp, the upper molar rudimentary. Because of the reduction in the number and size of the cheek teeth, a space remains between the canines and premolars in all cats except the cheetah. Felids form the most strictly carnivorous group in the order Carnivora, and the highly developed carnassial teeth reflect this specialized food habit. There is little if any specialization in the teeth for grinding or chewing. The strong masseter muscles, which raise the lower jaw, restrict lateral movement. The jaw primarily moves vertically for holding the prey in a viselike grip and for slicing off pieces of meat with the carnassials. Meat is thus cut off and swallowed in relatively unchewed chunks that are broken down by strong enzymes and acids in the digestive tract.

Evolution and Classification

The history of the cat family can be traced through the fossil record to the Late Eocene Epoch (about 37 million years ago). The "cat pattern" seems to have been established very early in the evolution of mammals, for the early cats were already typical cats at a time when the ancestors of most other modern mammalian species were scarcely recognizable. Cats of the subfamily Felinae appeared in western Eurasia about 10 million years ago and have continued almost unchanged into modern times. Genetic studies examining living and fossil pantherines—cats of the subfamily Pantherinae—suggest that the pantherine lineage emerged in central Asia some 16 million years ago and subsequently spread to other continents.

Canine and Feline Emergency protocol

Donor selection

Canine blood donors

Canine donors should be healthy, well-tempered, large breed dogs weighing at least 25 kg to allow collection of blood in standard human collection bags. Many blood donor programmers set an age limit of 1–8 years, with use of dogs older than the age limit at the discretion of the veterinary surgeon after careful evaluation of the donor. The dogs should receive routine veterinary preventative health care, including vaccination according to practice protocols. They should not be receiving any medication at the time of donation with the exception of flea preventive, routine worming medication or heartworm preventative (location specific). As blood is most frequently obtained from the jugular vein, consideration should be given to the conformation of the dog and venous access. It is preferable to use dogs that will remain still with minimal restraint during the blood collection procedure, avoiding sedation and possible adverse consequences of its use.

Feline blood donors

Feline donors should be clinically healthy cats between the ages of 1 and 8 years, receiving routine veterinary preventative health care. They should weigh at least 4 kg. Unlike canine donors, cats usually require sedation for the donation; however, they should still be of an agreeable temperament to allow transportation to the veterinary surgery and handling for administration of the sedative. Given the problems with naturally occurring alloantibodies in cats (see Feline blood types) it is essential that all feline donors as well as recipients be blood typed prior to collecting blood to prevent incompatibility of mismatched transfusions. To ensure that feline donors are in good health, haematology, serum biochemistry and infectious disease screening for feline leukaemia virus (FeLV) (serology), feline immunodeficiency virus (FIV) (serology) and Mycoplasma haemofelis (polymerase chain reaction (PCR)) are evaluated each year. Cats that are positive for infectious diseases should not be used as donors. Furthermore, to have confidence in the maintenance of a negative disease status, it is preferable to use only cats that are confined to living indoors.

Blood types

Red blood cell types are determined by speciesspecific, inherited antigens present on the cell surface. Blood type incompatibility is observed clinically as transfusion reactions or neonatal isoerythrolysis, the occurrence and severity of which is variable between individuals and species. The frequency of canine and feline blood types varies with geographical location and breed. Although the published population incidence of various blood types may offer the verterinary surgeon guidance, it is based on surveys with limited animal numbers and may not be applicable to the individual animal in question.

Canine blood types

Many systems are used to describe the blood groups of dogs; however, the dog erythrocyte antigen (DEA) nomenclature is most widely in use in the current literature. Typing antisera exist for 6 DEAs (1.1, 1.2, 3, 4, 5 and 7). For all of the DEA groups, a dog may be positive or negative. The DEA 1 group has at least two subtypes, DEA 1.1 and 1.2. A third subtype, DEA 1.3, has been described but not yet extensively evaluated due to lack of typing antisera. A dog may be positive for only one of these DEA 1 subtypes, or it may be negative for all three. The relevance of blood type is related to its antigenic potential. The most antigenic blood type is DEA 1.1; however there are no naturally occurring alloantibodies against DEA 1.1. As such, most dogs will not experience a severe transfusion reaction from a first transfusion of DEA 1.1-incompatible blood. However, sensitization occurs in DEA 1.1-negative dogs that receive DEA 1.1-positive cells. Antibodies (strong haemolysins and agglutinins) are produced which can cause an acute haemolytic transfusion reaction following repeated antigen exposure (e.g. a second transfusion with DEA 1.1-positive blood). Additionally in some of these dogs a delayed haemolytic transfusion reaction may occur more than 9 days after the first transfusion, as antibody production increases. Production of antibodies to other red cell antigens may develop in a sensitized recipient as early as 4 days after transfusion, emphasizing the importance of crossmatching donor and recipient samples prior to a second blood transfusion.

Feline blood type

Blood groups in cats are described by the A–B system, which includes three blood types: A, B and AB. The blood types are inherited as a simple dominant trait, with A being dominant over B. Genotypically type A cats are either homozygous a/a or heterozygous a/b; whereas type B cats are homozygous b/b. Type AB is a rare blood type in which a third allele is present, recessive to the a allele but dominant to the b allele, leading to expression of both A and B antigens. Mating studies have shown that type AB is not simply the result of mating a type A to a type B cat, but rather the type A cat must carry the rare allele for type AB blood. However this genetic pattern has not applied in all AB cats, and there is likely to be more than one mechanism for inheritance of this blood type

Collection, processing and storage of blood

Blood collection systems

All whole blood collection should take place in an aseptic manner and should use an appropriate anticoagulant. The anticoagulant solutions most often used are ACD (acid–citrate–dextrose), CPD (citrate–phosphate– dextrose) or CPDA-1 (citrate–phosphate–dextrose– adenine). Most of the commercially available blood collection systems contain either CPD or CPDA-1. ACD is more often used in open systems when collecting smaller volumes of blood. The volume of anticoagulant used and the duration of time for which the blood product can be stored varies depending on the composition of the anticoagulant and the collection method. ACD is used at a ratio of 1 ml of anticoagulant to 7–9 ml of blood and CPD and CPDA-1 are typically used in a ratio of 1 ml anticoagulant to 7 ml of blood. Use of other anticoagulants (e.g. sodium citrate, heparin) is not recommended. Whole blood may be collected using a closed or open collection system. A closed system is one in which the only exposure of the collection bag or its contents to air prior to administration is when the needle is uncapped to perform venipuncture during collection. Examples of a closed system are commercially available 450 ml blood collection bags containing 63 ml of CPD or CPDA-1 anticoagulant with an attached 16 gauge needle. These are most commonly used to collect blood from donor dogs weighing >25 kg. Multibag systems with empty transfer satellite bags and red cell preservative may be used for component processing. Packed red blood cells prepared from CPDA-1 closed-collection system processing have a storage life of 20 days when maintained at 1–6°C. Whole blood collected into CPD or CPDA-1 in a similar manner has a storage life of 28 days or 35 days respectively.

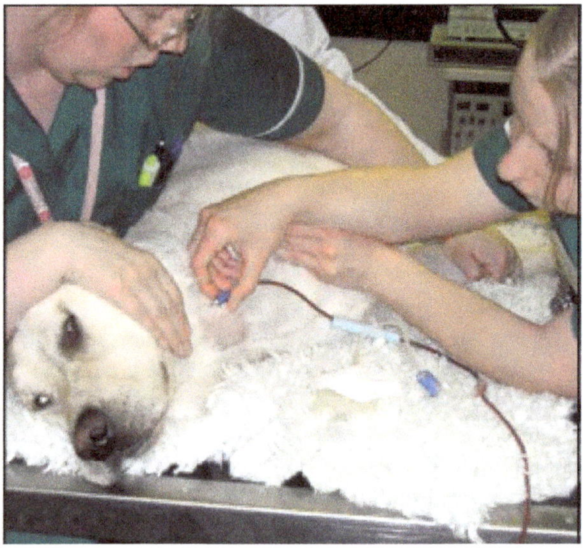

Monitoring transfusions

The following parameters should be measured prior to (baseline), every 15–30 minutes during, and 1, 12 and 24 hours after transfusion:

- Attitude
- Rectal temperature
- Pulse rate and quality
- Respiratory rate and character
- Mucous membrane color and CRT
- Plasma and urine color

The PCV/TP should also be monitored prior to, upon completion and at 12 and 24 hours after transfusion. It is helpful to design a transfusion monitoring sheet, with time points and monitoring parameters noted, to encourage diligent recording during and after the transfusion. Careful monitoring will allow for prompt recognition and treatment of transfusion reactions as well as evaluation of transfusion efficacy

Adverse reactions

Any undesired side effect noted as a consequence of a blood product transfusion is considered a transfusion reaction. The reported frequency of transfusion reactions is variable, as is their severity. Transfusion reactions may be classified as immunological (haemolytic or non-haemolytic) and non-immunological, as well as acute or delayed. Preventative measures necessary to minimize the risk of transfusion reactions include appropriate donor screening, collection, preparation, storage and administration of products. Adherence to standard protocols helps to ensure safety and efficacy of transfusions in practice.

Immunological transfusion reactions

The most concerning type of transfusion reaction is an acute haemolytic reaction with intravascular haemolysis. These are antigen–antibody, type II hypersensitivity reactions. This type of reaction is seen in type B cats receiving type A blood as well as DEA 1.1-negative dogs sensitized to DEA 1.1 upon repeated exposure. Clinical signs may include fever, tachycardia, dyspnoea, muscle tremors, vomiting, weakness, collapse, haemoglobinaemia and haemoglobinuria. These reactions may lead to shock, DIC, renal damage and, potentially, death.

Non-immunological transfusion reactions

Many non-immunological transfusion reactions have been described. Anaphylactoid reactions, which often result from too rapid an infusion rate, may be seen. They tend to subside after discontinuation of the transfusion or reduction of the infusion rate. Circulatory overload may occur in any patient receiving excessive volumes of blood products, or those with cardiac or renal disease. Treatment with diuretics may be required. Hypocalcaemia is identified most commonly following administration of large volumes of plasma or whole blood and is a result of citrate intoxication. Patients with impaired liver function are at greatest risk. Clinical signs of hypocalcaemia may be noted (vomiting, muscle tremors, tetany, electrocardiograph (ECG) changes) and treatment includes supplementation with calcium chloride or calcium gluconate. Other recognized non-immunological reactions include polycythaemia and hyperproteinaemia, hypothermia, coagulopathy, thrombosis, microbial contamination, hyperammonaemia, hypophosphataemia, hyperkalaemia, acidosis, pretransfusion (in vitro) haemolysis, haemosiderosis, air embolus and infectious disease transmission.

1
CHAPTER

COLD INTERMITTENT PNEUMATIC COMPRESSION: APPLICATION IN THE REHABILITATION OF MULTIPLE TRAUMA DOGS AND CATS OR AFTER SURGERY

Alice Critti, João Requicha and Ângela Martins

Keywords: Cold intermittent pneumatic compression technique, Rehabilitation, Cryotherapy, Postoperative, Multiple trauma, Dog, Cat, Pain management, Swelling

INTRODUCTION

Cryotherapy is one of the cheapest therapies and most used on postoperative inflammations, musculoskeletal trauma and muscle spasms, endorsing as well, structural and functional reconstruction, enhancing the rehabilitation process. However, this technique has some limitations in efficacy and TCFPI, being the combination of cryotherapy and compression, can fill those gaps and enables patients to gather the necessary physical conditions to achieve the best results within a shorter period of time.

TCFPI is applied with GameRead Accelerated Recovery System (CoolSystems, Inc., Concord, California, USA) which is an exclusive control unit that delivers an Active Compression and Cold Exchange Loop (ACCEL) by pumping water and air at each time to a hose which is connected to a wrap that is applied to the injured area. To control the system temperature, the unit container must be filled completely with ice and at least half full with clean water which will be pumped through the hose. The temperature, time and pressure applied will be regulated by knobs that can be adjusted by the operator of the control unit. Therefore, the temperature of the wrap will never be colder than the water in the ice box.

The therapeutic wraps allows a better displacement of the interstitial fluids removing them from the injured area, reducing swelling and muscle spasm and achieving a faster healing process. The appliance of those wraps also extends the application area for a better cold distribution and comfort for the patient during the treatment.

Citation: Critti A, Requicha J, Martins A (2016) Cold Intermittent Pneumatic Compression: Application in the Rehabilitation of Multiple Trauma Dogs and Cats or After Surgery. J Comm Pub Health Nurs 2:121. doi:10.4172/jcphn.1000121.

Hence, TCFPI, enables the temperature management during treatment, which can control the patients better at pain management, unlike any other techniques, also allowing a deeper cold penetration in a shorter time, letting cellular metabolism to lower secondary injuries.

Cold Appliance Effects in Rehabilitation

Cold is used on acute injury treatment since it minimizes the inflammatory process, stimulating analgesia [1-3].

The center responsible for controlling body temperature is located in the pre-optic region of the anterior hypothalamus which has cold sensitive neurons in quadruped animals. When the blood temperature is below than the regular levels, the cells located in the pre-optic region of the anterior hypothalamus will be inhibited, activating the hypothalamus producing heat which leads to trigger mechanisms that increase body temperature. In response , vasoconstriction occurs dropping skin temperature to room temperature and allowing a reduced heat loss which will result in temperature rising [4-6].

Tissues with high concentration of water, such as muscles, are excellent cold conductors unlike fat that has low conductivity. Ice has better penetration capacity (2 to 4 centimeters) and longer action when applying heat [7-10]. The reason lies in the thermodynamic properties and the impact of these when there is a physical change of state, in this case from solid to liquid. The heat transferred by contact with ice will be the amount of heat which is directly transferred to it and the heat exchange from the transition of physical state when ice melts into water. This leads to a decreased intramuscular temperature due to a greater heat transfer by ice that changes its state to liquid [11].

Cold Appliance Effects in Inflammation Control

Cold reduces the acute inflammatory process mostly in acute trauma, preventing blood leakage from capillaries and resulting in reduced synthesis of collagen and scar tissue [5,12].

Cold Appliance Effects in the Musculoskeletal System

In musculoskeletal injury during the acute inflammatory response due to vessel injury and swelling, occurs a drop of oxygen supply to healthy cells near the affected tissues. Thus, the cold's role is to reduce the metabolic rate of hypoxic tissues, allowing better survival odds in this period and minimizing secondary injury [5,12].

Multiple trauma patients are those with multiple injuries from the same incident. Young animals, both dogs and cats, are much more likely to be affected by traumatic processes because those individuals are more active, therefore, more liable to accidents. The application of cold in musculoskeletal injuries and multiple trauma patients aim to reduce pain, inflammation and the release of inflammatory mediators, helping tissue recovery after trauma and reducing the need for medicine consumption [1,13].

Cold Appliance Effects in Pain Control

Pain during ice massage is not as intense because the cold is applied in the form of scanning. Due to the temperature decrease, there is a reduced muscle activity and muscle relaxation, improving spasticity reduction and easing the kinesiotherapy exercises execution, neuroanatomically speaking, active cold inhibits Alpha motor neurons (α-MNs) contraction of the intrafusal fibers, allowing relaxation, avoiding pathological muscle co-contraction which may lead to hypertonicity and spasticity [1,11,14].

Cold Appliance Effects in the Circulatory System

When cold is applied to the affected area, heat transfers, induces vasoconstriction, reducing the amount of blood carried [12,13,15]. When vasoconstriction occurs the body responds with a dilatation of these vessels to maintain blood circulation. This phenomenon is called cold-induced vasodilation, improving metabolites removal and increasing gas exchange [12].

Cold Appliance Effects in Swelling Control

Cold application reduces vascular permeability, restraining leukocyte migration which means that there is contention on the liberation of free proteins process, avoiding edema formation [1].

Cold Appliance Effects in the Neuromuscular System

To reduce spasticity it is recommended cold application for 25 to 30 minutes, which is the time required to decrease excitatory impulses, promote muscle relaxation and reach deeper tissues. The relaxation effect lasts between 30 minutes to 2 hours and during this time, some kinesotherapy exercises workout can be performed, for example, cycling motion exercises, gait stimulation and hydrotherapy, to provide the patient a greater range to move out of the spastic pattern [16]. However, as cold acts directly on the muscle spindle and the Golgi tendon organ, it reduces the response of voluntary muscle contraction so, we must be especially careful with exercises and gait to avoid a new muscle injury due to the rupture of fibers [5,16,17].

PROCEDURES

Study Population

The study population comprised 61 animals, including cats and dogs. On 33 was applied TCFPI and 28 were subject of cryotherapy used as control of TCFPI.

Animals included in the study were those who (i) were presented in a critical situation, multiple trauma (pubic fractures and sacroiliac dislocation) and musculoskeletal disorders (edema), (ii) had undergone orthopedic surgery and had motor limitations (dislocation of the femoral head, dislocation of the humeral radio-ulnar joint and ruptured cruciate ligament), (iii) were submitted to soft tissue surgery at risk of hypovolemic shock due to hemorrhage (eg. splenectomy, mastectomy), and (iv) were submitted to neurological surgery to remove thoracolumbar hernias.

Protocol of TCFPI Application

TCFPI was held in an isolated room in order to calm down the patient for treatment and during execution the patient could never be unattended.

In post-surgical patients, TCFPI started only when the body temperature returned to stable values (minimum temperature of 37.4°C) then evaluate the degree of pain to determine the machine's application temperature. In multiple trauma patients, the TCFPI began immediately.

After surgery on the same day or the day of admission of multiple trauma patients, treatment was performed four times within a 6 hours interval. After this treatment period in the following week, this technique was carried out 3 times per day over a 6 hour interval. After the first week a reassessment of the patient's condition and a protocol adjustment if necessary, were made.

Orthopedic patients underwent longer treatments due to the fact that the surgeries are more invasive than the rest of the cases. With this it was possible to control the pain and reduce swelling in a gradual manner.

PAIN ASSESSMENT

Pain assessment was performed using the Glasgow Composite Measure Pain (GCMP) scale. After withdrawing the degree of pain, this value was crossed with the Glasgow abbreviated scale to know qualitatively the real pain. This procedure was performed before, immediately after and last 2/7 days of surgery (some patients did last measurement 7 days after having been submitted to more invasive surgeries) or the application of TCFPI/cryotherapy. The purpose of collecting these data is the validation of TCFPI in reducing the degree of pain and comparison of improvements over the cryotherapy. This review was also important to adjust the temperature, pressure and duration of application of TCFPI for maximum patient comfort.

RESULTS

Pain Assessment

The assessment of degree of pain was performed for all patients who underwent TCFPI and cryotherapy.

Orthopedic patients undergoing TCFPI, decreased approximately 4 degrees on the scale of pain and those who underwent cryotherapy decreased approximately 2 degrees.

Surgical patients undergoing TCFPI, decreased approximately 4 degrees on the scale of pain and those who underwent cryotherapy decreased approximately 2 degrees.

Emergency patients undergoing TCFPI decreased approximately 3 degrees on the scale of pain and those who underwent cryotherapy decreased approximately 3 degrees.

Pain Evolution within the Fields of Veterinary Medicine

For a better understanding on how the pain decreases, two samples, TCFPI and cryotherapy, were considered and the sample values were gathered for defined days (day 1 being the first measurement made during triage) and for each field of Veterinary Medicine. It was calculated two trend lines for each one of the techniques, which correspond to an estimation of the degree of pain to a certain day of measurement.

In Orthopedics, the average value for the degree of pain in TCFPI was 8.14 ± 1.07 and in the cryotherapy technique was 8.50 ± 0.93. There are no significant differences (p-value=0.500 t=0694).

Pain Evolution According Hospitalization Days

As for the evolution of the degree of pain according to the number of hospitalization days for Orthopedic patients, the TCFPI trend line has a bigger slope when compared to the cryotherapy trend line, implying a greater decrease in pain level using TCFPI in the same period of time (Figure 1). After 10 hospitalization days, the pain level declined two values more compared to those treated with cryotherapy.

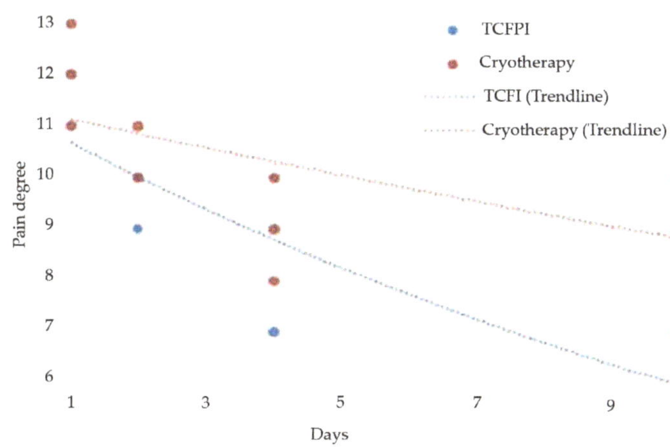

Figure 1: Evolution of pain degree in emergency patients to the cold intermittent pneumatic compression technique and cryotherapy.

In Surgical patients, the average value of the degree of pain with TCFPI was 7.90 ± 1.52, while for cryotherapy it was 7.50 ± 0.55. There are no significant differences (p-value=0.550 and t=-0612). It was not possible to obtain meaningful results for Surgery patients in the evolution of pain degree according to the hospitalization days.

In Emergency, the average value of pain for TCFPI was 9.92 ± 0.29, while for cryotherapy was 10.50 ± 0.52. There are significant differences (p-value=0.002 t=3,457).

As for the evolution of pain degree according to the hospitalization days in Emergency patients, the trend line for TCFPI has a greater slope than the line of cryotherapy, implying a greater decrease in pain in the same period of time when compared with cryotherapy, after 10 days, patients decreased 2 more levels compared to cryotherapy. In terms of time, the same results were achieved in approximately 2 days of treatment with TCFPI and in 10 days with cryotherapy.

DISCUSSION

This study allowed to visualize the positive effects of TCFPI in terms of reducing the amount of pain and therefore in hospitalization days in post-surgical and multiple trauma patients who used GameReady for their rehabilitation.

Regarding the age of patients treated using TCFPI and cryotherapy, there was a predominance of adults and geriatric, being the young animals the smallest age group in this study. This result is interesting due to the fact that, one of the factors for the owners not to invest in the rehabilitation of their animals, lies in the prejudice that age is a prediction and a drawback in their recovery, which was not observed in this study. The average age of TCFPI samples and cryotherapy were very similar although there is a wide dispersion of ages, from young patients to geriatric ones, justifying the high standard deviation value. Regardless the patient's age, there were improvements, which overcome the study by Drygas, which only observed the positive effect of TCFPI in significantly different animal samples, those patients who underwent TCFPI were significantly younger than animals that have not undergone any therapy [18].

Regarding the evolution of pain within the considered Veterinary Medicine fields, it was observed that in Orthopedic and Emergency patients that used TCFPI, it decreased significantly more than with cryotherapy. This data opposes to a human study in which orthopedic patients that applied TCFPI had empirical improvements, but not significant ones when compared to other techniques, such as cryotherapy [19]. The mentioned study shows no positive results for the appliance of TCFPI due to the small sample of patients used for this study and the assessment of the degree of pain being self-made, is not the most assertive method. Thus, it is recommended that a new comparative study is made in humans, specifically in Orthopedic patients, with a higher number of subjects and the assessment of pain must be performed by qualified professionals using scales for this purpose.

In dogs and cats, orthopedic patients, that used TCFPI, it was observed that the degree of pain decreased the most, verifying that it requires substantially less time for recovery than the cases that used cryotherapy. In Emergency patients, improvements from the use of TCFPI become more evident. In terms of time, TCFPI achieves the same results in approximately 2 days of treatment while cryotherapy takes 10 days. These results were positive, however, only the sample of Emergency patients contains significant results, which corroborates the results obtained when compared with the hospitalization days. This corroborates a study in humans by Nick C. Leegwater in which there was improvements in reducing the degree of pain and days of hospitalization in Orthopedic patients [20].

The Emergency patients sample was composed by cats who jumped from buildings or trees and fractured the basin and, although they have not undergone any surgery, they recovered using TCFPI only. It can be assumed that TCFPI may be a supplement or a valuable alternative to more invasive procedures such as surgery, as suggested by Kim in a study of a treatment in dog patients with ruptured cruciate ligaments in which it was used conservative management instead of surgery [21]. Most Emergency dogs that were hit by a car or unknown causes showed swelling in the limbs. In these animals, it was found that TCFPI was able to reduce edema more effectively, corroborating the competition study in dogs [15]. In this study, multiple trauma or undergoing surgery dogs and cats, greatly reduced the degree of pain using TCFPI when compared to cryotherapy, for each one of the fields of Veterinary Medicine, with particular emphasis on Emergency animals. Regarding the recovery time, animals using TCFPI required fewer days of hospitalization.

CONCLUSION

TCFPI is an asset for Animal Rehabilitation because it accelerates the recovery of patients who have undergone surgery or have multiple trauma, so that these achieve the necessary physical conditions to perform rehabilitation exercises and consequently decrease a morbidity rate.

Due to the obtained results in this study and due to neuroanatomical and neurophysiological similarities between the human biped and the quadruped animal, grows the importance and potential of TCFPI applied to humans to accelerate the recovery process to begin rehabilitation exercises and decrease hospitalization days. Besides being a functional rehabilitation modality that controls muscle spasticity, which is a clinical symptom that stimulates the movement disorder in all Lower Motor Neuron Syndrome patients, it may still be interesting to relate this modality with the diseases in their pathophysiology that have a deficit of co-contraction and throughout the Neuro Motor plate and neuropathic pain, which is a complex in decreasing the quality of human life.

REFERENCES

1. Moreira NB, Artifon ES, Meireles A, Silva LI, Rosaet CT, et al. (2011) A influência da crioterapianador e edemainduzidosporsinovite experimental. Fisioterapia e Pesquisa 18: 79-83.
2. Knobloch K, Grasemann R, Spies M, Vogt PM (2007) Intermittent KoldBluecryotherapy of 3x10 min changes mid-portion Achilles tendon microcirculation. Br J Sports Med 41: e4.
3. Holwerda SW, Trowbridge CA, WomochelKS, Keller DM (2015) Effects of Cold Modality Application With Static and Intermittent Pneumatic Compression on Tissue Temperature and Systemic Cardiovascular Responses. Sports Health 5: 27-33.
4. Lundy-Ekman L (2008) Neurociência: Fundamentospara a reabilitação. Elsevier.
5. Felice TD, Santana L (2009) RecursosFisioterapêuticos (Crioterapia e

Termoterapia) naespasticidade: revisão de literatura. RevistaNeurociências, pp: 57-62.

6. Klein BG (2013) Cunningham's Textbook of Veterinary Physiology. Saunders, pp: 1-624.
7. Dragone L (2011) Fisioterapiariabilitativa del cane e del gatto. Elsevier, pp: 1-286.
8. Behr S, Green R(2012) Small Animal Neurological Emergencies. CRC Press, London: Manson.
9. Carver D (2012) Musculoskeletal Conditions: Case Studies. Nursing Program - BSAVA Congress.
10. Zink MC, Dyke JBV (2013) Canine Sports Medicine and Rehabilitation. Wiley-Blackwell.
11. Dykstra JH, Hill HM, Miller MG, Cheatham CC, Michael TJ, et al. (2009) Comparisons of cubed ice, crushed ice, and wetted ice on intramuscular and surface temperature changes. J Athl Train 44: 136-141.
12. Oliveira NML, Gava AD, Salvini TF (2007) O Efeito da Crioterapia e CompressãoIntermitente no MúsculoLesado de Ratos: umaanálisemofométrica. RevistaBrasileira de Fisioterapia.
13. Drygas KA (2012) Post-operative management of the canine athlete. 28th Annual International Canine Sports Medicine Symposium.
14. Janwantanakul P (2009) The effect of quantity of ice and size of contact area on ice pack/skin interface temperature. Physiotherapy 95: 120-125.
15. Jones SC (2015) Cranial cruciate ligament insufficiency in performance dogs: New perspectives in the management 31st International Canine Sports Medicine Symposium.
16. Cameron MH (2009) Agentesfísicosnareabilitação: da pesquisa à prática. Elsevier Brasil, pp: 131-172.
17. Thomson C, Hahn C (2012) Veterinary Neuroanatomy: A Clinical Approach. Saunders Ltd, pp: 1-178.
18. Drygas KA, McClure SR, Goring RL, Pozzi A, Robertson SA, et al. (2011) Effect of cold compression therapy on postoperative pain, swelling, range of motion, and lameness after tibial plateau leveling osteotomy in dogs. J Am Vet Med Assoc 238: 1284-1291.
19. Kraeutler MJ, Reynolds KA, Long C, McCarty EC (2015) Compressive cryotherapy versus ice - a prospective, randomized study on postoperative pain in patients undergoing arthroscopic rotator cuff repair or subacromial decompression. J Shoulder Elbow Surg 24: 1-6.
20. Leegwater NC, Willems JH, Brohet R, Nolte PA (2012) Cryocompression therapy after elective arthroplasty of the hip. Hip Int 22: 527-533.
21. Kim, SE (2013) Advances in the treatment of cranial cruciate ligament insufficiency in dogs. 29th annual international canine sports medicine symposium.

2
CHAPTER

SPONTANEOUS OSTEOSARCOMA IN DOGS: DIAGNOSIS THROUGH CYTOPATHOLOGICAL AND HISTOPATHOLOGICAL ASSAYS

Marcela da Costa Gomes and Noeme Sousa Rocha

Keywords: Osteosarcoma, Dogs, Cytopathology, Histopathology

INTRODUCTION

Osteosarcomas (OSAs) or osteogenic sarcomas are, among bone neoplasms, the primary tumors with the highest incidence in dogs, as well as in human children, despite being about ten times more frequent in the canine species. This biological similarity has been turning dogs into a clinic model for the study of this type of cancer in humans [1,2], with several advantages over the study model in mice [3].

Most OSAs in dogs are malignant, as they may usually cause death through local infiltration, with about 80% of the dogs afflicted by OSA dying due to pulmonary metastases [4]. Over 15% of the patients with the clinical symptomatology are detected with pulmonary metastasis and it is estimated that over 80% present micrometastases [5].

Characteristically, OSA is found in the metaphyses of long bones and in the appendicular skeleton, with about 25% of the cases in dogs affecting the axial skeleton [6]. This neoplasms appear primarily in dogs with long limbs, such as the Irish Wolfhound, the Scottish Wolfhound and the Great Dane breeds [2,7,8], as well as in other large and giant breeds such as St. Bernard, Irish Setter, Dobermann, Rottweiler, German Shepherd and Labrador Retriever [2,6,8,9], including mixedbreeds [3,10,11].

OSAs afflict dogs from middle to old age, with an average age of seven to eight years old. Moreover, males tend to be afflicted more than females, but this statement is not a consensus among researchers, and some studies have not noticed any gender predisposition [8,12].

Citation: Gomes MC, Rocha NS (2016) Spontaneous Osteosarcoma in Dogs: Diagnosis through Cytopathological and Histopathological Assays. J Cytol Histol 7: 404. doi:10.4172/2157-7099.1000404.

The biologic behavior of OSAs is an aggressive local infiltration of the adjacent tissues and a fast hematogenic spread, usually to the lungs. Appendicular OSAs usually appear in the distal radius metaphysis, in the distal femur metaphysis and in the proximal humerus metaphysis, although other metaphyses may also be affected [13].

At the imaging exams, we can observe a mixed lytic-proliferative pattern at the metaphysis of the afflicted bone and an adjacent periosteal bone formation, which leads to the development of Codman's triangle, formed by the cortex of the afflicted area and the periosteal proliferation. Just like in humans, pulmonary metastases are the main causes of terminal morbidity, suggesting that over 90% of the canine patients may present microscopic metastases undetectable on imaging techniques during the routine [14].

Aside from the patient's clinical history, a detailed physical examination and radiographic examinations, the diagnosis is also based on a cytological assay, with the confirmation often being made through biopsy and histopathological assay [1,15]. The case study representativeness of this tumor is low in the Brazilian territory, due mainly to owners' choice for euthanasia given the high cost of the treatment. Therefore, records regarding the disease and other information regarding its clinic and pathologic manifestations are lost, both ante and post-mortem [14,16].

According to Ribeiro et al. [17], the early diagnosis of jaw OSA in humans favorably influences the treatment and prognosis of the disease, as, with a fast diagnosis and a precise assessment of the tumoral involvement, it is possible to conduct a conservative treatment with curative goals and minimal sequelae.

The treatment of OSA consists of amputation or limb-sparing surgery followed with adjuvant chemotherapy with doxorubicin, platinum-based drugs, or a combination of both, as well as cisplatin and carboplatin. The average survival of these animals with amputation and chemotherapy without metastasis ranges from 165 to 470 days [4,18-21]. With advances in the treatment and multi-agent chemotherapy, the prognosis has improved during the last few decades, with an increased survival rate, but the prognosis remains bad for patients with pulmonary metastasis or patients with refractory tumors [5].

Canine OSAs share many traits with human OSAs, including wounds of identical appearance, with dogs possibly being used as a comparative model [13,14]. Given the frequency in dogs, the canine model for spontaneous OSA has been offering unique opportunities towards comprehending the genomic origins of this tumor. This allows both studies regarding the role of metastases in the disease and tests with new research drugs that would otherwise take too long to provide results in humans [9].

Regarding morphological microscopic characterization, OSA cells are usually round or elliptical, with defined cytoplasmic borders, a bright blue granular cytoplasm and eccentric nucleus with or without nucleoli. Giant, multinucleated cells are common and often there is an amorphous pinkish material (osteoid) at the slide background or in the osteoblastic cytoplasm [22,23]. If the round cells cannot be identified with confidence as osteoblasts, it is possible to conduct, in non-stained slides, a cytochemical stain for alkaline phosphatase (ALP) as osteoblasts are usually ALP positive [15].

The Fine Needle Aspiration Cytology (FNAC) was created in the 1930s with the purpose of diagnosing malignant tumors in humans. In animals, the technique began to be employed in the 1980s, aiding in the distinction between hyperplasia, inflammations, neoplasms and degenerations [23-26]. OSA FNAC is usually conducted using a bone marrow aspiration needle. In most cases, a blunt percutaneous FNAC may be conducted with only manual containment – if the operator cannot penetrate the cortex, the ultrasound guide usually allows the visualization of a "window" through which the needle is inserted. The FNAC method potentially perfects the cytological sample due to architectural preservation, allowing the creation of paraffin blocks for later processing, similarly to a histological sample, which enables the use of histochemical and immunohistochemical adjuvant techniques [27].

Although this approach is seldom explored in veterinary medicine, the role of cytology as a diagnostic tool continues to expand [1]. The technique has several advantages, such as reliability, a minimally invasive diagnosis, reduced cost in comparison to histopathology and fast results [22,28], which enables the surgical and therapeutic approach. Despite the more specific and definitive characteristics related to the diagnosis through histopathology, several authors consider that cytopathology may be used as a definitive diagnosis [23,29-31], or at least be considerably helpful [32]. However, there are still several restrictions regarding the sensitivity of this method [25], as the irregular staining and the presence of precipitate or other refracting artifacts [26].

Ultimately, both techniques continue to be used in complementary diagnoses, illustrating an option between the low degree of invasion during sample collection for cytopathology and the higher level of information available to assess tissue architecture for histopathology [22].

This study aimed at verifying the morphologic expression of parameters used in the cytopathological diagnosis of spontaneous OSAs in dogs of several breeds, including mixed-breeds. It also aimed at analyzing the possible concordance between cytopathological and histopathological parameters of these bone neoplasms.

MATERIALS AND METHODS

For this experiment, we used canine OSAs diagnosed at the Veterinary Hospital and Veterinary Pathology Service at FMVZ – UNESP, Botucatu Campus, Brazil. Patients have, in order to reach a diagnosis, undergone clinical, radiologic, surgical and pathological examinations. The presumptive diagnosis was reached by cytological findings and confirmed by histopathological findings, as recommended by the World Health Organization – Histological Classification of Bone and Joint Tumors of Domestic Animals [32].

All owners received explanations regarding the procedures of this study, signing a Free, Prior and Informed Consent term. The project was approved in a favorable decision at the Ethics Council at FMVZ – UNESP, Botucatu Campus, Brazil.

The samples were collected from dogs with defined breeds and mixed-breeds with definitive diagnosis of OSA, totaling twenty animals. These animals firstly underwent FNAC of the lesion, followed by excision of the tumor, cytopathological and histopathological slides processing and their reading. The final diagnosis of OSA was given by distinct pathologists, and the slides were then archived in our Department of Veterinary Pathology. They were once more analyzed in behalf of this study.

In the cytopathological exam, each tumor was firstly divided in four quarters, followed by FNAC of each one. At least three microscope slides were used by quarter. The slides were first fixed through methanol and then stained by Giemsa; in those stained by Papanicolaou, 95% alcohol was used instead. All these proceedings were performed by different operators.

Surgical specimens were obtained from animals that underwent amputation or tumor excision. The tumor fragments were fixated in 10% neutral buffered formalin by at least 72 hours. They were then decalcified in 10% nitric acid and processed by the usual histological techniques of dehydration, diafanization and embedded in paraffin, cut with a maximum thickness of four micrometers, and stained with Hematoxylin-Eosin.

In this study, we first verified the quality of the samples, observing staining pattern and cellularity. Then, we then detailed the cellular characteristics for the diagnosis of OSA using previously established malignancy criteria for neoplasms as recommended by the World Health Organization – Histological Classification of Bone and Joint Tumors of Domestic Animals [33].

RESULTS

Twenty dogs participated in this study, with thirteen pure breeds (65%) and seven mixed breeds (35%). The average age of the animals was 9.5 years old, and the average weight was 34.8 kg (Tables 1 and 2).

Table 1: Information regarding weight, gender and age of the twenty dogs with OSA

Characteristics		Number of cases	% Total
Weight	Small (<10 kg)	1	5.0%
	Average (10 - 25 kg)	2	10.0%
	Large (25 - 45 kg)	11	55.0%
	Giant (45 - 90 kg)	2	10.0%
	Not weighted	4	20.0%
Gender	Female	11	55.0%
	Male	9	45.0%
Age (years)	0 to 5	1	5.0%
	5 to 7	3	15.0%
	≥ 7	16	80.0%

Table 2: Percentage of each breed affected with OSA, based on the thirteen pure breeds found in this study (65% of the twenty animals). There were seven (35%) mixed breed dogs in this study

Pure Breeds	Number of cases	% Total
Rottweiler	7	53.8%
Labrador Retriever	2	15.4%
Weimaranner	1	7.7%
Belgian Shepherd	1	7.7%
Dalmatian	1	7.7%
English Setter	1	7.7%
Total	13	100.0%

In the present study, we have analyzed the morphological expression of several diagnostic parameters for OSA in dogs for comparison between diagnosis techniques through cytopathology and histopathology. The malignancy criteria included cellularity (low, moderate and high) and cellular arrangement (isolated or cohesive), as well as characteristics of the nucleus: presence of a nuclear halo, uniform hyperchromasia, prominent and single nucleolus versus multiple nucleoli, nuclear molding, pseudoinclusion, multinucleation, atypical mitosis, enlarged nuclei (karyomegaly), chromatin aspect (finely or coarsely aggregated), presence of macronucleoli and nuclear morphology (rounded, oval and fibrillate). The criteria also consider cytoplasmic characteristics such as broad or scarce cytoplasm, presence of vacuoles and pseudopodia, cannibalism, basophilia, eosinophilia and cytoplasmic morphology (fibrillate or fusiform); anisocytosis and anisocariosis (discrete, moderate or marked); environmental characteristics such as inflammation, immature or mature bone matrix; distribution of mesenchymal cells (chondrocytes, osteoblasts and osteoclasts) and presence of platelets. Some of the aforementioned criteria are represented in (Figures 1 and 2).

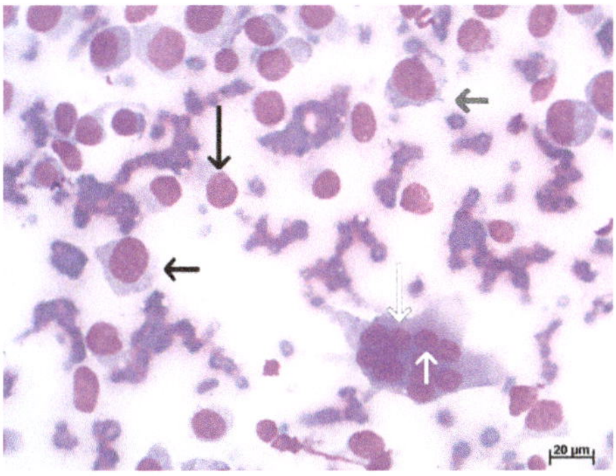

Figure 1: Dog osteosarcoma: atypical osteoclast (long white arrow), evident nucleoli (short white arrow), cytoplasm vacuolization (short black arrow), large nucleus-cytoplasm ratio (long black arrow), pseudopodium (gray arrow). Giemsa / 20 µm.

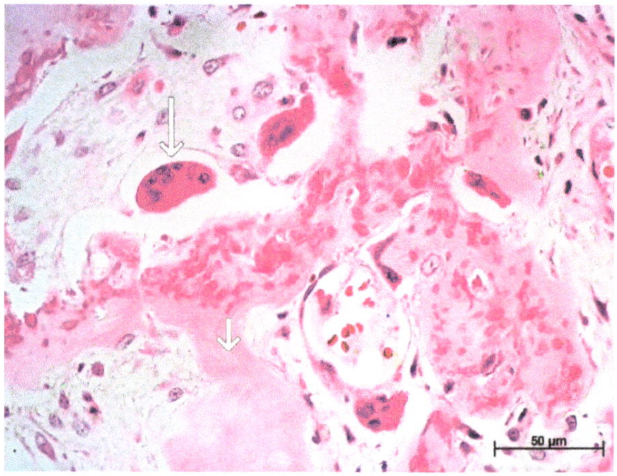

Figure 2: Dog osteosarcoma: disorganized bone trabeculae (short arrow) and atypical osteoclast (long arrow). Hematoxylin-Eosin / 50 μm.

We first conducted a quality test on the microscope slides, with none being considered inadequate for analysis. The staining techniques used in the cytology slides were Giemsa and Papanicolaou.

Criteria such as nuclear halo and pseudo inclusion have not been found in a relevant number, as occurred with criteria such as cannibalism and presence of fibroblasts in the microenvironment.

Due to the low number of cases with an OSA diagnosis in the routine of the veterinary hospital at FMVZ – Botucatu, the number of histopathology slides available for the study did not reach twenty, limiting the comparison study between histopathology and cytopathology to seven cases.

The same steps taken in the examination of the cytopathology slides of OSAs have been employed for the histopathology slides, first with a quality examination followed by an analysis of the malignancy criteria. All samples were previously stained with Hematoxylin-Eosin (Table 3).

Table 3: Anatomical parts afflicted by OSA of twenty dogs. It shows the percentage relating each affected part to its corresponding category (appendicular or axial skeleton)

Location	Number of cases	% Category	% Total
APPENDICULAR	16	100.0%	80,0%
Forelimb	11	68.8%	55.0%
Scapulo-humeral joint	1	6.3%	5.0%
Humerus	6	37.5%	30.0%
Radius/ ulna	2	12.5%	10.0%

Radius/ ulna and carpal bones	2	12.5%	10.0%
Hindlimbs	5	31.3%	25.0%
Femur	2	12.5%	10.0%
Tibia	2	12.5%	10.0%
Femur/ Tibia	1	6.3%	5.0%
AXIAL	4	100.0%	20.0%
Head	3	75.0%	15.0%
Hard palate	2	50.0%	10.0%
Jaw	1	25.0%	5.0%
Isquium	1	25.0%	5.0%
TOTAL	20	---	100%

Due to the nature of the technique employed in the creation of the histopathology slides, it was not possible to clearly establish the criteria related to the cytoplasm, which is much more marked in cytopathological assays with Giemsa staining. Therefore, the analysis of cytoplasmic vacuolization and of the nucleus-cytoplasm ratio were not included. What could be noticed was fibrillate cytoplasmic shape in 57% (4) of the cases and eosinophilia in 85.7% (6).

We have noted a discrepancy between the diagnosis in the system and the findings of this study. Two cases previously diagnosed as osteoblastic OSAs were, in fact, chondrosarcomas, due to the large number of pleomorphic chondrocytes and the marked proliferation of the cartilaginous matrix, characteristics of this kind of neoplasm. Another diagnostic discrepancy was a wound that was revealed a bone remodeling process, in which cells did not present the expected malignancy criteria such as disorganized proliferation of the bone matrix and evident nucleolus.

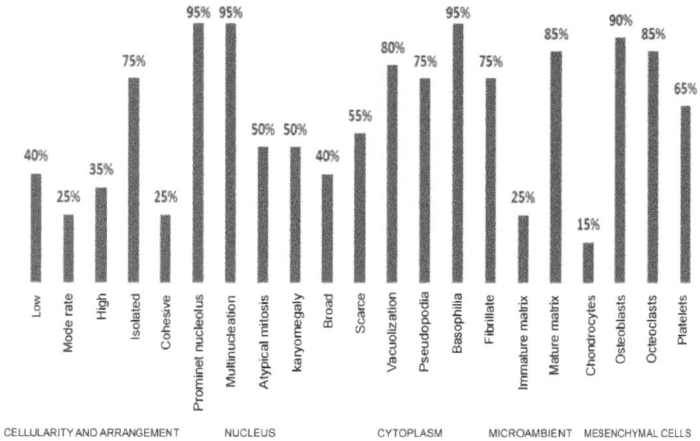

Figure 3: Percentage of the malignancy criteria analyzed in cytopathology slides of osteosarcoma.

This study observed that some malignancy criteria for canine OSAs are present both in cytopathology and in histopathology. Upon analyzing(Figures 3 and 4), we may note that the prominent nucleolus criteria is frequent in both techniques (95% in cytology and 85.7% in histology). The same happens with multinucleation (95% and 71.4%, respectively); fibrillate nucleus (50% and 42.9%), high number of osteoblasts (90% and 100%), high number of osteoclasts (85% and 85.7%) and mature bone matrix (85% and 85.7%).

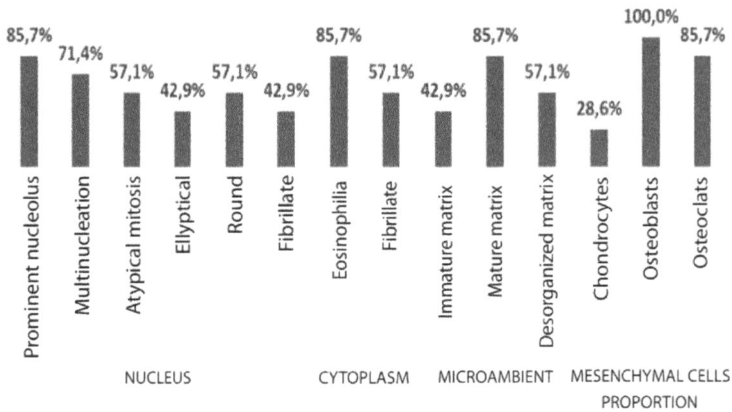

Figure 4: Percentage of the malignancy criteria analyzed in histopathology slides of osteosarcoma.

DISCUSSION

As previously mentioned, only seven histopathologic samples were analyzed instead of the twenty anticipated originally due to their scarcity. One hypothesis explaining this fact is the prominent position of the Veterinary Hospital at FMVZ-UNESP, Botucatu Campus, which is located in near the geographic center of the State of São Paulo, one of the most economically relevant states in Brazil. The hospital receives patients from several nearby regions and is considered a reference hospital for veterinary medicine in the country.

It is possible that owners of animals afflicted by this disease will choose not to conduct the treatment due to the distance between their hometowns and the hospital, transportation difficulties and traveling time, which makes the treatment unfeasible to some owners. Of all cases analyzed, seven (35%) animals belonged to residents of Botucatu. The cities of Rio Claro, Cerquilho and Tatuí presented two cases each (10% each), with the remaining seven belonging to residents of the cities of Atibaia, Brotas, Buri, Jaú, São Manuel, São Paulo and São Pedro (5% each).

We may also hypothesize that there is a chance that the studied OSA cases did not receive a surgical indication: there are situations in which the animal is not in good enough health to undergo a surgical procedure. It is also possible that the owners chose euthanasia instead of the treatment due to the low quality of life caused by metastases in vital organs or situations in which the owner does not authorize the surgery. According to Bersano [16], the non-representativeness of OSA in dogs is justified by the owners' decision for euthanasia instead of proceeding with the treatment, mainly due to the high costs involved.

According to the literature, large breeds like Rottweilers, Irish Setters and Labrador Retrievers show great predisposition for OSA [2,6,8]. Moreover, OSA has more often afflicted bones in the limbs or long bones, representing 85% of the cases, as well as the metaphyses [6]. In addition, 55% of the affected animals were large-sized and 10% were giant-sized.

Females have been more afflicted than males, with rates of 55% and 45% respectively. Despite the literature stating that males are more afflicted, there is still no clear consensus among researchers in this respect [8,12]. The average age of the dogs in this study was 9.5 years old. According to Vanel [8] and Morello [12], the average age of animals afflicted by OSAs was between seven and eight years old. The discrepancy between literature and this study may be explained by the increase in life expectancy of pets due to several factors. Among them, we can mention the higher availability of vaccines, the increasing awareness of owners regarding the geriatric issues of their pets and an improvement in the nutritional quality of pet foods [21]. Moreover, an early diagnosis of neoplastic diseases through cytopathological and histopathological assays enables increasingly efficient treatments, as well as higher life expectancy of patients [17].

According to Vanel et al. [8], chondrosarcomas are the main differential diagnosis for OSAs in dogs, being the second most common primary bone tumor in dogs, representing up to 10% of the cases. This study has found two cases of chondrosarcoma among six histopathological samples (33%). This difference can be explained due to the limited number of samples in the study, which is not representative of the described reality. Therefore, further studies regarding the incidence of chondrosarcomas in the State of São Paulo, Brazil, would be recommended, perhaps encompassing larger areas in order to reach an adequate representativeness of the population.

The results have shown that the cytopathological assay may indeed be used as a definite diagnosis for spontaneous OSA in dogs, as corroborated by several authors [23,29-31], since the malignancy criteria expressed through this technique coincide with those expressed in histopathological assays for this type of neoplasms, such as the presence of osteoids, giant multinucleated cells and single or multiple evident nucleolus [32,33]. However, in order to emphasize the morphological criteria, further research with large enough sample sizes to achieve representativeness is needed.

CONCLUSION

According to the results obtained in this study, we may conclude that cytopathological assays are viable as a diagnostic method for canine spontaneous OSA, being an equally adequate method for grading the malignancy of the neoplasm. Such factors allow the surgeon to conduct a more adequate and fast therapeutic protocol, which may significantly improve the prognosis of the animal in the face of a naturally aggressive neoplasm with low survival rates.

ACKNOWLEDGEMENTS

I thank the support of ISB - UNESP for the realization of this project, FAPESP and CNPq for the financial resources.

REFERENCES

1. Mueller F, Fuchs B, Kazer-Hotz BC (2007) Comparative biology of human and canine osteosarcoma. Anticancer Res 27: 155-164.
2. Fenger JM, London CA, Kisseberth WC (2014) Canine Osteosarcoma: a naturally occurring disease to inform pediatric oncology. ILAR J 55: 69-85.
3. Shahi MH, York D, Gandour-Edwards R, Withers SS, Holt R, et al. (2015) BMI1 is expressed in canine osteosarcoma and contributes to cell growth and chemotherapy resistance. PloS One 10: e 0131006.
4. Szewczyk M, Lechowski K, Zabielska K (2014) What do we know about canine osteosarcoma treatment? Review. Vet Res Commun 39: 61-67.
5. Jaffe N (2009) Adjuvant chemotherapy in osteosarcoma: An odyssey of rejection and vindication. Cancer Treat Res 152: 219-237.
6. Selvarajah GT, Kirpensteijn J (2010) Prognostic and predictive biomarkers of canine osteosarcoma. Vet J 185: 28-35.
7. Davis BW, Ostrander EA (2014) Domestic dogs and cancer research: a breed-based genomics approach. ILAR J 55: 59-68.
8. Vanel M, Blond L, Vanel V (2012) Imaging of primary bone tumors in veterinary medicine: Which differences? Eur J Radiol 82: 2129-2139.
9. Schiffman JD, Breen M (2015) Comparative oncology: what dogs and other species can teach us about humans with cancer. Philos Trans R Soc B BiolSci 370.
10. Trost ME, Kommers GD, Brown CC, Barros CSL, Irigoyen LF, et al. (2012) Primary bone neoplasms in dogs: 90 cases. Pesq Vet Bras 32: 1329-1335.
11. Arthur EG, Arthur GL, Keeler MR, Bryan JN (2016) Risk of osteosarcoma in dogs after open fracture fixation. Vet Surg 45: 30–35.
12. Morello E, Martano M, Buracco P (2011) Biology, diagnosis and treatment of canine appendicular osteosarcoma: Similarities and differences with human osteosarcoma. Vet J 189: 268-277.
13. Osborne TS, Khanna C (2012) A review of the association between osteosarcoma metastasis and protein translation. J Com Pathol 146: 132-142.
14. Dernell WS, Ehrhart NP, Straw RC, Vail DM (2007) Tumors of the skeletal system: Withrow and MacEwen's small animal clinical oncology (4th edn.), Saunders Elsevier, St. Louis, Missouri. pp: 540-567.
15. Ryseff JK, Bohn AA (2012) Detection of alkaline phosphatase in canine cells previously stained with Wright-Giemsa and its utility indifferentiating osteosarcoma from other mesenchymal tumors. Vet ClinPathol 41: 391-395.
16. Bersano PRO (2011) In vitroexpression of cyclooxygenase-2 (Cox2) for

osteosarcoma exposed to a Cox2 selective inhibitor. Doctorate Thesis - UniversidadeEstadualPaulista "Júlio de MesquitaFilho" School of Veterinary Medicine and Animal Science. Botucatu, São Paulo, Brazil.

17. Ribeiro ALR, Nobre RM, AlvesJr SM, Souza PARS, Silva Jr NG, et al. (2010) The importance of early diagnosis and an accurate tumoral evaluation in the treatment of mandibular osteossarcoma. RevistaOdontoCiência 25: 319-324.
18. Bacon NJ, Ehrhart NP, Dernell WS, Lafferty M, Withrow SJ (2008) Use of alternating administration of carboplatin and doxorubicin in dogs with microscopic metastases after amputation for appendicular osteosarcoma: 50 cases (1999-2006). J Am Vet Med Assoc 232: 1504-1510.
19. Spodnick GJ, Berg J, Rand WM, Schelling SH, Couto G, et al. (1992) Prognosis for dogs with appendicular osteosarcoma treated by amputation alone: 162 cases. J Am Vet Med Assoc 200: 995-999.
20. Regan RC, GogalJr RM, Barber JP, Tuckfield RC, Howerth EW, et al. (2014) Cytotoxic effects of LoperamideHydrocloride on Canine Cancer Cells. J Vet Med Sci 76: 1563-1568.
21. Hoskins JD, Fortney WF (2003) Geriatrics and aging: geriatrics and gerontology of the dog and cat (2nd edn.), WB Saunders, Philadelphia.
22. Fielder SE, Mahaffey EA (2008) The Musculoskeletal system:diagnostic cytology and hematology of the dog and cat (3rd edn.), Elsevier Mosby, St. Louis, Missouri.
23. Teixeira LV, Lopes STA, Martins DB, França RT, Fighera RA (2010) Punçãoasp irativaporagulhafinacomométodo de coleta de material para a histopatologia no osteossarcomacanino. PesquisaVeterináriaBrasileira 30: 145-148.
24. Thompson KG, Pool RR (2002) Tumors of bones: tumors of domestic animals (4thedn.). Iowa State Press, Iowa.
25. Sanchez N, Selvaggi SM (2006) Utility of cell blocks in the diagnosis of thyroid aspirates. Diagnostic Cytopathology 34: 89-92.
26. Magalhães AM, Ramadinha RR, Barros CSL, Peixoto PV (2001) Estudocomparativo entre citopatologia e histopatologia no diagnóstico de neoplasiascaninas. Pesq Vet Bras 21: 23-32.
27. Masserdotti, C (2006) Architectural patterns in cytology: Correlation with histology. Vet ClinPathol 35: 388-396.
28. Goldschmidt M, Peña L, Rasotto R, Zappulli V (2011) Classification and grading of canine mammary tumors. Vet Pathology 48: 117-131.
29. Wellman ML (1990) Thecytologic diagnosis of neoplasia. Vet Clin North Am Small AnimPract 20: 919-938.
30. Ghisleni G, Roccabianca P, Ceruti R, Stefanello D, Bertazzolo W, etal. (2006) Correlation between fine-needle aspiration cytology and histopathology in the evaluation of cutaneous and subcutaneous masses from dogs and cats. Vet ClinPathol 35:24-30.
31. Sharkey LC, Dial SM, Matz ME (2007) Maximizing the diagnostic value of

cytology in small animal practice. Vet Clin North Am Small AnimPract 37: 351-372.

32. Reinhardt S, Stockhaus C, Teske E, Rudolph R, Brunnberg L(2005) Assessment of cytological criteria for diagnosing osteosarcoma in dogs. J Small AnimPract 46: 65-70.

33. Slayter MV, Boosinger TR, Dammrich K, Misdorp W, Larsen S (1994) Histological classification of bone and joint tumors of domestic animals. World Health Organization. Armed Forces Institute of Pathology, American Registry of Pathology, Washington D.C.

3

CHAPTER

COMPARATIVE ASPECTS OF CANINE MELANOMA

Adriana Tomoko Nishiya, Cristina Oliveira Massoco, Claudia Ronca Felizzola , Eduardo Perlmann , Karen Batschinski, Marcello Vannucci Tedardi, Jéssica Soares Garcia, Priscila Pedra Mendonça, Tarso Felipe Teixeira and Maria Lucia Zaidan Dagli

Keywords: Melanoma, canine, cancer, histopathology, therapy

INTRODUCTION

Melanoma is a malignant neoplasm originating from melanocytes. Melanocytic neoplasms have been described in men and in most domesticated animal species, including dogs, cats, horses, and also in wild terrestrial and marine animals [1].

Since dogs live in close proximity to humans, they are influenced by similar environmental factors that may lead to chronic diseases and cancer. In fact, the domestic dog (*Canis familiaris*) reportedly presents more naturally inherited chronic diseases than any other animal species. Hence, those aspects have to be considered in the selection of an animal model for a multifactorial human disease, and the dog appears to be the one with the best characteristics [2,3,4]. Dogs are considered recommended models due to their relatively high susceptibility to cancers, including melanomas, and many behavioral similarities [5]. While many genetic alterations of melanomas have recently been discovered and studied, control of this disease is still challenging in both humans and animals, particularly in dogs and cats. The aim of this review is to report a comparative approach of the etiological, epidemiological, pathological, and molecular aspects of melanomas in dogs.

Citation: Adriana Tomoko Nishiya, Cristina Oliveira Massoco, Claudia Ronca Felizzola, Eduardo Perlmann, Karen Batschinski, Marcello Vannucci Tedardi, Jéssica Soares Garcia, Priscila Pedra Mendonça, Tarso Felipe Teixeira and Maria Lucia Zaidan Dagli, Comparative Aspects of Canine Melanoma, doi:10.3390/vetsci3010007.

CANINE MELANOMA EPIDEMIOLOGY

Melanoma is one of the most devastating types of cancer, killing around 50,000 people worldwide every year [6,7]. In 2015, according to the American Cancer Society, it is estimated that about 73,870 new melanoma cases will be diagnosed (about 42,670 in men and 31,200 in women), and 9940 people are expected to die of melanoma (about 6640 men and 3300 women).

Human malignant mucosal melanoma of the head and neck is increasing rapidly in incidence in the United States. It is an uncommon and fatal malignancy that does not appear to have the same etiologic basis as cutaneous melanoma. In 452 observed cases, the majority of patients had sino-nasal location (72.6%) and white women ages 70 or older were most affected [8]. This kind of human malignant melanoma is uncommon and has aggressive behavior with increasing rates of recurrence and regional and distant metastasis [9]. Regional lymphatic metastasis occurred in 57.9% to 21% of patients and recurrence rates were 57.9% to 26.3% for patients treated with surgery alone and for those treated with surgery and radiotherapy, respectively. Distant metastases occurred in 52.6% receiving surgery alone and in 47.3% receiving both therapies [10].

Canine oral malignant melanomas in dogs accounted for 0.99% of all (338/33826) canine pathology cases received from 1992 through 1999 at the University of Missouri—Veterinary. The most common sites are the gingiva and labial mucosa [11].

In a retrospective study of neoplasms in domestic animals (data collected between 1993 and 2002 at the School of Veterinary Medicine and Animal Science of the University of São Paulo, Brazil), of 1813 cases of neoplasms in dogs, 58 were melanocytic neoplasms, accounting for 3% of the total in this species [12]. In another retrospective study, 2154 neoplasms were diagnosed at the University of São Paulo between 2000 and 2006. A total of 193 cases (8.9%) were melanocytic neoplasms, of which 186 cases occurred in dogs (96.4%), and only seven in cats (3.6%). Male mixed-breed dogs with black hair coats, with ages varying from 8 to 11 years, were the most commonly affected animals [13].

Canine malignant melanomas are located at different anatomical sites, such as the mouth (Figure 1A,B), lips, skin (Figure 1C), eyes, and digits (Table 1). Studies are controversial about the most common location for this disease in dogs; however, most studies point to the oral cavity and skin as the most common sites [14,15,16,17]. In a survey of 384 melanocytic canine tumors, oral, cutaneous, lips/feet, and eye sites comprised 19%, 59%, 19%, and 3%, respectively [18]. In another study considering malignant melanomas, oral cavity and cutaneous localization were the most common in 40%–62% and 27%–31%, respectively [13,19].

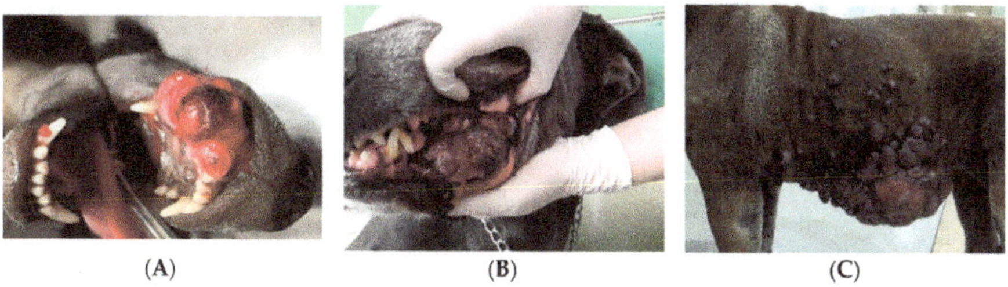

Figure 1: Clinical aspect of malignant oral melanomas (A) in maxilla; (B) in mandible. Clinical aspect of malignant cutaneous melanoma (C) in thoracic and abdominal wall (*Adriana Nihiya*).

Table 1: Common sites of malignant melanomas in dogs

Sites/Total Number of Cases	n = 1652	n = 143	n = 209
Oral	1026	57	67
Cutaneous	448	44	88
Scrotum	-	4	-
Digit	94	21	-
Ungual	60	-	-
Ocular	24	17	-
Lips/Feet	-	-	54
Reference	Gillard *et al.*, 2014 [19]	Teixeira *et al.*, 2010 [13]	Spangler and Kass, 2006 [18]

Data obtained from historical studies indicated that the following breeds of dogs are considered at risk to develop melanocytic tumors: Airedale Terrier, Boston Terrier, Boxer, Chihuahua, Chow Chow, Cocker Spaniel, Doberman Pinscher, English Springer Spaniel, Golden Retriever, Irish Setter [20], Miniature Schnauzer, Scottish Terrier [19,20], Poodles, Beauce Shepherds, Rottweilers, and Labrador Retrievers [19]. Some breeds of dogs, specifically the Schnauzer family (miniature and standard), Scottish Terriers, and Irish Setters are at risk for developing digital malignant melanomas [21,22].

Malignant melanomas typically occur in middle-aged to older dogs, as Miller *et al.* [23] found an average age of nine years, and with no gender predilections.

Teixeira *et al.* [24] studied 25 canine oral melanomas, including 16 melanotic and nine amelanotic specimens. In this study, 25% of the melanotic melanoma-bearing dogs were eight-year old animals, and 22.2% of amelanotic melanoma-bearing group were younger, with ages varying from four to eight years.

Most information on animal cancer epidemiology in the literature comes from laboratories or hospitals, usually from a unique center and using non-standard coding protocols. This may lead to epidemiological bias, and the data rarely generate reliable information useful to establish comparisons. Cancer registries are the most important source of epidemiological data for neoplasms [25]. There are some animal cancer registries around the world, situated mostly in Europe and the USA. In 2013, the São

Paulo Animal Cancer Registry was created at the University of São Paulo, Brazil, serving as the first animal cancer registry in Latin America [25,26]. This system will allow for better and more accurate epidemiologic studies in domestic animals in this region.

CANINE MALIGNANT MELANOMA ETIOLOGY

In humans, malignant melanoma is the most aggressive, therapy-resistant, and deadly form of skin cancer [27]. The major risk factors for human melanoma include family history, skin and mucosal pigmentation characteristics, sun exposure, particularly to UVB light, and skin reactions to sun exposure. Another type of melanoma, oral malignant melanoma, is a rare aggressive neoplasm usually seen in middle-aged adults.

Several etiological factors are supposed to be involved in canine malignant melanomas, including consanguinity, trauma, chemical exposure, hormones, and genetic susceptibility [28]. However, there is no consensus regarding the etiology of malignant melanomas in dogs [29]. Sunlight may be involved in the development of this disease in the sun-exposed skin areas of the body, such as the face and pinnae; however, sunlight probably is not involved in mucosal melanomas, like the ones found in the canine buccal cavity. Other factors, like the presence of pigmented cells, trauma, chemical agents, or even the buccal microbiota, and inflammation may be associated with the etiology of these tumors [30].

Although melanomas can arise in any dog, the prevalence of this disease is higher in purebred dogs, especially Standard and Miniature Schnauzers, Doberman Pinschers, Scottish Terriers, Irish and Gordon Setters, and Golden Retrievers. This fact supports the theory that melanomas in dogs could have a genetic basis [28]. Genetic and epigenetic modifications in melanocytes that lead to alterations in expression or function of genes and proteins involved in cell cycle control and apoptosis are certainly involved in the development of melanomas.

CANINE MELANOMA PATHOLOGICAL ASPECTS AND PROGNOSIS

Melanocytic neoplasms can be classified as benign or malignant tumors [31]. Malignant melanomas are considered malignant neoplasms arising from melanocytes, while melanocytomas are the benign counterparts [31].

Melanocytes, which are dendritic cells derived from the neuroectoderm and melanoblasts of the neural crest, migrate during embryogenesis to the dermis and epidermis, mucous membranes, and eyes [29,32]. These dendritic cells in melanoma development have demonstrated altered expression of cell–cell adhesion molecules, such as decreased expression of E-cadherin and V-CAM 1 and increased expression of N-cadherin, Mel-CAM 1, ICAM 1, and $\alpha\beta$ integrins [33]. The development of malignant melanoma is generally characterized by a series of transitions that are outlined in [34], and arises from melanocytes that normally reside within the basal layer of epidermis [35].

According to Head *et al.* [36], a melanocytoma is a benign tumor composed of melanocytes in the basal region of the epithelium and extending into the submucosa (junctional melanocytoma) or in the sub-epithelial connective tissue under normal epithelium (dermal melanocytoma). Malignant melanoma can be subdivided into three patterns on the basis of cell shape [36]:

- -epithelioid—round and polygonal cells (Figure 2)

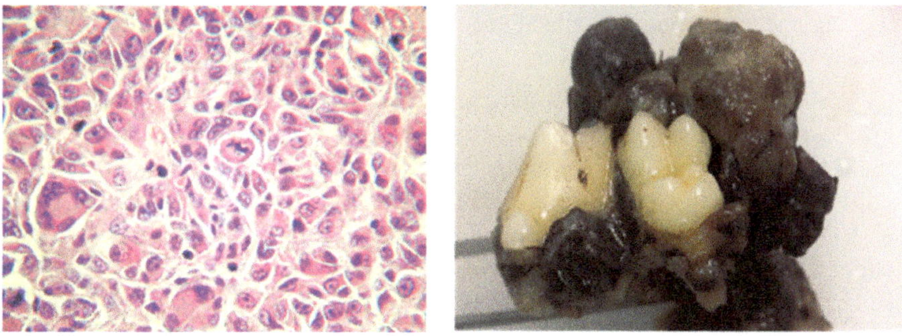

(A) (B)

Figure 2: Photomicrograph of the most common histopathology type of malignant melanoma (epithelioid), showing formation of cell nests, with the presence of multinucleated giant cells and atypical mitotic figures, HE, Objective 40 × (A). Canine oral malignant melanoma, pigmented, exophytic mass protruding from the gingiva (B). Formalin-fixed tissue. Photographs are courtesy of Professor Dr. José Guilherme Xavier.

- -spindle cell—tumor resembles fibroblasts
- -mixed tumors—show both cell types

Malignant melanoma histologically can be the highly melanotic type or the highly anaplastic amelanotic type. Anaplastic melanocytes can be large with abundant cytoplasm with one or more oval or elongated nuclei, with obvious nucleoli. These are frequently characterized to form nests in the submucosa by a mixed structure of epithelial-like cells and fusiform cells and junctional infiltration between basal cells and in the submucosa [36] (Figure 3).

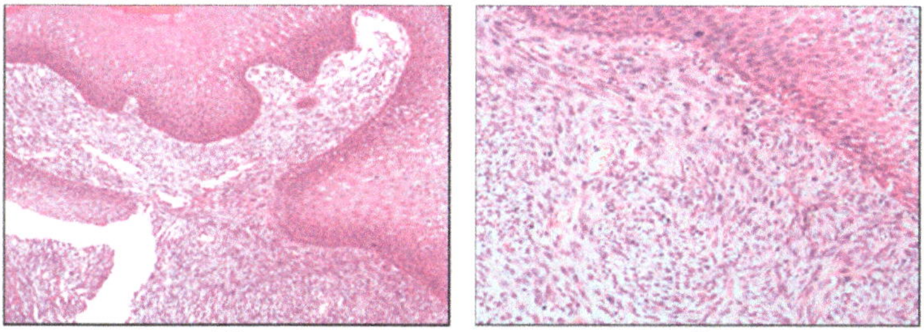

(A) (B)

Figure 3: Photomicrograph of oral amelanotic melanoma ((A), Objective 10 ×; (B), Objective 20 ×). Hematoxylin and eosin.

The most prominent biological property of melanoma cells is the ability to produce melanin [37]. The disruption of homeostasis of close association between melanocytes and basal keratinocytes may trigger a continuous proliferation of the melanocytes, which may lead to the development of a malignant melanoma [7]. Once malignant melanoma cells have escaped from the keratinocyte control, they become able to invade the tissue by the degradation of extracellular matrix through the action of metalloproteinases [38].

The histopathological diagnosis of melanoma may be difficult if the tumor does not contain melanin. Amelanotic malignant melanomas may represent one third of all melanoma cases in dogs.

Their histopathological aspect may resemble carcinomas, sarcomas, lymphomas, and osteogenic tumors. For this reason, the diagnosis of malignant melanoma should be made with the use of immunohistochemistry [11,39,40]. Teixeira *et al.* [13] used two different antibodies to confirm the diagnosis of malignant melanoma in amelanotic cases: HMB 45 (Mouse monoclonal anti-human HMB45, from Dako) and Melan A (Monoclonal mouse anti-human Melan-A, from Dako), and both were considered suitable to immunostain canine melanocytes. Ramos-Vara *et al.* [11] considered Melan A as a specific and sensitive marker for malignant melanomas. Smedley *et al.* [41] evaluated 49 amelanotic melanomas and created a cost-effective and efficient immunodiagnostic cocktail panel containing antibodies against PNL2, Melan-A, TRP-1, and TRP-2 that had 100% specificity and 93.9% sensitivity in identifying canine oral amelanotic melanocytic neoplasms. In addition, malignant melanomas are positive for vimentin and variably positive for S-100 protein and neuron-specific enolase (NSE) [42].

In order to use immunohistochemical techniques to study melanoma cell characteristics, it is frequently necessary to remove melanin from the histopathological specimen. There are several methods to do bleaching in melanoma cells, but the one described by Silva *et al.* [43] is one of the most effective, in which slides were immersed only in 10% hydrogen peroxide in pH 7.4 0.2 mol/L Tris-HCl buffer solution for 24 h in the dark at room temperature.

CANINE MELANOMA: MOLECULAR ASPECTS

Melanomas in humans seem to arise from normal melanocytes that suffer a number of molecular events that lead to their transformation. The progression from normal melanocytes to melanoma sometimes involves its transformation to melanocytic nevus. The genetic alterations involved in this progression are still under study. Several genes/genetic pathways were identified in human melanomas, and these are important for the diagnosis, establishment of prognosis, and drug targeting [44]. Some of these genes are described below:

- CDKN2A Locus—about 70% of melanomas harbor mutations or deletions in this locus on chromosome 9p21.
- Genes that are altered when normal melanocytes generate a nevus: BRAF, NRAS, and INK4a/ARF.

- Genes that are mutated or deregulated when a nevus is transformed to a melanoma: BRAF, NRAS, INK4a/ARF, PTEN, c-kit, NEDD9, and MITF.

Genetic alterations in canine malignant melanomas from mucosal or acral sites have not been fully described. Activating mutations in BRAF exon 15 have not been found [6,45]. Activating mutations of NRAS and c-kit appear to be absent in canine mucosal melanoma, in contrast to human mucosal melanoma, where these genes are mutated in 15% of tumors [44,46,47]. Further studies are necessary to understand the molecular basis of canine malignant melanomas.

Genetic alterations in canine malignant melanomas from human mucosal melanomas have not been fully studied (Table 2). Mutations in exon 15 of BRAF are not found [6], similar to human mucosal malignant melanoma [48]. Activating mutations of NRAS are presented in three of 77 cases [19] and c-kit appears absent in canine mucosal melanomas [49], in contrast to human mucosal melanoma, where these genes are mutated in 4% and 14% of tumors, respectively [50].

Table 2: Genes altered by mutations in canine and human mucosal malignant melanomas

	Human	**Dog**
BRAF	4% [50], 2% [48], 6% [14]	0% [6,19]
C-KIT	12.5% [16], 4% [50]	0% [49]
NRAS	22% [15], 14% [50], 10% [14]	6% [19]
PTEN	48.1% [15]	4% [19]
GNAQ	0% [16]	0% [19]
CDK4	0% [17]	0% [19]

In 2014, Gillard *et al.* [19] compared the histopathology and genetic alterations of canine and human melanomas. They observed that dog malignant melanomas present cytological characteristics similar to human melanoma simulating “nevus” and “animal type,” suggesting a new melanoma classification. They also studied six genes in canine melanomas that are recurrent mutations in human melanomas, BRAF, NRAS, PTEN, KIT, GNAQ, and CDK4. In total, out of the 95 cases (77 oral and 18 cutaneous melanomas), no mutations were found in BRAF, KIT, GNAQ, and CDK4 genes; only three had a positive NRAS mutation and two had a PTEN gene mutation, of which one case had both changes [19]. BRAF mutations were seen in 57% of human cutaneous melanomas and NRAS was mutated in 17% of samples. Both changes were seen in 15.4% [51].

The low frequency of BRAF mutations associated with UV-independent carcinogenesis and oral anatomical distribution of canine melanomas supports the dog as a spontaneous model for investigation of non-UV-associated human melanomas [52].

Human and canine melanoma share differential gene expression patterns of MAPK, but similar sensitivity in cell culture to therapeutic inhibitors of MAPK (AZD6244) and PI3K/AKT (rapamycin) [6].

Dog malignant melanomas share numerous immunohistochemistry similarities (KIT, PTEN, and phosphorylated forms of AKT and ERK1/2) with human melanoma subtypes; particularly with mucosal, digital and ungual localizations that usually show high growth and aggressive behavior [5].

CANINE ORAL MELANOMAS

Melanoma is considered the most common oral malignancy in dogs [53], accounting for 14.4% to 45.5% of all oral tumors [54,55,56,57,58,59]. Some studies describe melanomas as the second most frequent oral cancer in dogs [54,56]. Oral malignant melanoma may also occur in cats and humans, but it is infrequent [60,61].

Malignant melanoma can be located in any portion of the oral cavity, but the gingival mucosa is the most common site [54,62]. The mandibular labial mucosa was the most common area, affected in 53% of cases, as described by Ramos-Vara *et al.* [11]. Although malignant melanoma rarely affects the tongue, it is considered the most common tumor type of this anatomic site as described by Dennis *et al.* [63], and large-breed dogs, particularly Chow Chow and Shar Pei, are at increased risk for malignant lingual melanoma [62,63].

Small-breed dogs and dogs with pigmented oral mucosa appear to be at increased risk for the development of oral malignant melanoma [61,62]. Cocker Spaniel, Poodle, Pekinese, Gordon Setter, Chow Chow, Golden Retriever, mixed-breed dogs, and Dachshund are the most commonly affected breeds [11,61]. Boxers and German Shepherds appear to be less affected by the disease, as described by Ramos-Vara *et al.* [11].

Dogs with oral malignant melanoma are usually 10.5 to 12 years old, with an average age of 11.4 years [11,54,61]. Males are supposed to be more predisposed to oral malignant melanomas, as verified by Todoroff *et al.* [54] and Vos *et al.* [55]; however, Ramos-Vara *et al.* [11], in a study of 328 dogs diagnosed with oral melanoma, and Teixeira *et al.* [13] found no such predisposition.

Oral malignant melanoma is a highly locally aggressive disease, with local invasion into bones occurring in 57% of lesions, with metastasis to regional lymph nodes (Figure 4) in 30.3% to 74% of cases, and to the lungs and other distant organs in 14% to 92% of affected dogs [11,61,64].

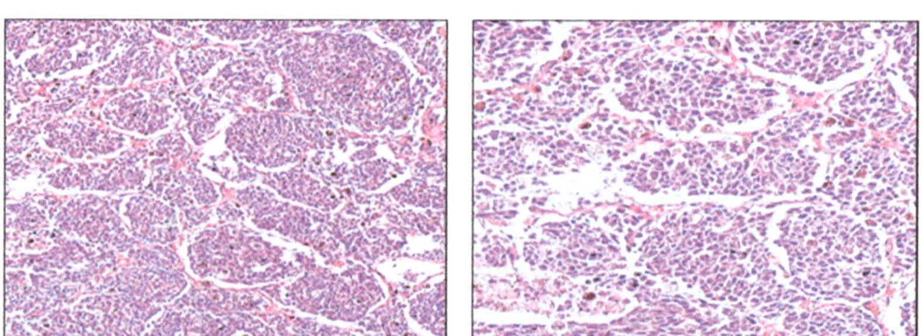

(A) (B)

Figure 4: Photomicrograph of lymph node metastasis from oral melanocytic neoplasm ((A), Objective 10x; (B), Objective 20x). Hematoxylin and eosin.

Melanoma is one of the few neoplasms in animals for which location is an important prognostic indicator [65]. The statement that all oral melanocytic neoplasms should be considered malignant is commonly found throughout the literature and has become dogma [41]. The prognosis for oral melanoma varies from favorable to unfavorable, with an overall median survival time (MST) of less than 36 months, depending on the intrinsic characteristics of the tumor, and the stage of the disease [61,66,67,68,69].

Historically, many studies confirm that oral and lip melanomas have a poorer prognosis when compared to skin melanomas. The differences concerning the results of different studies of lip melanomas are directly related to the real site of the tumor, that is, either in the skin or in the mucocutaneous junction. In one study, oral melanomas had an MST of 147 days, while the MST of melanoma of the lips and digits were 676 days and 725 days, respectively [18]. Large and poorly or non-pigmented tumors, necrosis, ulceration, high rate of cell proliferation (PCNA expression), and p53 expression are considered poor prognostic factors [29]. Amelanotic melanomas showed a significantly higher amount of mitotic cells when compared to melanotic melanomas [24]. The PCNA (proliferating cell nuclear antigen) in pigmented and non-pigmented melanomas was also assessed. It was demonstrated that cells of all samples stained positive for PCNA, confirming the proliferative activity of this tumor.

The World Health Organization (WHO) staging scheme for dogs with oral melanoma is based on the size of the tumor and the presence of regional and distant metastasis (Table 3) [70]. These staging systems are old and size is not considered a prognostic factor for malignant melanoma [18,28,36], but they are still cited in veterinary practice.

Table 3: TNM classification of tumors in domestic animals, WHO, Geneva, 1980.

Clinical Staging System for Oral Tumor	
Primary Tumor (T)	
Tis	Tumor *in situ*
T1	Tumor <2 cm in diameter at greatest dimension
T1a	Without evidence of bone invasion
T1b	With evidence of bone invasion
T2	Tumor 2–4 cm in diameter at greatest dimension
T2a	Without evidence of bone invasion
T2b	With evidence of bone invasion
T3	Tumor >4 cm in diameter at greatest dimension
T3a	Without evidence of bone invasion
T3b	With evidence of bone invasion
Regional Lymph Nodes (N)	
N0	No regional lymph node metastasis
N1	Movable ipsilateral lymph nodes
N1a	No evidence of lymph mode metastasis
N1b	Evidence of lymph mode metastasis
N2	Movable contralateral lymph nodes
N2a	No evidence of lymph mode metastasis
N2b	Evidence of lymph mode metastasis
N3	Fixed lymph nodes
Metastasis (M)	
M0	No distance metastasis
M1	Distance metastasis

Stage Group	**Tumor (T)**	**Nodes (N)**	**Metastasis (M)**
I	T1	N0, N1a, N2a	M0
II	T2	N0, N1a, N2a	M0
III	T3	N0, N1a, N2a	M0
	Any T	N1b	M0
IV	Any T	N2b, N3	M0
	Any T	Any N	M0

Dogs with stage I melanomas have tumors smaller than 2 cm in diameter, while dogs with stage II and III have tumors measuring between 2 to 4 cm, and more than 4 cm, respectively. Dogs with lymph node metastasis are also classified as stage III disease, and dogs with distant metastasis are classified as stage IV disease. Median survival times for dogs with oral melanoma treated with surgery are approximately 17–18 months, 5–6 months, and 3 months for stage I, II, and III disease, respectively [67].

In a study of 70 dogs with oral melanoma, Tuohy *et al.* [71] observed that 11.4% of dogs had mandibular lymph node metastasis and 1.4% of dogs had lung metastasis at the time of diagnosis. After 821 days (mean time of follow-up), 8.6% of mandibular lymph node metastasis, 17.1% of lung metastasis, 5.7% of metastasis to both sites, and 4.2% of metastasis to lung and other locations were observed. Williams *et al.* [64] reported that 70% of canines with melanomas had metastasis when lymphadenomegaly was present, and that 40% had metastasis in the absence of lymphadenomegaly. Harvey *et al.* [72] observed that dogs with untreated oral melanomas have a median survival time of 65 days.

Gillard *et al.* [19] performed clinical and histopathological analyses of 153 malignant canine melanomas with a four-year follow-up. These samples were histopathological characterization by human classification and showed that most canine tumors are intradermal and homologous to human nevocytoid (72%) type, animal type (16.5%), composite type (6.5%), pleomorphic type (4.5%), and superficial spreading melanoma type (0.5%) [19]. Figure 5 shows a representative histology of canine oral malignant melanoma on which local invasion, sparsely pigmented cells, and pleomorphism with variation in shape and cell or nuclear size can be seen.

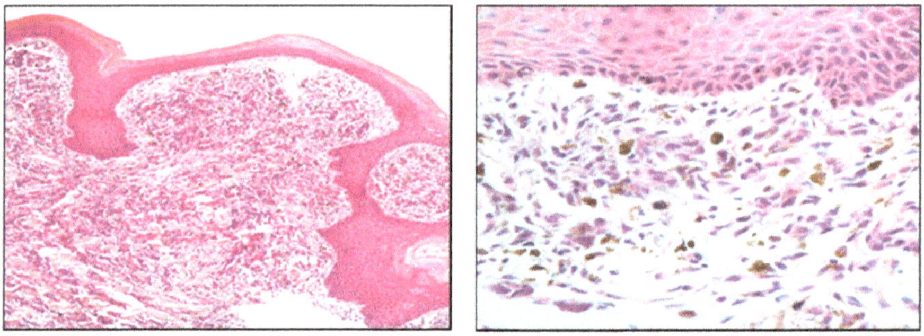

(A) (B)

Figure 5: Photomicrograph of oral melanocytic neoplasm ((A), Objective 4 ×; (B), Objective 40 ×); Hematoxylin and Eosin.

A recent study of over 382 canine oral melanomas did not find statistically significant differences in survival among different sites or mitotic indices [11].

CANINE OCULAR MELANOMAS

Ocular melanocytic tumors, benign or malignant, may occur in humans and domestic animals. These tumors may affect the eyelids, conjunctiva, orbit, limbo, and uvea [73,74]. Melanomas have different biological behaviors depending on the location in the eye [75]. In general, canine ocular melanomas are less aggressive than oral melanomas. Within the ocular melanoma group, the uveal melanoma is characterized by being more aggressive than the epibulbar melanoma [75].

Eyelid tumors in dogs are usually benign, such as sebaceous adenomas and sebaceous epitheliomas. Among all eyelid tumors, the melanocytic neoplasms account for 20%, and only 8% of these are melanomas [73]. Most, if not all, eyelid skin melanomas are benign [75]. Eyelid melanomas in dogs are usually pedunculated with nodular internal infiltration [73]. They are generally non-aggressive tumors, but occasionally some pigmented melanomas act aggressively and become locally invasive with the development of metastasis [73]. When compared to dogs, melanomas of the eyelid in humans carry a worse prognosis, especially when the tumor is located on the lid margin [76].

Conjunctival melanomas generally affect the nictitating membrane and the bulbar and/or eyelid conjunctiva [77]. Rottweilers and Cockers Spaniels are predisposed [74]. Lesions appear as dark, raised solid masses. Metastasis is rarely seen, but when it occurs it is typically associated with melanomas of the conjunctival eyelid. Complete surgical removal is warranted in early-diagnosed cases [77]. Due to the high risk of local recurrence, enucleation should be considered for invasive tumors [74]. Although conjunctival melanomas in humans are unusual, they have the potential to cause vision impairment and reduce life expectancy, with a mortality rate varying from 18% to 44% [74,78].

Canine and feline limbal melanomas have a benign biological behavior. They appear as raised, well-circumscribed heavily pigmented masses that arise from scleral and subconjunctival connective tissue melanocytes. Most of them develop slowly and are located closely to the superior aspect of the limbus. Labrador Retrievers are genetically predisposed [79].

Among the intraocular melanocytic tumors in the dog, melanocytomas are the most common tumors encountered, representing approximately 80% of the neoplasms. Melanomas account for only 20% of tumors [74]. It is difficult and unreliable to clinically differentiate between melanocytomas and melanomas, since melanocytomas can be locally aggressive and even invade the drainage angle and adjacent tissues [73,80]. Therefore, histopathological analysis is indispensable for a definitive diagnosis [81]. Despite the fact that melanocytomas are benign, when located in the iris, they can spontaneously cause necrosis and pigment dispersion, which may lead to obstruction of drainage and cause glaucoma in dogs and humans [82] (Figure 6).

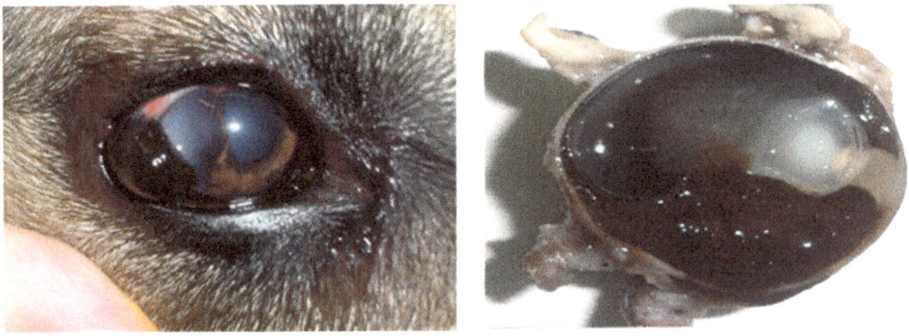

(A) (B)

Figure 6: Photographs showing: blackened mass in the iris with extraocular extension (A) and sagittal section of the eyeball revealing melanocytic neoplasia of iris, ciliary body, and choroid (B) (*Eduardo Perlmann*).

Melanocytomas most commonly affect the anterior uvea in dogs, but rarely affect the choroid [29]. When located in the uvea, they may cause several changes, such as intraocular hemorrhage, uveitis, and secondary glaucoma. Despite the fact that human intraocular melanocytomas are commonly located at the level of the optical disk or adjacent tissues, this location was never described in dogs [74]. An early diagnosis and rapid surgical treatment increase the chances of a favorable prognosis [83]. Wilcock *et al.* [75] studied 91 canine uveal melanocytic neoplasms, and only three developed metastatic disease. These data emphasize the low metastatic rate of uveal melanoma in dogs. Giuliano *et al.* [84], however, showed that animals affected by uveal melanomas had a lower life expectancy when compared with patients diagnosed with uveal melanocytomas. Tumors located in the uvea most frequently are consistent with primary neoplasia; however, animals presenting with intraocular-pigmented tumors should have a complete diagnostic work-up and physical exam to rule out metastasis [85].

In general, when tumors are only confined to the intraocular space, the recommended treatment is enucleation. Exenteration is indicated when the tumor extends to the extraocular space [83]. Other treatment options include iridectomy or diode laser photocoagulation in small-pigmented tumors of the iris [86]. There is no evidence that chemotherapy is effective in the treatment of ocular melanomas [87], but long-term follow-up evaluation would be needed. Ocular malignant melanoma had significantly shorter survival time than benign melanocytomas [84].

CANINE DIGITAL MELANOMAS

Melanoma is considered the second most common type of cancer of the digits in dogs [22,29,88]. Local invasion is a common feature of digital melanomas and 5%–58% of dogs with this disease have evidence of bone lysis [22,88,89,90]. Tumors of the footpad and interdigital region are less likely to invade into the bone [22,90]. Besides possible local invasion, regional and distant metastasis via lymphatics is frequently noted. It is estimated that 30%–40% of dogs have metastasis at the time of presentation and that even after appropriate local treatment with surgery, subsequent metastasis is frequently seen [22,88].

Due to its aggressive behavior, canine digital melanomas often require digital amputation. The median survival time for dogs without metastasis at the time of diagnosis treated with digital amputation is approximately 12 months, with 42%–57% of dogs surviving one year, and 11%–13% surviving two years [22,88,90,91].

Canine Cutaneous Melanomas

In contrast to digital melanomas, cutaneous melanomas typically have benign behavior in dogs, with the exception of melanomas that develop on the mucocutaneous junctions [18,92]. They account for 0.8%–2% of all canine cutaneous tumors [64] and are more commonly seen in dogs with heavily pigmented skin. Predisposed breeds include Scottish Terrier, Poodle, Golden Retriever, Dachshund, Cocker Spaniel, Miniature Poodle, Chow Chow, and Gordon Setter [93]. Benign skin melanomas are usually solitary, small, pigmented, firm, and freely moveable over deeper structures. Malignant melanomas tend to be fast-growing tumors, and often are ulcerated, and pigmented (grey, brown, or black) [21].

The most common sites for benign cutaneous melanomas are the face (near the eyelids), trunk, and extremities. Malignant melanoma is found most frequently on the head, ventral abdomen, and scrotum. When metastases occur, lymph nodes, followed by lungs, are the main organs involved [29].

Brockley *et al.* [94] studied 63 dogs diagnosed with melanomas at different locations. Surgery was performed in 24 cutaneous melanomas, with 88% of dogs alive a year after treatment.

Most dogs are cured with complete surgical excision, although some characteristics of the tumor, such as a mitotic index of ≥3/10 HPF, the presence of ≥20% of nuclear atypia, a Ki67 index ≥15%, ulceration, lymphatic invasion, and tumors extending beyond dermis, may have a negative influence on prognosis [18,41,92].

TREATMENT MODALITIES FOR CANINE MELANOMAS

Surgery

Surgery is the most common and main treatment option for local management of all melanomas, including oral [69], ocular [74], cutaneous, and digital melanomas [90,92]. Due to its high metastatic potential, systemic therapy should also be considered [61,62].

Tuohy *et al.* [71] studied 70 cases of canine oral malignant melanomas treated with curative intent surgery. Surgical resections were done with wide margins, including 2 to 3 cm of bone margins, and 1 cm of soft tissue margins. Histopathological analysis showed that 72.9% of tumors were completely excised, with 10% of these patients developing local tumor recurrence. In this study, dogs that had surgery as their sole treatment option had a progression-free interval (PFI) longer than 567 days, and an

MST of 874 days. In a survey performed by Boston *et al.* [69], among wide-margin surgeries performed, 79.3% (73/92) were completely excised based on histologic evaluation, and the recurrence rate was 8.3% (6/73) in this group. The MST of these dogs was 354 days. Esplin [65] studied 61 dogs diagnosed with well-differentiated oral melanomas that were surgically excised, and reported an MST of 34 months with 3.2% of local recurrence.

Regional lymph node resection has been studied in maxillofacial tumors. The analysis of sentinel lymph nodes provides essential information regarding the clinical stage of disease, and also helps determine the appropriate treatment plan [95,96]. As previously shown, in a survey of 100 dogs with oral malignant melanoma, 53% had cytological or histopathological evidence of mandibular lymph node metastasis, even in normal sized nodes [64]. Therefore, regional lymph node removal is warranted, especially in dogs with oral melanomas.

Radiation Therapy

Radiation therapy is effective for malignant melanomas in dogs and may be useful for the control of local disease and involved regional lymph nodes [97]. Response rates are generally best for smaller tumors rather than for salvage therapy against large tumor burdens late in their clinical progression [98]. Another prognostic factor that appears to affect therapy outcome includes the presence of bone lysis. Proulx *et al.* [97] found that dogs without evidence of radiologic bone destruction experienced longer disease-free intervals and overall survival when compared to dogs with bone invasion.

Although melanoma has traditionally been viewed as a "radio-insensitive" disease, many studies suggest a significant role for radiation therapy in the treatment of melanoma [99]. Optimal fractionation schedules have not yet been established for canine malignant melanoma; however, hypofractionated protocols have been utilized with some success [93]. Overall response rates range from 82% to 94.4%, with the complete and partial resolution of tumors in 51% to 69% and 25% to 31% of cases, respectively [91,92,93,94,95,96,97,98,99,100,101,102]. The reported median time to progression ranges from 3.6 to 7.9 months with a median survival time varying from 5.3 to 11.9 months [97,98,100,101,102,103].

Chemotherapy alone has generally offered little benefit in terms of clinical outcome for the control of local canine melanomas; however, a few published studies have shown that the association of radiation with chemotherapy may potentially slow local progression and/or improve overall survival. Cancedda *et al.* [102] compared the efficacy of radiation therapy (5 × 6 Gy) alone and radiation therapy with post-radiation temozolamide (60 mg/m^2 PO for five consecutive days every 28 days) in dogs with measurable malignant melanoma. Dogs treated with temozolamide had a significantly longer median time to progression (6.8 months) than dogs treated only with radiation (3.6 months). Freeman *et al.* [103] retrospectively looked at dogs with incompletely resected oral melanoma treated with either cisplatin (10–30 mg/m^2 IV) or carboplatin (90 mg/m^2 IV) given once weekly 1 h before receiving radiation therapy (6 × 6 Gy). The reported median survival time was 11.9 months, representing the longest survival time when compared to the survival time previously reported for dogs with incompletely resected oral malignant melanoma [103]. Other studies combining radiation with chemotherapy agents, such as carboplatin, cisplatin, or melphalan, did not have a significant impact on either time to progression or overall survival [97,101,104].

Chemotherapy

Despite treating dogs with appropriate local therapies, such as surgery and/or radiation therapy, the ultimate cause of death, especially in oral melanomas, is metastasis. Therefore, the use of systemic therapies is typically recommended. Many chemotherapy protocols have been published in the veterinary literature with minimal improvement in survival times when compared to local treatment alone.

Many chemotherapy protocols using platinum agents have been studied. Rassnick *et al.* [104] reported an overall response rate of 28% using carboplatin as a single agent (300 to 350mg/m^2/IV/ every 21 days) prior to surgery in dogs with oral (25/27) and cutaneous melanomas (2/27). Boria *et al.* [105] reported an overall response rate of 18% and a MST of 119 days using cisplatin (50 to 55 mg/m^2/IV/ every three weeks) in combination with piroxicam (0.3 mg/kg/PO/24 hs) in oral melanomas.

Brockley *et al.* 2013 [94] evaluated the effect of carboplatin on the survival of 63 canine patients diagnosed with oral, cutaneous, or digital malignant melanomas. In this survey, carboplatin was administered at 300 mg/m^2 IV every 21 days for a total of 4–6 cycles. The addition of carboplatin after local therapy did not lead to a significant increase in survival times, and the anatomic site was significantly associated with survival. The overall median survival time for patients with oral, digital, and cutaneous melanomas were 389 days, 1350 days, with a median follow-up of 776 days, respectively.

In another survey, Dank *et al.* [106] compared the outcome of 17 dogs treated with surgery, adjuvant carboplatin (150 to 300 mg/m^2/IV every three weeks), with or without radiation therapy. The MST was 387 days for the group treated with radiotherapy and 440 days for the group without the addition of radiotherapy.

In a comparative study reported by Tuohy *et al.* [71], surgery with or without any adjuvant therapy (carboplatin, cyclophosphamide as a metronomic therapy, radiotherapy, or xenogeneic canine melanoma vaccine) did not improve overall survival time in dogs with oral melanoma. The MST reported was 874 and 396 days for dogs that had surgery or surgery plus adjuvant therapy, respectively. Boston *et al.* [69] treated 151 dogs with oral melanoma and also concluded that there were no benefits in survival times among dogs that had surgery alone (MST of 335 days for 98 dogs) *versus* dogs that had surgery followed by systemic adjuvant therapy (MST of 352 for 53 dogs). Carboplatin, lomustine, dacarbazine, doxorubicin, metronomic chemotherapy, or commercial melanoma vaccine were the adjuvant therapies used in this study. Postoperative radiation therapy was associated with a longer survival time (MST of 1747 days), but was not significant in the multivariate analysis of this study.

Immunotherapy

Many researchers are currently using and developing therapies to activate the immune system of dogs. The immune responses by therapeutic vaccine represent a potential and powerful strategy for the treatment of melanomas [107]. There is wide evidence that the immune system could modulate the progression and metastasis of melanoma.

Many biological agents have the capacity to demonstrate antitumor activation, such as BCG, IFN-alpha, IL-2, and immunization activators, using an anticancer vaccine [108].

Bacillus Calmette–Guérin (BCG) is used intralesionally in melanomas to activate an immune response and induce tumor regression; however, there may be some complications, such as granulomas and hypersensitivity reactions [109].

Corynebacterium parvum is a bacterial substance that has antitumor activity in humans and canines with melanoma. MacEwen *et al.* [67] used *C. parvum* in dogs with stage II and III oral melanomas and compared the outcomes between surgical excision alone and surgery plus *C. parvum* immunotherapy. Animals who received *C. parvum* and surgery had a better prognosis than those with surgery only.

In rodents, dogs, and men, a liposome-encapsulad muramyl tripeptide phosphatidyl ethanolamine (L-MTP-PE), when used *in vivo*, actives monocytes and macrophages, resulting in antitumor activity, which can lead to melanoma metastasis tumor regression or at least stable disease. According to MacEwen *et al.* [108], when L-MTP-PE was used alone or in combination with GM-CSF the antitumor response was minimal, and only prolonged the survival time in dogs with stage I melanoma.

Bianco *et al.* [110], demonstrated that peripheral blood mononuclear cells with apoptotic melanoma cells significantly increased the antitumor immune response, leading to a reduction of the melanoma in three out of five dogs treated intralesionally with FasL-DNA.

Alexander *et al.* [111] used an allogeneic melanoma vaccine in combination with human a glycoprotein 100 (hgp 100), which is a xenogeneic melanoma protein. The vaccine was well tolerated in dogs, and the tumor response rate was 35% for six weeks (including complete response and stable disease).

Hogge *et al.* [112] used an autologous vaccine made of lysate cells transfected with GM-CSF in dogs with soft tissue sarcoma or melanoma. There was a large concentration of inflammatory cells at the site of vaccine administration, different from the ones that received a vaccine placebo only.

A xenogeneic human DNA-encoding tyrosinase protein vaccine (Oncept®) has been developed and used in dogs with stage II and III oral malignant melanoma [113]. This vaccine was generally well tolerated in a study of 111 dogs. No systemic reactions occurred, only local hematomas and pain at the injection site [114]. In another retrospective study, medical records from 45 dogs were reviewed, including 30 dogs with stage II and III disease, treated with the Oncept® vaccine after appropriate achievement of loco-regional cancer control. The review found that dogs that received the vaccine did not achieve a greater progression-free survival, disease-free interval, or median survival time than dogs that did not receive the vaccine [115].

The role of dendritic cells (DCs) as a biological adjuvant against malignant melanoma through the induction of an active immune response in the oncologic patient has been explored. Dendritic cells, as professional antigen-presenting cells with an ability to initiate the immune response, could therefore qualify for vaccination strategies to treat human or canine cancers. Compared with the human clinical trials using DC-based vaccines, reports of testing in dogs are scarce.

For humans, at least 13 clinical trials conducted in the United States have been registered using *ex vivo* autologous DCs [116] and, for dogs, only a few reports have been published to strengthen the rational use of DC vaccination for canine malignant melanoma [117,118]. Both protocols used bone marrow-derived DC of dogs with or without malignant melanoma. Gyorffy *et al.* [117] conducted a study using a few canine melanoma bearers and employed DC transduced with an adenovirus vector encoding a xenoantigen, human melanoma antigen gp100, as a coadjuvant of radiation therapy. One dog had an antigen-specific cytotoxic T lymphocyte (CTL) activity in peripheral blood lymphocytes, with no clinical signs, either locally or systemically, with melanoma recurrence 48 months after initial DC injection. However, another dog, which had a negative CTL activity, relapsed 22 months after vaccination. Tamura *et al.* [118], using an autologous DC pulsed with canine melanoma CMM2 cell lysate, efficiently elicited T cell-mediated immunity against CMM-2 cells *in vivo*, reinforcing the rationale to use DC as a therapeutic vaccine.

Although the immunotherapeutic approach using a DC vaccine to drive tumor-specific immune responses appears to be a promising strategy to control malignant melanoma, there are limitations, such as the cost of vaccine production for veterinary use as well as the very fragmentary designed strategies available.

Outcomes after Treatment

Table 4 describes the reported outcomes for canine oral malignant melanoma treated with different protocols.

Table 4: Outcomes for canine oral malignant melanoma after different therapeutic protocols

Summary of Treatment Outcome for Canine Oral Malignant Melanoma
Radiation Therapy (RT)
- Response Rate = 82%–94.4% - Local Recurrence = 11%–27% - MST (Median Survival Time) = 5.3–11.9 months
References: Theon *et al.*, 1997 (98); Bateman *et al.*, 1994 (100); Murphy *et al.*, 2005 (101); Cancedda *et al.*, 2014 (102); Proulx *et al.*, 2003 (97); Freeman *et al.*, 2003 (103).
Surgery (SX) with Wide Margins
- Local Recurrence = 3.2%–10% - MST = 11.8–34 months
References: Tuohy *et al.*, 2014 (71); Boston *et al.*, 2014 (69); Esplin *et al.*, 2008 (65).
Chemotherapy (CT) for Macroscopic Disease
- Carboplatin response rate = 28% - Cisplatin + piroxicam response rate = 18%
References: Rassnick *et al.*, 2001 (104); Boria *et al.*, 2004 (105).
Adequate Local Treatment + Systemic Therapy
- SX ± RT + adjuvant carboplatin: MST = 14.6 months - SX ± RT + adjuvant carboplatin, metronomic therapy, or melanoma vaccine: MST = 13.2 months (adjuvant therapy did not improve overall MST) - SX + adjuvant carboplatin, lomustine, dacarbazine, doxorubicin, or melanoma vaccine: MST = 11.7 months (adjuvant therapy did not improve overall MST) - RT + post-RT temozolamide: CT did not improve MST, but was associated with a longer median time to progression when compared to dogs treated with RT alone (6.8 months *versus* 2.6 months) - SX + RT + cisplatin or carboplatin once weekly 1 h before RT: MST = 11.9 months
References: Dank *et al.*, 2012 (106); Tuohy *et al.*, 2014 (71); Boston *et al.*, 2014 (69); Cancedda *et al.*, 2014 (102); Freeman *et al.*, 2003 (103).

Abbreviations: RT = radiotherapy, SX = surgery, CT = chemotherapy, MST = median survival time.

New Perspectives for the Treatment of Canine Melanomas

The aggressive nature of melanomas in canines and humans, with short survival times and minimal clinical outcome benefits after surgery and adjuvant therapy, emphasizes the importance of new studies to find an effective therapy for treatment and prevention of melanomas metastasis.

A canine therapeutic vaccine has been commercially available since 2007. The Merial melanoma vaccine for dogs (Oncept®) consists of DNA encoding the gene for the human melanocyte protein tyrosinase but apparently seems not to cure all melanoma cases. Published studies evaluating the survival times in dogs with melanoma in the mouth undergoing surgery and treatment with the Merial melanoma vaccine report average survival times of 599 days (20 months) or longer [113,114]. These results, though not from randomized studies, are promising and have prompted many veterinary oncologists to recommend the vaccine for patients with stage II and III melanoma despite the lack of FDA-standard clinical trials. The vaccine is well tolerated and has not been reported to be associated with side effects requiring medical intervention. In patients with very large and aggressive melanoma, there may not be sufficient time for an immune response to be mounted against the tyrosinase protein to prevent progression of the melanoma. In fact, 15% of patients treated with the vaccine reportedly die within three months of initiation of treatment, presumably due to the aggressive nature of the melanoma and insufficient time for the vaccine to be effective [119].

Lupeol [120] is among the new therapies under study. Lupeol is a triterpene extracted from various fruits and vegetables that reportedly inhibits melanoma cell proliferation *in vitro* and *in vivo*. A total of 11 dogs bearing buccal melanomas (three, five, and three dogs diagnosed with clinical stage I, II, and III melanoma, respectively) were evaluated. Subcutaneous lupeol (10 mg/kg) was administered postoperatively at various time points. Of the 11 subjects, seven exhibited no local recurrence 180 days postoperatively and no severe adverse effects were observed in any of these cases. Furthermore, no metastases have been detected during the period of the trial.

The current and promising immunotherapy to further augment the options for treatment in malignant melanomas, at least in humans, has been based on checkpoint–blocking antibodies, which can restore anticancer immune responses. Immune checkpoint molecules regulate the immune response avoiding autoimmunity and deleterious effects of an inflammatory response, but when expressed on tumors cells they work as a mechanism of immune evasion. Good examples of immune checkpoint molecules include PD-1 immune checkpoint inhibitor antibody (Pembrolizumab-humanized IgG4; Nivolumab- human IgG4), which was the first drug to gain FDA approval to a phase I trial in patients with BRAF inhibitor-resistant advanced melanoma and BRAFV600 mutation-positive melanoma [121]; and a checkpoint inhibitor (ipilimumab) directed against the cytotoxic T lymphocyte Antigen (CTLA-4). Data from clinical trials has demonstrated the important role this therapeutic approach can play—even with the development of immune-related side effects—since it has been proved a meaningful clinical improvement and an impressive increase in overall survival in melanoma patients [122] when compared to conventional chemotherapy. In the veterinary medicine field, the perspective of this therapy was described by Maekawa*et al.* [123], who demonstrated that an antibovine PD-L1 monoclonal antibody effectively blocked the binding of recombinant PD-1 with PD-L1-expressing tumor cells in a dose-dependent manner, including canine melanoma cells.

Other therapy as future treatment strategy for canine malignant melanoma can be based on oncolytic virotherapy. Basically, the virus infects and kills tumor cells when replication, lysis, and release of viruses occur. Tumor oncolysis by reovirus infection that was related in Ras-transformed cells was studied in six canine malignant melanoma cell lines CMeC1, CMeC2, KMeC, LMeC, CMGD2, and CMGD5. All of them were susceptible to reovirus infection, although Ras activation was not related in these cells, and only one of them (CMGD2) demonstrated more than 50% of cell death [124].

All efforts are geared toward better characterization of malignant melanomas in dogs, for the benefit of these companion animals, and also in an attempt to benefit the treatment of melanoma in humans.

CONCLUSIONS

Melanomas are very aggressive tumors and dogs are considered good models to study this disease. All efforts are geared toward better characterization and control of malignant melanomas in dogs, for the benefit of these companion animals, and also in an attempt to benefit the treatment of human melanomas.

ACKNOWLEDGMENTS

Karen Batschinski is the recipient of a fellowship from Fundação de Amparo a Pesquisa do Estado de São Paulo, FAPESP, Proc. Number 2013/16423-8. The authors are grateful to Jose Guilherme Xavier for supplying photos of canine melanomas.

AUTHOR CONTRIBUTIONS

Adriana Tomoko Nishiya, Claudia Ronca Felizzola, Eduardo Perlmann, Claudia Ronca Felizzola, Priscila Pedra Mendonça, Jéssica Soares Garcia, Tarso Felipe Teixeira, Maria Lucia Zaidan Dagli and Maria Lucia drafted the manuscript, Karen Batschinski, Marcello Vannucci Tedardi and the others revised the manuscript. All authors read and approved the final manuscript.

REFERENCES

1. Sweet, M.; Kirkham, N.; Bendall, M.; Currey, L.; Bythell, J.; Heupel, M. *PLoS ONE* 2012.
2. Starkey, M.P.; Scase, T.J.; Mellersh, C.S.; Murphy, S. Dogs really are man's best friend—Canine genomics has applications in veterinary and human medicine! *Brief. Funct. Genomic. Proteomic.* 2005, *4*, 112–128.
3. Paoloni, M.; Khanna, C. Translation of new cancer treatments from pet dogs to humans. *Nat. Rev. Cancer* 2008, *8*, 147–156. [Google Scholar]
4. Nowend, K.L.; Starr-Moss, A.N.; Murphy, K.E. The function of dog models in developing gene therapy strategies for human health. *Mamm. Genome* 2011, *22*, 476–485.
5. Khanna, C.; Lindblad-Toh, K.; Vail, D.; London, C.; Bergman, P.; Barber, L.; Breen, M.; Kitchell, B.; McNeil, E.; Modiano, J.F.; *et al.* The dog as a cancer model. *Nat. Biotechnol.* 2006, *24*, 1065–1066.
6. Fowles, J.S.; Denton, C.L.; Gustafson, D.L. Comparative analysis of MAPK and PI3K/AKT pathway activation and inhibition in human and canine melanoma. *Vet. Comp. Oncol.* 2015, *13*, 288–304.
7. Haass, N.K.; Smalley, K.S.; Herlyn, M. The role of altered cell–cell communication in melanoma progression. *J. Mol. Histol.* 2004, *35*, 309–318.
8. Marcus, D.M.; Marcus, P.M.; Prabhu, R.S.; Owonikoko, T.K.; Lawson, D.H.; Switchenko, J.; Beither, J. Rising incidence of mucosal melanoma of the head and neck in the United States. *J. Skin Cancer* 2012, 231693.
9. Gavriel, H.; McArthur, G.; Sizeland, A.; Henderson, M. Review: Mucosal

melanoma of the head and neck. *Melanoma Res.* 2011, *21*, 257–266.

10. Meleti, M.; Leemans, C.R.; De Bree, R.; Vescovi, P.; Sesenna, E.; van der Waal, I. Head and neck mucosal melanoma: Experience with 42 patients, with emphasis on the role of postoperative radiotherapy. *Head Neck* 2008, *30*, 1543–1551.
11. Ramos-Vara, J.A.; Beissenherz, M.E.; Miller, M.A.; Johnson, G.C.; Pace, L.W.; Fard, A.; Kottler, S.J. Retrospective study of 338 canine oral melanomas with clinical, histologic, and immunohistochemical review of 129 cases. *Vet. Pathol.*2000, *37*, 597–608.
12. Kimura, K.C.; Garate, A.P.; Dagli, M.L.Z. Retrospective study of neoplasms in domestic animals: A survey between 1993 and 2002 of the service of animal pathology, department of pathology, school of veterinary medicine and animal science, University of Sao Paulo, Southeast Brazil. *Braz. J. Vet. Pathol.* 2012, *5*, 60–69.
13. Teixeira, T.F.; Silva, T.C.; Cogliati, B.; Nagamine, N.K.; Dagli, M.L.Z. Retrospective study of melanocytic neoplasms in dogs and cats. *Braz. J. Vet. Pathol.* 2010, *3*, 100–104.
14. Omholt, K.; Grafström, E.; Kanter-Lewensohn, L.; Hansson, J.; Ragnarsson-Olding, B.K. KIT pathway alterations in mucosal melanomas of the vulva and other sites. *Clin. Cancer Res.* 2011, *17*, 3933–3942.
15. Zanoni, M.T.; Medicina, D.; Lombardi, D.; Ungari, M.; Balzarini, P.; Rossini, C.; Pellegrini, W.; Battaglia, P.; Capella, C.; Castelnuovo, P.; *et al.* Sinonasal mucosal melanoma: Molecular profile and therapeutic implications from a series of 32 cases. *Head Neck* 2013, *35*, 1066–1077.
16. Lyu, J.; Wu, Y.; Li, C.; Wang, R.; Song, H.; Ren, G.; Guo, W. Mutation scanning of BRAF, NRAS, KIT, and GNAQ/GNA11 in oral mucosal melanoma: A study of 57 cases. *J. Oral Pathol. Med.* 2015.
17. Curtin, J.A.; Fridlyand, J.; Kageshita, T.; Patel, H.N.; Busam, K.J.; Kutzner, H.; Cho, K.H.; Aiba, S.; Bröcker, E.B.; LeBoit, P.E.; *et al.* Distinct sets of genetic alterations in melanoma. *N. Engl. J. Med.* 2005, *353*, 2135–2147.
18. Spangler, W.L.; Kass, P.H. The histologic and epidemiologic bases for prognostic consideration in canine melanocytic neoplasia. *Vet. Pathol.* 2006, *43*, 136–149.
19. Gillard, M.; Cadieu, E.; De Brito, C.; Abadie, J.; Vergier, B.; Devauchelle, P.; Degorce, F.; Dreano, S.; Primot, A.; Dorso, L.; *et al.* Naturally occurring melanomas in dogs as models for non-UV pathways of human melanomas. *Pigment Cell Melanoma Res.* 2014, *27*, 90–102.
20. Priester, W.A. Skin tumors in domesticated animals. Data from 12 United States and Canadian Colleges of Veterinary Medicine. *J. Natl. Cancer Insit.* 1973, *50*, 457–466.
21. Goldschmidt, M.H. Pigmented lesions of the skin. *Clin. Dermatol.* 1994, *12*, 507–514.
22. Marino, D.J.; Matthiesen, D.T.; Stefanacci, J.D.; Moroff, S.D. Evaluation of dogs with digit masses: 117 cases (1981–1991). *J. Am. Vet. Med. Assoc.* 1995, *207*,

726–728. [PubMed]

23. Miller, W.H.; Griffin, I.; Campbell, K.L. *Muller and Kirk's Small Animal Dermatology*, 7th ed.; Elsevier Mosby: St. Louis, MO, USA, 2013; pp. 774–843.
24. Teixeira, T.F.; Gentile, L.B.; Silva, T.C.; Mennecier, G.; Chaible, L.M.; Cogliati, B.; Roman, M.A.; Gioso, M.A.; Dagli, M.L.Z. Cell proliferation and expression of connexins differ in melanotic and amelanotic canine oral melanomas. *Vet. Res. Commun.* 2014, *38*, 29–38.
25. Tedardi, M.V.; Biondi, L.R.; Kimura, K.C.; Pedra Mendonça, P.; Grandi, F.; Latorre, A.M.; Dagli, M.L.Z. Comparative oncology in Sao Paulo, Brazil—What to learn from cancer registry. *Source J. Vet. Sci.* 2014, *1*, 1–8.
26. Tedardi, M.V.; Veneziano, D.B.; Kimura, K.C.; Pedra Mendonça, P.; Biondi, L.R.; Grandi, F.; Latorre, A.M.; Dagli, M.L.Z. Sao Paulo animal cancer registry, the first in Latin America. *Vet. Comp. Oncol.* 2015, *13*, 154–155.
27. Haass, N.K.; Ripperger, D.; Wladykowski, E.; Dawson, P.; Gimotty, P.A.; Blome, C.; Fischer, F.; Schmage, P.; Moll, I.; Brandner, J.M. Melanoma progression exhibits a significant impact on connexin expression patterns in the epidermal tumor microenvironment. *Histochem. Cell Biol.* 2010, *133*, 113–124.
28. Modiano, J.F.; Ritt, M.G.; Wojcieszyn, J. The molecular basis of canine melanoma: Pathogenesis and trends in diagnosis and therapy. *J. Vet. Intern. Med.* 1999, *13*, 163–174.
29. Smith, H.; Goldschmidt, H.; Mcmanus, P.M. A Comparative review of melanocytic neoplasms. *Vet. Pathol.* 2002, *39*, 651–678.
30. Dzutsev, A.; Goldszmid, R.S.; Viaud, S.; Zivtogel, L.; Trinchieri, G. The role of the microbiota in inflammation, carcinogenesis, and cancer therapy. *Eur. J. Immunol.* 2015, *45*, 17–31.
31. Goldschmidt, M.H.; Hendrick, M.J. Tumors of the skin and soft tissues. In *Tumors in Domestic Animals*, 4th ed.; Meuten, D.J., Ed.; Iowa State Press: Ames, IA, USA, 2002; pp. 78–82.
32. Scott, D.W.; Miller, W.H., Jr.; Griffin, C.E. *Muller & Kirk's Small Animal Dermatology*, 6th ed.; Elsevier Saunders: Philadelphia, PA, USA, 2001; pp. 1–70.
33. Li, G.; Herlyn, M. Dynamics of intercellular communication during melanoma development. *Mol. Med. Today* 2000, *6*, 163–169.
34. Chin, L. The genetics of malignant melanoma: Lessons from mouse and man. *Nat. Rev. Cancer* 2003, *3*, 559–570.
35. Gaggioli, C.; Sahai, E. Melanoma invasion—Current knowledge and future directions. *Pigment Cell Res.* 2007, *20*, 161–172.
36. Head, K.W.; Else, R.W.; Dubielzig, R.R. Tumors of the Alimentary Tract. In *Tumors in Domestic Animals*, 4th ed.; Meuten, D.J., Ed.; Iowa State Press: Ames, IA, USA, 2002; pp. 426–430.
37. Tajima, S.; Ura-Ishiko, A.; Hayashi, A. Melanogenesis, biosynthetic phenotype of fibronectin and collagen, and migrating activity in cloned B16 mouse melanoma cells. *J. Dermatol. Sci.* 1996, *12*, 24–30.

38. Simonetti, O.; Lucarini, G.; Brancorsini, D.; Nita, P.; Bernardini, M.L.; Biagini, G.; Offidani, A. Immunohistochemical expression of vascular endothelial growth factor, matrix metalloproteinase 2 and matrix metalloproteinase 9 in cutaneous melanocytic lesions. *Cancer* 2002, *95*, 602–624.

39. Nakhleh, R.E.; Wick, M.R.; Rocamora, A.; Swanson, P.E.; Dehner, L.P. Morphologic diversity in malignant melanomas. *Am. J. Clin. Pathol.* 1990, *93*, 731–740.

40. Chénier, S.; Doré, M. Oral Malignant Melanoma with Osteoid Formation in a Dog. *Vet. Pathol.* 1999, *36*, 74–76.

41. Smedley, R.C.; Spangler, W.L.; Esplin, D.G.; Kitchell, B.E.; Bergman, P.J.; Ho, H.Y.; Bergin, I.L.; Kiupel, M. Prognostic markers for canine melanocytic neoplasms: A comparative review of the literature and goals for future investigation.*Vet. Pathol.* 2011, *48*, 54–72.

42. Sandusky, G.E.; Carlton, W.W.; Wightman, K.A. Diagnostic immunohistochemistry of canine round cell tumors. *Vet. Pathol.* 1987, *24*, 495–499.

43. Silva, A.P.; Silva, R.G.; Cogliati, B.; Dias, A.S.M.; Le Bas, A.E.; Hernandez-Blazquez, F.J. Bleaching of melanin in the epidermis of South American fur seal and its application on enzyme immunohistochemistry. *Pesqui. Vet. Bras.* 2011,*31*, 267–270.

44. Fisher, D.E.; Kwong, L.N.; Chin, L. Melanoma. In *DeVita VT, Hellman and Rosenberg's Cancer Principles & Practice of Oncology*, 8th ed.; De Vita, V.T., Jr., Lawrence, T.S., Rosenberg, S.A., Eds.; Lippincott Williams & Wilkins: Philadelphia, PA, USA, 2008; pp. 1889–1951.

45. Shelly, S.; Chien, M.B.; Yip, B.; Kent, M.S.; Theon, A.P.; McCallan, J.L.; London, C.A. Exon 15 BRAF mutations are uncommon in canine oral malignant melanomas. *Mamm. Genome* 2004, *16*, 211–217.

46. Chu, P.Y.; Pan, S.L.; Liu, C.H.; Lee, J.; Yeh, L.S.; Liao, A.T. KIT gene exon 11 mutations in canine malignant melanoma.*Vet. J.* 2013, *196*, 226–230.

47. Curtin, J.A.; Busam, K.; Pinkel, D.; Bastian, B.C. Somatic activation of KIT in distinct subtypes of melanoma. *J. Clin. Oncol.* 2006, *24*, 4340–4346.

48. Maldonado, J.L.; Fridlyand, J.; Patel, H.; Jain, A.N.; Busam, K.; Kageshita, T.; Ono, T.; Albertson, D.G.; Pinkel, D.; Bastian, B.C. Determinants of BRAF mutations in primary melanomas. *J. Natl. Cancer Inst.* 2003, *95*, 1878–1890.

49. Murakami, A.; Mori, T.; Sakai, H.; Murakami, M.; Yanai, T.; Hoshino, Y.; Maruo, K. Analysis of KIT expression and KIT exon 11 mutations in canine oral malignant melanomas. *Vet. Comp. Oncol.* 2011, *9*, 219–224.

50. Zebary, A.; Jangard, M.; Omholt, K.; Ragnarsson-Olding, B.; Hansson, J. KIT, NRAS and BRAF mutations in sinonasal melanoma. *Br. J. Cancer* 2013, *109*, 559–564.

51. Goel, V.K.; Lazar, A.J.; Warneke, C.L.; Redston, M.S.; Haluska, F.G. Examination of mutations in BRAF, NRAS, and PTEN in primary cutaneous melanoma. *J. Investig. Dermatol.* 2006, *126*, 154–160.

52. Mochizuki, H.; Kennedy, K.; Shapiro, S.G.; Breen, M. BRAF Mutations in Canine Cancers. *PLoS ONE* 2015.
53. Bergman, P.J. Canine Oral Melanoma. *Clin. Tech. Small Anim. Pract.* 2007, *22*, 55–60.
54. Todoroff, R.J.; Brodey, R.S. Oral and pharyngeal neoplasia in the dog: A retrospective survey of 361 cases. *J. Am. Vet. Med. Assoc.* 1979, *175*, 567–571.
55. Vos, J.H.; Gaag, I.V.D. Canine and feline oral-pharyngeal tumours. *J. Vet. Med.* 1987, *34*, 420–427.
56. Guerra, J.L.; Dagli, M.L.; Godoy, L.F.; Birman, E.G. A retrospective study of oral neoplasms in dogs: A survey from 1941 to 1986. *Rev. Fac. Med. Vet. Zootec. Univ. S. Paulo* 1989, *26*, 207–212.
57. Stopiglia, A.J.; Felizzola, C.R.; Dagli, M.L.Z.; Xavier, J.G.; Guerra, J.L.; Birman, E. Estudo clínico e anátomo-patológico das formações neoplásicas e não neoplásicas da cavidade bucal de cães. *Comun. Cient. Fac. Med. Vet. Zootec. USP* 1992,*16*, 33–39.
58. Ghirelli, C.D.O. In Biblioteca Digital USP. Available online: http://www.teses.usp.br/teses/disponiveis/10/10137/tde-22072008-090727/pt-br.php (assecced on 15 November 2015).
59. Requicha, J.F.M.F. Repositório Universidade de Trás-os-Montes e Alto Douro. Available online: https://repositorio.utad.pt/bitstream/10348/711/1/MsC_jfmfrequicha.pdf (accessed on 15 November 2015).
60. Bronden, L.B.; Eriksen, T.; Kristensen, A.T. Oral malignant melanomas and other head and neck neoplasms in Danish dogs-data from the Danish Veterinary Cancer Registry. *Acta Vet. Scand.* 2009, *51*, 1–6.
61. Liptak, J.M.; Withrow, S.J. Cancer of gastrointestinal tract. In *Small Animal Clinical Oncology*, 5th ed.; Withrow, S.J., Vail, D.M., Page, R.L., Eds.; Elsevier Saunders: St. Louis, MO, USA, 2013; pp. 381–395.
62. McEntee, M.C. Clinical behavior of nonodontogenic tumors. In *Oral and Maxillofacial Surgery in Dogs and Cats*; Verstraete, F.J.M., Lommer, M.J., Eds.; Elsevier Saunders: Pennsylvania, PA, USA, 2012; pp. 387–402.
63. Dennis, M.; Ehrhart, N.; Duncan, C.; Barnes, A.; Ehrhart, E. Frequency of and risk factors associated with lingual lesions in dogs: 1196 cases (1995–2004). *J. Am. Vet. Med. Assoc.* 2006, *228*, 1533–1537.
64. Williams, L.E.; Packer, R.A. Association between lymph node size and metastasis in dogs with oral malignant melanoma: 100 cases (1987–2001). *J. Am. Vet. Med. Assoc.* 2003, *222*, 1234–1236.
65. Esplin, D.G. Survival of dogs following surgical excision of histologically well-differentiated melanocytic neoplasms of the mucous membranes of the lips and oral cavity. *Vet. Pathol.* 2008, *45*, 889–896.
66. White, R.A.S.; Jefferies, A.R.; Freedman, L.S. Clinical staging for oropharyngeal malignancies in the dog. *J. Small Anim. Pract.* 1985, *26*, 581–594.
67. MacEwen, E.G.; Patnaik, A.K.; Harvey, H.J.; Hayes, A.A.; Matus, R. Canine

oral melanoma: Comparison of surgery*versus* surgery plus Corynebacterium parvum. *Cancer Investig.* 1986, *4*, 397–402.

68. Hahn, K.A.; Denicola, D.B.; Richardson, R.C.; Hahn, E.A. Canine oral malignant melanoma: Prognostic utility of an alternative staging system. *J. Small Anim. Pract.* 1994, *35*, 251–256.
69. Boston, S.E.; Lu, X.; Culp, W.T.N.; Montinaro, V.; Romanelli, G.; Dudley, R.M.; Liptak, J.M.; Mestrinho, L.A.; Buracco, P. Efficacy of systemic adjuvant therapies administered to dogs after excision of oral malignant melanomas: 151 cases (2001–2012). *J. Am. Vet. Med. Assoc.* 2014, *245*, 401–407.
70. Owen, L.N. *TNM Classification of Tumours in Domestic Animals*; World Health Organization: Geneve, Switzerland, 1980.
71. Tuohy, J.L.; Selmic, L.E.; Worley, D.R.; Ehrhart, N.P.; Withrow, S.J. Outcome following curative-intent surgery for oral melanoma in dogs: 70 cases (1998–2011). *J. Am. Vet. Med. Assoc.* 2014, *245*, 1266–1273.
72. Harvey, H.J.; MacEwen, E.G.; Braun, D.; Patnaik, A.K.; Withrow, S.J.; Jongeward, S. Prognostic criteria for dogs with oral melanoma. *J. Am. Vet. Med. Assoc.* 1981, *178*, 580–582.
73. Mould, J.R.B.; Petersen-Jones, S.M.; Peruccio, C.; Ratto, A.; Sassani, J.W.; Harbour, J.W. Uveal melanocytic tumors. In*Ocular Tumors in Animals and Humans*; Peiffer, R.L., Jr., Simons, K.B., Eds.; Iowa State Press: Ames, IA, USA, 2002; pp. 225–282.
74. Dubielzig, R.R.; Ketring, K.L.; Mclellan, G.J.; Albert, D.M. *Veterinary Ocular Pathology: A Comparative Review*; W.B. Saunders: Philadelphia, PA, USA, 2010; p. 472.
75. Wilcock, B.P.; Peiffer, J.R. Morphology and behavior of primary ocular melanomas in 91 dogs. *Vet. Pathol.* 1986, *23*, 418–424.
76. Garner, A.; Koornneef, L.; Levene, A.; Collin, J.R. Malignant melanoma of the eyelid skin: Histopathology and behaviour. *Br. J. Ophthalmol.* 1985, *69*, 180–186.
77. Conceição, L.F.; Ribeiro, A.P.; Piso, D.Y.T.; Laus, J.L. Considerations about ocular neoplasia of dogs and cats. *Cienc. Rural* 2010, *40*, 2235–2242.
78. Lim, L.A.; Madigan, M.C.; Conway, R.M. Conjunctival melanoma: A review of conceptual and treatment advances.*Clin. Ophthalmol.* 2013, *7*, 521–531.
79. Donaldson, D.; Sansom, J.; Scase, T.; Adams, V.; Mellersh, C. Canine Limbal melanoma: 30 cases (1992–2004). Part 1. Signalment, clinical and histological features and pedigree analysis. *Vet. Ophthalmol.* 2006, *9*, 115–119.
80. Perlmann, E.; Barros, P.S.M.; Fernandez, L.; Di Cesare, S.; Bakalian, S.; Burnier, M.N., Jr. Histopathological evaluation of pigmented intraocular tumors in dogs. *Investig. Ophthalmol. Vis. Sci.* 2010, *5*, 5159.
81. Esson, D.; Fahrer, C.; Zarfoss, M.K.; Dubielzig, R.R. Suspected uveal metastasis of a nail bed melanoma in a dog. *Vet. Ophthalmol.* 2007, *10*, 262–266.
82. Fineman,M.S.;Eagle,R.C.;Shields,J.A.;Shields,C.L.;Potter,P.Melanocytomalytic glaucoma in eyes with necrotic iris melanocytoma. *Ophthalmology* 1998, *105*,

492–496.

83. Ryan, A.M.; Diters, R.W. Clinical and pathologic features of canine ocular melanomas. *J. Am. Med. Assoc.* 1984, *184*, 60–67.

84. Giuliano, E.A.; Chappell, R.; Fischer, B.; Dubielzig, R.R. A matched observational study of canine survival with primary intraocular melanocytic neoplasia. *Vet. Ophthalmol.* 1999, *2*, 185–190.

85. Konrade, K.A.; Hoffman, A.; Schubert, C.S.; Dubielzig, R.R. A histologic series of secondary uveal melanomas in eleven dogs. In Proceedings of the 40th Annual Meeting of the American College of Veterinary Ophthalmologist, Chicago, IL, USA, 4–7 November 2009.

86. Willis, A.M.; Wilkie, D.A. Ocular oncology. *Clin. Tech. Small Anim. Pract.* 2001, *16*, 77–85.

87. Cazalot, G.; Raymond-Letron, I.; Regnier, A. Choroidal melanoma presented as glaucoma in a dog: Case report and review of the literature. *Rev. Med. Vet.* 2008, *159*, 74–78.

88. Henry, C.J.; Brewer, W.G.; Whitley, E.M.; Tyler, J.W.; Ogilvie, G.K.; Norris, A.; Fox, L.E.; Morrison, W.B.; Hammer, A.; Vail, D.M.; *et al.* Canine digital tumors: Veterinary cooperative oncology group retrospective study of 64 dogs. *J. Vet. Intern. Med.* 2005, *19*, 720–724.

89. Aronsohn, M.G.; Carpenter, J.L. Distal extremity melanocytic nevi an malignant melanomas in dogs. *J. Am. Anim. Hosp. Assoc.* 1990, *26*, 605–612.

90. Wobeser, B.K.; Kidney, B.A.; Powers, B.E.; Withrow, S.J.; Mayer, M.N.; Spinato, M.T.; Allen, A.L. Diagnosis and clinical outcomes associated with surgically amputated canine digit submitted to multiple veterinary diagnostic laboratories. *Vet. Pathol.* 2007, *44*, 355–361.

91. Manley, C.A.M.; Leibman, N.F.; Wolchok, J.D.; Riviere, I.C.M.; Bartido, S.; Craft, D.M.; Bergman, P.J. Xenogeneic Murine Tyrosinase DNA Vaccine for Malignant Melanoma of the Digit of Dogs. *J. Vet. Intern. Med.* 2011, *25*, 94–99.

92. Bostock, D.E. Prognosis after surgical excision of canine melanoma. *Vet. Pathol.* 1979, *16*, 32–40.

93. Bergman, P.J.; Kent, M.S.; Farese, J.P. Melanoma. In *Small Animal Clinical Oncology*, 5th ed.; Withrow, S.J., Vail, D.M., Page, R.L., Eds.; Elsevier Saunders: St. Louis, MO, USA, 2013; pp. 321–334.

94. Brockley, L.K.; Cooper, M.A.; Bennett, P.F. Malignant melanoma in 63 dogs (2001–2011): The effect of carboplatin chemotherapy on survival chemotherapy on survival. *N. Z. Vet. J.* 2013, *61*, 25–31.

95. Smith, M.M. Surgical approach for lymph node staging of oral and maxillofacial neoplasms in dogs. *J. Am. Anim. Hosp. Assoc.* 1995, *31*, 514–518.

96. Herring, E.S.; Smith, M.M.; Robertson, J.L. Lymph node staging of oral and maxillofacial neoplasms in 31 dogs and cats. *J. Vet. Dent.* 2002, *19*, 122–126.

97. Proulx, D.R.; Ruslander, D.M.; Dodge, R.K.; Hauck, M.L.; Williams, L.E.; Horn, B.; Price, G.S.; Thrall, D.E. A retrospective analysis of 140 dogs with oral

melanoma treated with external beam radiation. *Vet. Radiol. Ultrasound.*2003, *44*, 352–359.

98. Théon, A.P.; Rodriguez, C.; Madewell, B.R. Analysis of prognostic factors and patterns of failure in dogs with malignant oral tumors treated with megavoltage irradiation. *J. Am. Vet. Med. Assoc.* 1997, *210*, 778–784.

99. Khan, N.; Mohammad, K.K.; Almasan, A.; Singh, A.D.; Macklis, R. The evolving role of radiation therapy in the management of malignant melanoma. *Int. J. Radiat. Oncol. Biol. Phys.* 2011, *80*, 645–654.

100. Bateman, K.E.; Catton, P.A.; Pennock, P.W.; Kruth, S.A. 0-7-21 radiation therapy for the treatment of canine oral melanoma. *J. Vet. Intern. Med.* 1994, *8*, 267–272.

101. Murphy, S.; Hayes, A.M.; Blackwood, L.; Maglennon, G.; Pattinson, H.; Sparkes, A.H. Oral malignant melanoma: The effect of coarse fractionation alone or with adjuvant carboplatin therapy. *Vet. Comp. Oncol.* 2005, *3*, 222–229.

102. Cancedda, S.; Bley, C.R.; Aresu, L.; Dacasto, M.; Leone, V.F.; Pizzoni, S.; Gracis, M.; Marconato, L. Efficacy and side effects of radiation therapy in comparison with radiation therapy and temozolomide in the treatment of measurable canine malignant melanoma. *Vet. Comp. Oncol.* 2014.

103. Freeman, K.P.; Hahn, K.A.; Harris, F.D.; King, G.K. Treatment of dogs with oral melanoma by hypofractionated radiation therapy and platinum-based chemotherapy (1987–1997). *J. Vet. Intern. Med.* 2003, *17*, 96–101.

104. Rassnick, K.M.; Ruslender, D.M.; Cotter, S.M.; Al-Sarraf, R.; Bruyette, D.S.; Gamblin, R.M.; Meleo, K.A.; Moore, A.S. Use of carboplatin for treatment of dogs with malignant melanoma: 27 cases (1989–2000). *J. Am. Vet. Med. Assoc.* 2001,*218*, 1444–1448.

105. Boria, P.A.; Murry, D.J.; Bennett, P.F.; Glickman, N.W.; Snyder, P.W.; Merkel, B.L.; Schlittler, D.L.; Mutsaers, A.J.; Thomas, R.M.; Knapp, D.W. Evaluation of cisplatin combined with piroxicam for the treatment of oral malignant melanoma and oral squamous cell carcinoma in dogs. *J. Am. Vet. Med. Assoc.* 2004, *224*, 388–394.

106. Dank, G.; Rassnick, K.M.; Sokolovsky, Y.; Garrett, L.D.; Post, G.S.; Kitchell, B.E.; Sellon, R.K.; Kleiter, M.; Northrup, N.; Segev, G. Use of adjuvant carboplatin for treatment of dogs with oral malignant melanoma following surgical excision. *Vet. Comp. Oncol.* 2014, *12*, 78–84.

107. Bergman, P.J.; Mcknight, J.; Novosad, A.; Charney, S.; Farrelly, J.; Craft, D.; Wulderk, M.; Jeffers, Y.; Sadelain, M.; Hohenhaus, A.E.; *et al.* Long-term survival of dogs with advanced malignant melanoma after DNA vaccination with xenogeneic human tyrosinase: A phase I trial. *Clin. Cancer Res.* 2003, *9*, 1284–1290.

108. MacEwen, E.G.; Kurzman, I.D.; Vail, D.M.; Dubielzig, R.R.; Everlith, K.; Madewell, B.R.; Rodriguez, C.O., Jr.; Phillips, B.; Zwahlen, C.H.; Obradovich, J.; *et al.* Adjuvant therapy for melanoma in dogs: Results of randomized clinical trials using surgery, liposome-encapsulated muramyl triptide, and granulocyte

macrophage colony-stimulang factor. *Clin. Cancer Res.* 1999, *5*, 4249–4258.

109. Moff, S.L.; Corey, G.R.; Gottfredsson, M. Distant cutaneous granulomas after bacille Calmette-Guérin immunotherapy for malignant melanoma: Case for direct infection. *Clin. Infect. Dis.* 1999, *29*, 1569–1570.

110. Bianco, S.R.; Sun, J.; Fosmire, S.P.; Hance, K.; Padilla, M.L.; Ritt, M.G.; Getzy, D.M.; Duke, R.C.; Withrow, S.J.; Lana, S.;*et al.* Enhancing anti melanoma immune responses through apoptosis. *Cancer Gene Ther.* 2003, *10*, 726–736.

111. Alexander, A.N.; Huelsmeyr, M.K.; Mitzey, A.; Dubielzig, R.R.; Kurzman, I.D.; MacEwen, E.G.; Vail, D.M. Development of an allogenic whole-cell tumor vaccine expressing xenogenic gp100 and implementation in phase II clinical trial in canine patients with malignant melanoma. *Cancer Immunol. Immunother.* 2006, *55*, 433–442.

112. Hogge, G.S.; Burkholder, J.K.; Culp, J.; Albertini, M.R.; Dubielzig, R.R.; Keller, E.T.; Yang, N.S.; MacEwen, E.G. Development of human granulocyte-macrophage colony-stimulating factor- transfected tumor cell vaccines for treatment of spontaneous canine cancer. *Hum. Gene Ther.* 1998, *9*, 1851–1861.

113. Bergman, P.J.; Wolchok, J.D. Of mice and men (and dogs): Development of a xenogeneic DNA vaccine for canine oral malignant melanoma. *Cancer Ther.* 2008, *6*, 817–826.

114. Grosenbaugh, D.A.; Leard, A.T.; Bergman, P.J.; Klein, M.K.; Meleo, K.; Susaneck, S.; Hess, P.R.; Jankowski, M.K.; Jones, P.D.; Leibman, N.; *et al.* Safety and efficacy of a xenogeneic DNA vaccine encoding for human tyrosinase as adjunctive treatment for oral malignant melanoma in dogs following surgical excision of the primary tumor. *Am. J. Vet. Res.* 2011, *72*, 1631–1638.

115. Ottnod, J.M.; Smedley, R.C.; Walshaw, R.; Hauptman, J.G.; Kiupel, M.; Obradovich, J.E. A retrospective analysis of the efficacy of Oncept vaccine for the adjunct treatment of canine oral malignant melanoma. *Vet. Comp. Oncol.* 2013, *11*, 219–229.

116. Rotte, A.; Bhandaru, M.; Zhou, Y.; Mcelwee, K.J. Immunotherapy of melanoma: Present options and future promises.*Cancer Metastasis Rev.* 2015, *34*, 115–128.

117. Gyorffy, S.; Rodriguez-Lecompte, J.C.; Woods, J.P.; Foley, R.; Kruth, S.; Liaw, P.C.; Gauldie, J. Bone marrow-derived dendritic cell vaccination of dogs with naturally occurring melanoma by using human gp100 antigen. *J. Vet. Intern. Med.* 2005, *19*, 56–63.

118. Tamura, K.; Yamada, M.; Isotani, M.; Arai, H.; Yagihara, H.; Ono, K.; Washizu, T.; Bonkobara, M. Induction of dendritic cell-mediated immune responses against canine malignant melanoma cells. *Vet. J.* 2008, *175*, 126–129.

119. Elmslie, R. VRCC Veterinary Speciality & Emergency Hospital. Available online: http://www.vetcancerspecialists.com/blog/2013/1/31/the-controversy-surrounding-the-melanoma-vaccine-for-dogs/ (accesse on 15 November 2015).

120. Yokoe, I.; Azuma, K.; Hata, K.; Mukaiyama, T.; Goto, T.; Tsuka, T.; Imagawa, T.; Itoh, N.; Murahata, Y.; Osaki, T.; *et al.* Clinical systemic lupeol administration for

canine oral malignant melanoma. *Mol. Clin. Oncol.* 2015, *3*, 89–92.

121. Robert, C.; Ribas, A.; Wolchok, J.D.; Hodi, F.S.; Hamid, O.; Kefford, R.; Weber, J.S.; Joshua, A.M.; Hwu, W.J.; Gangadhar, T.C.; *et al.* Anti-programmed-death-receptor-1 treatment with pembrolizumab in ipilimumab-refractory advanced melanoma: A randomised dose-comparison cohort of a phase 1 trial. *Lancet* 2014, *384*, 1109–1117.
122. Schadendorf, D.; Hodi, F.S.; Robert, C.; Weber, J.S.; Margolin, K.; Hamid, O.; Patt, D.; Chen, T.T.; Berman, D.M.; Wolchok, J.D. Pooled analysis of long-term survival data from phase II and phase III trials of ipilimumab in unresectable or metastatic melanoma. *J. Clin. Oncol.* 2015, *33*, 1889–1894.
123. Maekawa, N.; Konnai, S.; Ikebuchi, R.; Okagawa, T.; Adachi, M.; Takagi, S.; Kagawa, Y.; Nakajima, C.; Suzuki, Y.; Murata, S.; *et al.* Expression of PD-L1 on canine tumor cells and enhancement of IFN-c production from tumor infiltrating cells by PD-L1 blockade. *PLoS ONE* 2014.
124. Igase, M.; Hwang, C.C.; Coffey, M.; Okuda, M.; Noguchi, S.; Mizuno, T. The oncolytic effects of reovirus in canine solid tumor cell lines. *J. Vet. Med. Sci.* 2015, *77*, 541–548.

4
CHAPTER

THERAPEUTIC INNOVATIONS: TYROSINE KINASE INHIBITORS IN CANCER

Nikolaos Dervisis and Shawna Klahn

Keywords: Tyrosine kinase inhibitors, comparative, cancer, chemotherapy, dog, cat, human

INTRODUCTION

Kinases are among the first oncogenes identified. Initial understanding of oncogene function originates from experiments utilizing retroviruses expressing oncogenic kinases. Murine, feline, and avian retroviruses were the first to demonstrate integration into the host genome, thereby transducing genes harbored at the insertion site. Src kinase is transduced within the avian genome by the Rous sarcoma virus and is the driving force behind Rous sarcoma. Similarly, Raf kinase is transduced by the same retrovirus. Activation of genes encoding kinases contribute to oncogenic transformation of the infected cell. An array of over 500 kinases have since been identified using animal tissue culture models and genetic methodologies [1,2]. Their role in tumorigenesis, tumor progression, and metastasis has been expanding, along with pharmacological attempts to therapeutically intervene the aberrant functions.

DIGITAL AGE IN CELLULAR BIOLOGY

Kinases catalyze the transfer of the gamma-phosphate group of ATP onto a substrate. Kinases mediate nearly all signal transductions, thereby regulating multiple cellular activities such as proliferation, survival, apoptosis, metabolism, transcription, differentiation [3,4]. Accumulating pharmacological and pathological evidence demonstrate that kinases are promising drug targets for the treatment of numerous

Citation: Nikolaos Dervisis and Shawna Klahn, Therapeutic Innovations: Tyrosine Kinase Inhibitors in Cancer, doi:10.3390/vetsci3010004.

diseases, such as cancer, inflammatory diseases, central nervous system disorders, cardiovascular diseases, and diabetes [5]. The catalytic activity depends on the phosphorylation status of specific amino-acid residues. Conformational and other changes induced by phosphorylation events result in dramatic shifts in the kinase catalytic activity, manifesting as a binary switch in functional behavior of the enzyme [6,7,8].

Kinases are located at key positions within the cell. Intercellular communication and the extracellular environment are monitored through signal receptors, while intracellular communication is conducted through secondary signaling molecules and at specific functional checkpoints. Individual subcircuits representing relative simplified functions, such as cellular growth and energy metabolism, have multiple interconnections and crosstalk, forming a functional signaling network that is characterized by higher-level complexity [9]. Kinases have an important role in the amplification and termination of signals, facilitating communication between integral parts of the cell, and between cells. Thus, kinases can be thought as the molecular receptors, amplifiers and transducers of extra and intracellular signals, facilitating the cell's response to the challenges of life.

A consequence of this complex and intricate signaling network is that kinases exhibit pleiotropy and locus heterogeneity. Mutations within the same gene may result in several phenotypes, while the same disease phenotype can sometimes result from mutations in different kinase genes. For example, gain-of-function mutations in the region of the immunoglobulin domain of fibroblast growth factor receptor 1 (FGFR1) result in Pfeiffer syndrome and osteoglophonic dysplasia, whereas loss-of-function mutations throughout the protein cause hypogonadotrophic hypogonadism [10,11].

DISEASE AS A KINASE DYSFUNCTION

Despite the enormous amount of research and rapid developments during the past decades, cancer continues to be a worldwide killer. In the USA, cancer accounts for 23% of the total deaths, and is the second most common cause of death after heart disease. It is expected to surpass heart disease as the leading cause of death in the next few years [12,13]. The intense research in the molecular biology of cancer resulted in an explosion of candidate genes that drive oncogenesis. Nearly simultaneous with the discovery of cancer-associated genes, strategies to repair them were explored. Early attempts focusing on gene replacement therapies were not translated into clinical use due to technological, ethical, and biological barriers. Efforts were soon turned towards pharmacologic methods of blocking specific aberrant oncogenic signaling.

Mutations in protein kinases are overrepresented approximately four-fold compared with a random selection of genes, and reportedly the most frequently mutated family of genes contributing to neoplastic diseases [14,15]. Protein kinases may act as tumor suppressors or proto-oncogenes in normal, healthy cells. Aberrations in protein kinase function can lead to tumorigenesis through numerous mechanisms, including the activation of proliferative pathways, genomic instability, reduction of the DNA damage response, deactivation of apoptotic pathways and/or the promotion of angiogenesis and cellular motility [15]. Gain-of-function mutations typically increase constitutive kinase activity, leading to unrestrained cellular signaling, while loss of-function mutations can lead to a loss in cell signaling. The combined signal aberrations can have a profound effect on the cell, leading to oncogenesis, tumor growth and metastasis.

KINASES AS AN ATTRACTIVE DRUG TARGET

Protein kinases are considered to be the second most important group of drug targets after G-protein-coupled receptors [16,17]. Aberrant kinase activity is implicated in a large variety of diseases, particularly those involving inflammatory or proliferative responses, such as cancer, rheumatoid arthritis, cardiovascular and neurological disorders, asthma and psoriasis. Directly or indirectly, hundreds of human diseases have been connected to protein kinase dysfunction. The ability to modulate kinase activity therefore represents an attractive therapeutic strategy for the treatment of human illnesses [18].

Kinase activity is typically regulated by interconverting between two structural conformations via phosphorylation of key amino acid residues, shifting the balance between active and inactive. These two states are characterized by movements in conformationally mobile loops that border or block the ATP binding site of the kinase. For this reason, the dissociation constant for ATP may be significantly higher for the inactive conformation than for the active conformation. This kinase activation model provides the framework for drugs designed to interact with specific kinase domains. A large number of kinase inhibitors selectively target the inactive conformation, whereas other compounds bind to both conformations with similar affinity [19,20,21]. Inhibitors that bind to the inactive conformation likely face weaker competition with cellular ATP. The potential result is enhanced activity *in vivo*, acting primarily to shift equilibria between conformational states to prevent kinase activation, indirectly inhibiting activity [22].

The modulation of kinase activity can be achieved through either direct or indirect strategies (Figure 1). Imatinib (Gleevec; Novartis) is the prototype of direct protein-tyrosine kinase inhibitors that inhibits the BCR-ABL phosphorylation activity through blocking ATP binding. Imatinib has been approved for the treatment of patients with BCR-ABL positive chronic myeloid leukemia (CML) and patients with Kit (CD117)-positive gastrointestinal stromal tumors. BCR-ABL is the constitutively active tyrosine kinase in CML and in certain forms of acute lymphoblastic leukemia. Imatinib also inhibits the kinase activity of platelet derived growth factor receptor, stem-cell factor receptor and c-kit. Indirect kinase inhibition involves disruption of protein-protein interactions. Cetuximab (Erbitux; ImClone/Bristol-Myers Squibb) is a monoclonal antibody that selectively binds to the extracellular domain of human epidermal growth factor receptor (EGFR), and competitively inhibits binding of epidermal growth factor (EGF) to its receptor tyrosine kinase. Bevacizumab (Avastin; Genentech) is the first anti-angiogenesis cancer drug approved by the FDA. Bevacizumab binds to human vascular endothelial growth factor A (VEGF-A), and prevents it from binding to its receptor tyrosine kinases, Flt-1/VEGFR1 and KDR/VEGRF2. Inhibition of VEGF signaling interferes with tumor blood vessel development, a process that is crucial for tumor growth and metastasis [23].

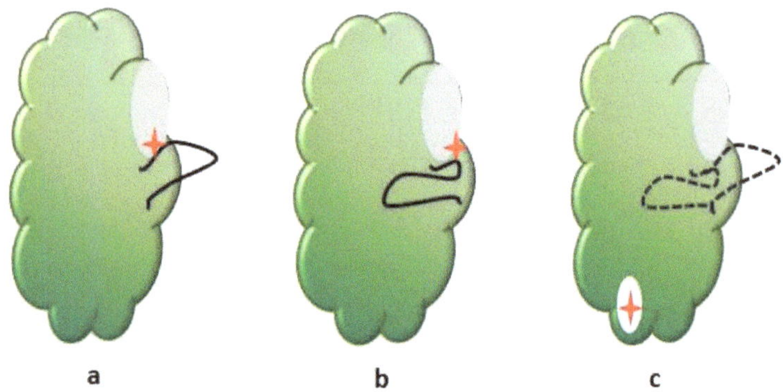

Figure 1: The activation loop of the protein kinase domain regulates access to the ATP binding site. The conformation of a conserved Asp-Phe-Gly (DFG) motif within the activation loop is used to categorize the binding mode of inhibitors. The common types of kinase—kinase inhibitor interactions include: (a) Type I inhibitors (red star) bind the ATP binding site (grey) of the protein kinase domain (green). The aspartate side chain in the conserved DFG motif at the beginning of the activation loop (black) faces into the active site; (b) Type II inhibitors bind a flipped conformation of the DFG motif in which the aspartate side chain faces outwards; (c) Allosteric ligands bind to binding pockets (white) that do not overlap with the active site of the kinase. The DFG motif conformation is not important. These binding pockets can be adjacent to the active site or distant from the active site.

Compounds that bind to protein kinases outside of the ATP-binding pocket may possess advantages over ATP-competitive counterparts. Drugs can be administered at concentrations closer to their biochemical inhibition constant, as inhibition is not affected by fluctuations in the cellular concentration of ATP. There is a potential for greater selectivity as residues outside the ATP binding pocket tend to be less conserved. In certain cases, noncompetitive inhibitors can be substrate selective, inhibiting the activity of a kinase against only a subset of its targets. Rapamycin, the first noncompetitive kinase inhibitor to be identified, is a cyclic macrolide that inhibits the protein kinase mammalian target of rapamycin (mTOR) [24]. MEK1 inhibitor PD098059, the first synthetic noncompetitive kinase inhibitor to be described, acts by binding to inactive MEK1 and preventing its phosphorylation by the upstream kinase Raf [25,26]. Several such inhibitors, termed allosteric, have been described, targeting kinases such as Akt, and inhibitor of nuclear factor kappa-B kinase (IKK-2) [27,28].

The target regions for most kinase inhibitors are intracellular. As small molecules, kinase inhibitors enter the cell by diffusion down the concentration gradient that exists across the membrane. The rate at which this process occurs, and the rate of active efflux, are important determinantsof the intracellular bioavailability of a kinase. How quickly the intracellular inhibitor concentration reaches a steady state and the relative concentrations of inhibitor inside and outside the cell at steady state rely on the relative lipophilicity *vs.* hydrophilicity characteristics of the drug. The rate that it permeates the cellular membrane and non-specific binding to proteins and may affect the route of administration and dosing schedule [29,30]. Expression of drug efflux pump transporters has been shown to reduce the steady-state intracellular drug concentration, although most mammalian cells in culture appear to have less efflux activity for kinase inhibitors compared to chemotherapeutics such as doxorubicin.

HITTING THE TARGET

The transition from cytotoxic chemotherapy to molecularly targeted cancer drug discovery and development has resulted in an increasing number of successful therapies that have impacted the lives of a large number of cancer patients. The BCR-ABL inhibitor imatinib is generally regarded as a trailblazer drug that most impressively validated the concept of designing a small molecule therapeutic. Imatinib is designed to treat a defined patient population with chronic myeloid leukemia in which the malignancy is driven by the BCR-ABL translocation. The improvement in survival has been dramatic [31]. These successes were followed by a number of other small molecule drugs inhibiting critical cancer targets, essentially changing the anti-neoplastic armamentarium of modern Oncology. There has been an explosion of approved kinase inhibitors, with nearly 20 drugs approved by the FDA in a four-year period (Table 1).Veterinary Oncology has been slowly following the fast pace of human Oncology, and there are currently three kinase inhibitors approved by FDA, and a number of small molecular inhibitors under various stages of development (Table 2).

The clinical success of such targeted therapeutics depends to a large degree to the availability of predictive markers. The specific histopathologic diagnosis may not be of such importance, as the presence of markers associated with specific genetic aberrations (mutations, internal tandem duplications, gene amplifications) [32,33,34,35]. For example, the anaplastic lymphoma kinase (ALK) was first implicated in the pathogenesis of an aggressive type of non-Hodgkin's lymphoma [36]. Rearrangements of the ALK gene were subsequently discovered to be are present in 3% to 5% of non-small-cell lung cancers (NSCLC) [37]. These genetic lesions define a distinct subgroup of NSCLC that typically occurs in younger patients who have never smoked or have a history of light smoking [38]. Knowing the presence of these rearrangements can guide the treatment protocol selection, alter the prognosis, and essentially result in a truly personalized approach in cancer therapy [29,35].

Table 1: Approved tyrosine kinase inhibitors in human medicine, 2011–2015 [a]

Drug	Target	Year Approved	Indication
Vandetanib (Caprelsa®)	Flt1, Flt4, KDR, EGFR, Ret	2011	MTC
Crizotinib (Xalkori®)	ALK, MET, EML4-ALK fusion protein	2011	NSCLC
Ruxolitinib (Jakafi®/Jakavi®)	JAK1, JAK2	2011	Myelofibrosis
Vemurafenib (Zelboraf®)	BRAF	2011	Melanoma
Bosutinib (Bosulif®)	BCR/ABL1	2012	CML
Axitinib (Inlyta®)	Flt1, Flt4, KDR, Kit, PDGF-Rα/β	2012	RCC
Cabozantinib (Cometriq®)	KDR, Mek	2012	MTC
Regorafinib (Stivarga®)	KDR, TEK	2012	CC, GIST
Ponatinib (Iclusig®)	BCR/ABL1	2012	CML, ALL
Dabrafenib (Tafinlar®)	BRAF	2013	Melanoma
Trametinib (Mekinist®)	MEK1, MEK2	2013	Melanoma
Afatinib (Gilotrif®)	ERBB2, EGFR	2013	NSCLC
Ibrutinib (Imbruvica®)	BTK	2013	MCL, CLL
Tofacitinib (Xeljanz®)	JAK3	2013	Rheumatoid arthritis
Idelalisib (Zydelig®)	PI3-K	2014	CLL
			Follicular B-cell NHL
Ceritinib (Zykadia®)	ALK	2014	ALK+ NSCLC
Lenvatinib (Lenvima®)	VEGFR2 and VEGFR3	2015	Radioactive iodine-refractory DTC
Palbociclib (Ibrance®)	CDK4 and CDK6	2015	Breast carcinoma

[a] Abbreviations: ALL, acute lymphoblastic leukemia; CC, colorectal cancer; CML, chronic myelogenous leukemia; DTC, differentiated thyroid cancer; GIST, gastrointestinal stromal tumor; MCL, mantle cell lymphoma; MTC, medullary thyroid carcinoma; NHL, Non-Hodgkin's lymphoma; NSCLC, non-small-cell lung carcinoma; RCC, renal cell carcinoma.

Table 2: Approved tyrosine kinase inhibitors in veterinary medicine, all drugs

Drug	Targets	Year Approved	Indication
Toceranib (Palladia®)	VEGF-R2 PDGF-Rα Kit Flt-3 *RET* *JAK family*	2009	Patnaik grade 2 or 3, recurrent, cutaneous mast cell tumors with or without regional lymph node involvement in dogs
Masitinib (Kinavet-CA1®)	Kit PDGF-Rα/β Lyn FGF-R3	2010 [a]	Nonresectable grade 2 and 3 cutaneous mast cell tumors in dogs that have not previously received radiotherapy and/or chemotherapy except corticosteroids
Oclacitinib (Apoquel®)	JAK1 JAK 2	2013	Control of pruritus associated with allergic dermatitis and control of atopic dermatitis in dogs at least 12 mos of age

[a] Conditional approval by the FDA expired in December 2015 and the drug is not commercially available in the US. The drug can only be obtained through the FDA's personal import mechanism.

MISSING THE POINT

The high specificity of the kinase inhibitors appears to be their Achilles heel. As many of the kinase inhibitors exert their tumoricidal effects primarily by inhibiting a specific kinase, there is a strong selective pressure for cells to acquire resistance through mutations in the kinase gene that abrogate drug binding. Additional non-mutation kinase inhibitor resistance mechanisms have been documented, including target amplification and upregulation of alternative kinase pathways such as hepatocyte growth factor receptor in the acquisition of resistance to EGFR kinase inhibitors in lung cancer [30,39,40]. The rapid proliferation of cancer cells and the acquisition of mutations conferring drug resistance has become a recurring theme in the clinic. To date the most extensive clinical and laboratory characterization of resistance-causing mutations has been performed for BCR–ABL in the context of imatinib and second-generation inhibitors. Furthermore, it has been shown in specific hematological tumors that quiescent stem cells are refractory to tyrosine kinase inhibitors, and these cell populations may be instrumentally involved in resistance mechanisms [41].

Inhibitor resistance conferred by mutations at the gatekeeper residue appears to be the common theme for a variety of kinases. The gatekeeper residue term refers to the amino acid side chain at the position that determines the relative accessibility of the hydrophobic pocket located near the ATP/drug binding site. Access to this pocket is important to many kinase inhibitors because hydrophobic interactions in this site are crucial for the binding affinity of the drug. Several strategies are being investigated to overcome kinase inhibitor resistance mutants. A first approach was to develop inhibitors that can tolerate diverse amino acids at the gatekeeper position [42,43]. A second approach is to target the kinase with inhibitors that bind at alternative binding sites [44]. A third approach involves targeting other molecules that may be required for signal transduction in the specific kinase pathway [45]. These approaches have been demonstrated to work in cell culture, and rodent models and clinical trials are currently underway.

UNANSWERED QUESTIONS

Considerable progress made with the new molecularly targeted therapies. Significant advances have occurred in the treatment of diseases in which few treatment options are available, such NSCLC and melanoma. However, for many patients the therapeutic options are still limited, and the process of bringing a new drug to patients is frustratingly slow with very high failure rates [46,47]. The point of failure between basic research and new drug approval has often referred to as the "Valley of Death" [48,49].

The current model of targeted drug development is severely flawed. The inefficiency of translating seemingly important discoveries from the lab to the clinic can be demonstrated by a simple comparison between the research publications on kinase function and the drug approvals. Multiple obstacles within the current framework severely restrict the timely exploration of combinatorial kinase inhibitor therapies. Regulatory, patent secrets, and risk-averse corporate cultures need to be quickly remedied in order to be prepared, as cancer is becoming the leading cause of death in both humans and veterinary patients.

Scientific questions potentially affecting patient clinical management and treatment options include:

- When to treat with kinase inhibitors?
- What is the biologically sound way to combine kinase inhibitors with cytotoxic chemotherapy?
- How to combine multiple kinase inhibitors in a treatment protocol
- How to determine efficacy when tumor size is not an appropriate measure
- How to manage treatment failure? Switch to different kinase inhibitors, or add different kinase inhibitors to the current therapy?

The canine cancer patient can help in answering some of these questions. Spontaneous cancers in pet dogs offer a unique and largely unexploited translational research opportunity for cancer imaging, device and drug development. Dogs suffer from spontaneous malignancies at similar rates and types as humans. Limitations with rodent models stem from development from inbred strains of mice kept in controlled environments. Companion animals, like humans, are genetically diverse and are exposed to many of the same environmental influences. Furthermore, purebred dogs represent unique gene pools, with genetic predisposition to cancers segregating within specific breeds. This provides the opportunity to study complex phenotypes in a relatively simplified genetic background, allowing the identification of critical genetic events that drive malignant behavior.

Dogs suffering from cancer have been successfully used in elegantly designed studies, providing useful and translatable pharmacokinetic/pharmacodynamic data [50,51,52,53,54,55]. Data from canine clinical trials have informed on the scheduling and dosing of small molecular inhibitors in human cancer patients [56]. The availability of the canine genome and growth of high throughput genomic technologies and informatics has enabled comparative oncology to describe canine cancer biology and define potential therapeutic targets in many of the same ways as human cancers [57,58]. Canine cancer patients offer an unparalleled resource for targeting the tumor stroma and tumor/host immune interactions, due to the presence of syngeneic host-tumor relationship and a competent immune function [50].

Using spontaneous pet dog oncology modeling does not require up-front treatment with specific cancer treatment regimens. Thus, novel therapeutic agents can be offered through clinical trials at any stage in cancer presentation. The disease progression times in pet dogs is compressed, allowing for evaluation of a variety of pharmacodynamics intervention outcomes and providing longitudinal endpoints of cancer response through serial sampling. Randomized controlled trials can be conducted in the newly-diagnosed, adjuvant, or metastatic settings, evaluating the utility of drug combinations and drug selection algorithms across a range of tumor and genetic background scenarios [51].

Finally, the infrastructure and resources to realize the potential of the canine cancer patient as an additional tool in conquering cancer exists. The National Cancer Institute's Comparative Oncology Trials Consortium (NCI-COTC;http://ccr.cancer.gov/resources/cop/COTC.asp) brings together study sponsors with academic veterinary oncology centers in North America to support multicenter clinical trials of investigational therapeutics [59]. High-quality biologic samples (tumor, normal, biologic fluids) from dogs with various malignancies are available via the Pfizer-Canine Comparative

Oncology and Genomics Consortium (CCOGC) biospecimen repository (www.ccogc.net) [60]. As a direct result of such mechanisms drugable target identification and signaling pathway similarities have been identified between canine and human cancer patients [61,62,63,64,65].

FUTURE DIRECTIONS

The use of pet dogs in translational medicine may be the "bridge" to the Death Valley [66]. Translational medicine is the process of applying knowledge gained from basic biomedical research to clinical practice. It involves bridging new research findings, scientific discoveries and new techniques to approaches in the prevention, diagnosis or treatment of diseases. The ultimate outcome is the patient's health. The paradigm shift is that scientific discoveries should not only be celebrated in basic laboratories and research institutes, or published (and archived) in prestigious medical journals—they need to make their way to hospitals, clinics, and into patients' lives to be real successes. Translational medicine involves a longer-term strategy for research that is beyond the immediate outcomes of a research project [67].

A major hurdle in therapeutic development is the translation of efficacy determined during the drug discovery phase into efficacy in the clinic. There are often discrepancies between drug efficacy, demonstrated in the current preclinical experimental models, and final efficacy, or lack thereof, in patients. Tissue culture and various rodent models have been and are used as potential predictive models for response in human cancers. It remains to be decided which model is most predictive, however, it is clear that none can reliably predict significant clinical efficacy.

CONCLUDING REMARKS

Veterinary cancer patients can provide the solution for some of the current limitations faced in targeted therapies. Several of the features that define human cancer, including long periods of latency, the complex biology of cancer recurrence and metastasis, the stromal interactions, and outcomes to novel therapies are frequently not adequately represented in murine cancer [68]. Dogs develop cancer and are diagnosed, staged, and treated in an almost identical manner to human cancer patients. Canine tumors develop in a complex genetic background, in the backdrop of intact immune system, and are exposed to the same environmental carcinogens as their human counterparts. Many dogs are essentially family members. Their owners are motivated to treat their pets, and as advocates for their pet, they actively seek participation in Clinical Trials. With the continuous improvement of the canine genomic annotation, dogs with cancer may represent an excellent opportunity for bridging the Valley of Death. One of the payoffs for human cancer patients is reduced exposure to ineffective clinical trials. The partnership under One Medicine of basic science researchers, veterinary and human oncologists, and pharmaceutical industry, has significant potential to advance drug discovery and approval. Ultimately, this ideal could result in improved cancer management, regardless of species.

AUTHOR CONTRIBUTIONS

Nikolaos Dervisis and Shawna Klahn equally contributed to the writing, revisions and editing of the paper. They are both veterinary oncologists with extensive experience in cancer chemotherapy.

REFERENCES

1. Zhang, J.; Yang, P.L.; Gray, N.S. Targeting cancer with small molecule kinase inhibitors. *Nat. Rev. Cancer* 2009, *9*, 28–39.
2. Tsatsanis, C.; Spandidos, D.A. Oncogenic kinase signaling in human neoplasms. *Ann. N. Y. Acad. Sci.* 2004, *1028*, 168–175.
3. Johnson, L.N.; Lewis, R.J. Structural basis for control by phosphorylation. *Chem. Rev.* 2001, *101*, 2209–2242.
4. Adams, J.A. Kinetic and catalytic mechanisms of protein kinases. *Chem. Rev.* 2001, *101*, 2271–2290.
5. Rask-Andersen, M.; Zhang, J.; Fabbro, D.; Schioth, H.B. Advances in kinase targeting: Current clinical use and clinical trials. *Trends Pharmacol. Sci.* 2014, *35*, 604–620.
6. Burnett, G.; Kennedy, E.P. The enzymatic phosphorylation of proteins. *J. Biol. Chem.* 1954, *211*, 969–980.
7. Cohen, P. The origins of protein phosphorylation. *Nat. Cell Biol.* 2002, *4*, 127–130.
8. UniProt, C. Uniprot: A hub for protein information. *Nucleic Acids Res.* 2015, *43*, 204–212. [Google Scholar]
9. Hanahan, D.; Weinberg, R.A. Hallmarks of cancer: The next generation. *Cell* 2011, *144*, 646–674.
10. Muenke, M.; Schell, U.; Hehr, A.; Robin, N.H.; Losken, H.W.; Schinzel, A.; Pulleyn, L.J.; Rutland, P.; Reardon, W.; Malcolm, S.; *et al.* A common mutation in the fibroblast growth factor receptor 1 gene in Pfeiffer syndrome. *Nat. Genet.*1994, *8*, 269–274.
11. Pitteloud, N.; Acierno, J.S., Jr.; Meysing, A.; Eliseenkova, A.V.; Ma, J.; Ibrahimi, O.A.; Metzger, D.L.; Hayes, F.J.; Dwyer, A.A.; Hughes, V.A.; *et al.* Mutations in fibroblast growth factor receptor 1 cause both kallmann syndrome and normosmic idiopathic hypogonadotropic hypogonadism. *Proc. Natl. Acad. Sci. USA* 2006, *103*, 6281–6286.
12. CDC. Leading Causes of Death. Available online: http://www.cdc.gov/nchs/fastats/leading-causes-of-death.htm(accessed on 19 January 2016).
13. Siegel, R.L.; Miller, K.D.; Jemal, A. Cancer statistics, 2015. *CA Cancer J.*

Clin. 2015, *65*, 5–29.

14. Futreal, P.A.; Coin, L.; Marshall, M.; Down, T.; Hubbard, T.; Wooster, R.; Rahman, N.; Stratton, M.R. A census of human cancer genes. *Nat. Rev. Cancer* 2004, *4*, 177–183.
15. Lahiry, P.; Torkamani, A.; Schork, N.J.; Hegele, R.A. Kinase mutations in human disease: Interpreting genotype-phenotype relationships. *Nat. Rev. Genet.* 2010, *11*, 60–74.
16. Vlahovic, G.; Crawford, J. Activation of tyrosine kinases in cancer. *Oncologist* 2003, *8*, 531–538.
17. Cohen, P. Protein kinases—The major drug targets of the twenty-first century? *Nat. Rev. Drug Discov.* 2002, *1*, 309–315.
18. Melnikova, I.; Golden, J. Targeting protein kinases. *Nat. Rev. Drug Discov.* 2004, *3*, 993–994.
19. Schindler, T.; Bornmann, W.; Pellicena, P.; Miller, W.T.; Clarkson, B.; Kuriyan, J. Structural mechanism for STI-571 inhibition of abelson tyrosine kinase. *Science* 2000, *289*, 1938–1942.
20. Wan, P.T.; Garnett, M.J.; Roe, S.M.; Lee, S.; Niculescu-Duvaz, D.; Good, V.M.; Jones, C.M.; Marshall, C.J.; Springer, C.J.; Barford, D.; *et al.* Mechanism of activation of the RAF-ERK signaling pathway by oncogenic mutations of β-RAF. *Cell* 2004, *116*, 855–867.
21. Frantz, B.; Klatt, T.; Pang, M.; Parsons, J.; Rolando, A.; Williams, H.; Tocci, M.J.; O'Keefe, S.J.; O'Neill, E.A. The activation state of p38 mitogen-activated protein kinase determines the efficiency of ATP competition for pyridinylimidazole inhibitor binding. *Biochemistry* 1998, *37*, 13846–13853.
22. Knight, Z.A.; Shokat, K.M. Features of selective kinase inhibitors. *Chem. Biol.* 2005, *12*, 621–637.
23. Ferrara, N.; Hillan, K.J.; Novotny, W. Bevacizumab (avastin), a humanized anti-VEGF monoclonal antibody for cancer therapy. *Biochem. Biophys. Res. Commun.* 2005, *333*, 328–335.
24. Benjamin, D.; Colombi, M.; Moroni, C.; Hall, M.N. Rapamycin passes the torch: A new generation of mTOR inhibitors.*Nat. Rev. Drug Discov.* 2011, *10*, 868–880.
25. Alessi, D.R.; Cuenda, A.; Cohen, P.; Dudley, D.T.; Saltiel, A.R. PD 098059 is a specific inhibitor of the activation of mitogen-activated protein kinase kinase *in vitro* and *in vivo*. *J. Biol. Chem.* 1995, *270*, 27489–27494.
26. Dudley, D.T.; Pang, L.; Decker, S.J.; Bridges, A.J.; Saltiel, A.R. A synthetic inhibitor of the mitogen-activated protein kinase cascade. *Proc. Natl. Acad. Sci. USA* 1995, *92*, 7686–7689.
27. Lindsley, C.W.; Zhao, Z.; Leister, W.H.; Robinson, R.G.; Barnett, S.F.; Defeo-Jones, D.; Jones, R.E.; Hartman, G.D.; Huff, J.R.; Huber, H.E.; *et al.* Allosteric AKT (PKB) inhibitors: Discovery and SAR of isozyme selective inhibitors. *Bioorg. Med. Chem. Lett.* 2005, *15*, 761–764.
28. Yang, J.; Amiri, K.I.; Burke, J.R.; Schmid, J.A.; Richmond, A. Bms-345541

targets inhibitor of κβ kinase and induces apoptosis in melanoma: Involvement of nuclear factor κβ and mitochondria pathways. *Clin. Cancer Res.* 2006, *12*, 950–960.

29. Shaw, A.T.; Kim, D.W.; Nakagawa, K.; Seto, T.; Crino, L.; Ahn, M.J.; de Pas, T.; Besse, B.; Solomon, B.J.; Blackhall, F.; *et al.* Crizotinib versus chemotherapy in advanced alk-positive lung cancer. *N. Engl. J. Med.* 2013, *368*, 2385–2394.
30. le Coutre, P.; Tassi, E.; Varella-Garcia, M.; Barni, R.; Mologni, L.; Cabrita, G.; Marchesi, E.; Supino, R.; Gambacorti-Passerini, C. Induction of resistance to the abelson inhibitor sti571 in human leukemic cells through gene amplification. *Blood* 2000, *95*, 1758–1766.
31. Druker, B.J.; Guilhot, F.; O'Brien, S.G.; Gathmann, I.; Kantarjian, H.; Gattermann, N.; Deininger, M.W.; Silver, R.T.; Goldman, J.M.; Stone, R.M.; *et al.* Five-year follow-up of patients receiving imatinib for chronic myeloid leukemia. *N. Engl. J. Med.* 2006, *355*, 2408–2417.
32. Yang, J.C.; Sequist, L.V.; Geater, S.L.; Tsai, C.M.; Mok, T.S.; Schuler, M.; Yamamoto, N.; Yu, C.J.; Ou, S.H.; Zhou, C.; *et al.* Clinical activity of afatinib in patients with advanced non-small-cell lung cancer harbouring uncommon EGFR mutations: A combined post-hoc analysis of LUX-Lung 2, LUX-Lung 3, And LUX-Lung 6. *Lancet Oncol.* 2015, *16*, 830–838.
33. Lorenzen, S.; Riera Knorrenschild, J.; Haag, G.M.; Pohl, M.; Thuss-Patience, P.; Bassermann, F.; Helbig, U.; Weissinger, F.; Schnoy, E.; Becker, K.; *et al.* Lapatinib *versus* lapatinib plus capecitabine as second-line treatment in human epidermal growth factor receptor 2-amplified metastatic gastro-oesophageal cancer: A randomised phase II trial of the arbeitsgemeinschaft internistische onkologie. *Eur. J. Cancer* 2015, *51*, 569–576.
34. London, C.A.; Malpas, P.B.; Wood-Follis, S.L.; Boucher, J.F.; Rusk, A.W.; Rosenberg, M.P.; Henry, C.J.; Mitchener, K.L.; Klein, M.K.; Hintermeister, J.G.; *et al.* Multi-center, placebo-controlled, double-blind, randomized study of oral toceranib phosphate (SU11654), a receptor tyrosine kinase inhibitor, for the treatment of dogs with recurrent (either local or distant) mast cell tumor following surgical excision. *Clin. Cancer Res.* 2009, *15*, 3856–3865.
35. Solomon, B.J.; Mok, T.; Kim, D.W.; Wu, Y.L.; Nakagawa, K.; Mekhail, T.; Felip, E.; Cappuzzo, F.; Paolini, J.; Usari, T.; *et al.* First-line crizotinib *versus* chemotherapy in ALK-positive lung cancer. *N. Engl. J. Med.* 2014, *371*, 2167–2177.
36. Duyster, J.; Bai, R.Y.; Morris, S.W. Translocations involving anaplastic lymphoma kinase (ALK). *Oncogene* 2001, *20*, 5623–5637.
37. Rikova, K.; Guo, A.; Zeng, Q.; Possemato, A.; Yu, J.; Haack, H.; Nardone, J.; Lee, K.; Reeves, C.; Li, Y.; *et al.* Global survey of phosphotyrosine signaling identifies oncogenic kinases in lung cancer. *Cell* 2007, *131*, 1190–1203.
38. Blackhall, F.H.; Peters, S.; Bubendorf, L.; Dafni, U.; Kerr, K.M.; Hager, H.; Soltermann, A.; O'Byrne, K.J.; Dooms, C.; Sejda, A.; *et al.* Prevalence and clinical outcomes for patients with ALK-positive resected stage I to III adenocarcinoma:

Results from the european thoracic oncology platform lungscape project. *J. Clin. Oncol.* 2014, *32*, 2780–2787.

39. Engelman, J.A.; Zejnullahu, K.; Mitsudomi, T.; Song, Y.; Hyland, C.; Park, J.O.; Lindeman, N.; Gale, C.M.; Zhao, X.; Christensen, J.; *et al.* Met amplification leads to gefitinib resistance in lung cancer by activating ERBB3 signaling. *Science* 2007, *316*, 1039–1043.
40. Cui, J.J. Targeting receptor tyrosine kinase met in cancer: Small molecule inhibitors and clinical progress. *J. Med. Chem.* 2014, *57*, 4427–4453.
41. Copland, M.; Hamilton, A.; Elrick, L.J.; Baird, J.W.; Allan, E.K.; Jordanides, N.; Barow, M.; Mountford, J.C.; Holyoake, T.L. Dasatinib (BMS-354825) targets an earlier progenitor population than imatinib in primary cml but does not eliminate the quiescent fraction. *Blood* 2006, *107*, 4532–4539.
42. Weisberg, E.; Manley, P.W.; Breitenstein, W.; Bruggen, J.; Cowan-Jacob, S.W.; Ray, A.; Huntly, B.; Fabbro, D.; Fendrich, G.; Hall-Meyers, E.; *et al.* Characterization of AMN107, a selective inhibitor of native and mutant BCR-ABL.*Cancer Cell* 2005, *7*, 129–141.
43. Shah, N.P.; Lee, F.Y.; Luo, R.; Jiang, Y.; Donker, M.; Akin, C. Dasatinib (BMS-354825) inhibits kitd816v, an imatinib-resistant activating mutation that triggers neoplastic growth in most patients with systemic mastocytosis. *Blood* 2006,*108*, 286–291.
44. Gumireddy, K.; Reddy, M.V.; Cosenza, S.C.; Boominathan, R.; Baker, S.J.; Papathi, N.; Jiang, J.; Holland, J.; Reddy, E.P. ON01910, a non-ATP-competitive small molecule inhibitor of Plk1, is a potent anticancer agent. *Cancer Cell* 2005, *7*, 275–286.
45. Copland, M.; Pellicano, F.; Richmond, L.; Allan, E.K.; Hamilton, A.; Lee, F.Y.; Weinmann, R.; Holyoake, T.L. BMS-214662 potently induces apoptosis of chronic myeloid leukemia stem and progenitor cells and synergizes with tyrosine kinase inhibitors. *Blood* 2008, *111*, 2843–2853.
46. Yap, T.A.; Workman, P. Exploiting the cancer genome: Strategies for the discovery and clinical development of targeted molecular therapeutics. *Annu. Rev. Pharmacol. Toxicol.* 2012, *52*, 549–573.
47. DiMasi, J.A.; Grabowski, H.G. Economics of new oncology drug development. *J. Clin. Oncol.* 2007, *25*, 209–216.
48. Adams, D.J. The valley of death in anticancer drug development: A reassessment. *Trends Pharmacol. Sci.* 2012, *33*, 173–180.
49. Wong, T.Y. How to bridge the "valley of death" between a research discovery and clinical application? *Ann. Acad. Med. Singap.* 2014, *43*, 422–424.
50. Paoloni, M.; Mazcko, C.; Selting, K.; Lana, S.; Barber, L.; Phillips, J.; Skorupski, K.; Vail, D.; Wilson, H.; Biller, B.; *et al.* Defining the pharmacodynamic profile and therapeutic index of NHS-IL12 immunocytokine in dogs with malignant melanoma. *PLoS ONE* 2015.
51. Paoloni, M.; Webb, C.; Mazcko, C.; Cherba, D.; Hendricks, W.; Lana, S.; Ehrhart,

E.J.; Charles, B.; Fehling, H.; Kumar, L.; *et al.* Prospective molecular profiling of canine cancers provides a clinically relevant comparative model for evaluating personalized medicine (PMed) trials. *PLoS ONE* 2014.

52. Paoloni, M.; Lana, S.; Thamm, D.; Mazcko, C.; Withrow, S. The creation of the comparative oncology trials consortium pharmacodynamic core: Infrastructure for a virtual laboratory. *Vet. J.* 2010, *185*, 88–89.
53. Paoloni, M.C.; Mazcko, C.; Fox, E.; Fan, T.; Lana, S.; Kisseberth, W.; Vail, D.M.; Nuckolls, K.; Osborne, T.; Yalkowsy, S.;*et al.* Rapamycin pharmacokinetic and pharmacodynamic relationships in osteosarcoma: A comparative oncology study in dogs. *PLoS ONE* 2010.
54. Gordon, I.; Paoloni, M.; Mazcko, C.; Khanna, C. The comparative oncology trials consortium: Using spontaneously occurring cancers in dogs to inform the cancer drug development pathway. *PLoS Med.* 2009.
55. Paoloni, M.C.; Tandle, A.; Mazcko, C.; Hanna, E.; Kachala, S.; Leblanc, A.; Newman, S.; Vail, D.; Henry, C.; Thamm, D.; *et al.* Launching a novel preclinical infrastructure: Comparative oncology trials consortium directed therapeutic targeting of TNFα to cancer vasculature. *PLoS ONE* 2009, *4*, e4972.
56. London, C.A.; Bernabe, L.F.; Barnard, S.; Kisseberth, W.C.; Borgatti, A.; Henson, M.; Wilson, H.; Jensen, K.; Ito, D.; Modiano, J.F.; *et al.* Preclinical evaluation of the novel, orally bioavailable selective inhibitor of nuclear export (SINE) KPT-335 in spontaneous canine cancer: Results of a phase I study. *PLoS ONE* 2014.
57. Lindblad-Toh, K.; Wade, C.M.; Mikkelsen, T.S.; Karlsson, E.K.; Jaffe, D.B.; Kamal, M.; Clamp, M.; Chang, J.L.; Kulbokas, E.J., 3rd; Zody, M.C.; *et al.* Genome sequence, comparative analysis and haplotype structure of the domestic dog. *Nature* 2005, *438*, 803–819.
58. Hoeppner, M.P.; Lundquist, A.; Pirun, M.; Meadows, J.R.; Zamani, N.; Johnson, J.; Sundstrom, G.; Cook, A.; FitzGerald, M.G.; Swofford, R.; *et al.* An improved canine genome and a comprehensive catalogue of coding genes and non-coding transcripts. *PLoS ONE* 2014.
59. LeBlanc, A.K.; Mazcko, C.N.; Khanna, C. Defining the value of a comparative approach to cancer drug development.*Clin. Cancer Res.* 2015.
60. Webster, J.D.; Simpson, E.R.; Michalowski, A.M.; Hoover, S.B.; Simpson, R.M. Quantifying histological features of cancer biospecimens for biobanking quality assurance using automated morphometric pattern recognition image analysis algorithms. *J. Biomol. Tech.* 2011, *22*, 108–118.
61. Simpson, R.M.; Bastian, B.C.; Michael, H.T.; Webster, J.D.; Prasad, M.L.; Conway, C.M.; Prieto, V.M.; Gary, J.M.; Goldschmidt, M.H.; Esplin, D.G.; *et al.* Sporadic naturally occurring melanoma in dogs as a preclinical model for human melanoma. *Pigment Cell Melanoma Res.* 2014, *27*, 37–47.
62. Bushell, K.R.; Kim, Y.; Chan, F.C.; Ben-Neriah, S.; Jenks, A.; Alcaide, M.; Fornika, D.; Grande, B.M.; Arthur, S.; Gascoyne, R.D.; *et al.* Genetic inactivation of TRAF3 in canine and human B-cell lymphoma. *Blood* 2015, *125*, 999–1005.

63. Elvers, I.; Turner-Maier, J.; Swofford, R.; Koltookian, M.; Johnson, J.; Stewart, C.; Zhang, C.Z.; Schumacher, S.E.; Beroukhim, R.; Rosenberg, M.; *et al.* Exome sequencing of lymphomas from three dog breeds reveals somatic mutation patterns reflecting genetic background. *Genome Res.* 2015, *25*, 1634–1645.

64. Mochizuki, H.; Kennedy, K.; Shapiro, S.G.; Breen, M. BRAF mutations in canine cancers. *PLoS ONE* 2015.

65. Decker, B.; Parker, H.G.; Dhawan, D.; Kwon, E.M.; Karlins, E.; Davis, B.W.; Ramos-Vara, J.A.; Bonney, P.L.; McNiel, E.A.; Knapp, D.W.; *et al.* Homologous mutation to human BRAF V600E is common in naturally occurring canine bladder cancer—Evidence for a relevant model system and urine-based diagnostic test. *Mol. Cancer Res.* 2015, *13*, 993–1002.

66. Butler, D. Translational research: Crossing the valley of death. *Nature* 2008, *453*, 840–842.

67. Jiang, F.; Zhang, J.; Wang, X.; Shen, X. Important steps to improve translation from medical research to health policy.*J. Transl. Med.* 2013.

68. Ranieri, G.; Gadaleta, C.D.; Patruno, R.; Zizzo, N.; Daidone, M.G.; Hansson, M.G.; Paradiso, A.; Ribatti, D. A model of study for human cancer: Spontaneous occurring tumors in dogs. Biological features and translation for new anticancer therapies. *Crit. Rev. Oncol. Hematol.* 2013, *88*, 187–197.

5
CHAPTER

A COMPARATIVE STUDY OF THE EFFICACY OF A CANARYPOX BASED RECOMBINANT LEUKEMIA VACCINE AGAINST A NATURAL CONTACT FELV CHALLENGE IN CATS

Sparkes AH, Tasker S, Thibault JC and Poulet H

Keywords: FeLV, vaccine, Canarypox virus, Efficacy, Contact challenge

INTRODUCTION

Feline leukaemia virus (FeLV) is a major pathogen of cats causing a wide range of clinical syndromes [1,2]. It has been described as the "most destructive of feline infectious diseases" [3] and an important cause of death. The prognosis for persistently viraemic cats is typically poor with over 80% dying within 3-5 years after diagnosis [4-6].

The prevalence of FeLV depends on the geography and the cat population, typically ranging from 2-3% to more than 10% p27 positive cats in high-risk environment [7-11]. Overall the prevalence has been reduced in some countries as a result of both vaccination and management of infected cats. Nevertheless, FeLV infection still remains a risk in some cat populations, such as certain free-roaming cats [9,12] or even client-owned cats in some geographical areas [13-15] which display higher prevalence rates. It is well recognized that FeLV p27 antigen negative status can occur following exposure to FeLV, as indicated by the presence of FeLV provirus in tissues or blood [16,17]. Since most studies are based on FeLV p27 antigen detection, it is therefore likely that FeLV exposure and infection are underestimated in such studies.

Citation: Sparkes AH, Tasker S, Thibault JC, Poulet H (2015) A Comparative Study of the Efficacy of a Canarypox Based Recombinant Leukemia Vaccine against a Natural Contact Felv Challenge in Cats. J Vaccines Vaccin 6:300. doi:10.4172/2157-7560.1000300.

Although they do not necessarily prevent infection [18,19], FeLV vaccines are potentially able to prevent persistent viraemia and thereby the diseases caused by FeLV as well as the shedding of the virus [20]. Most vaccines available on the market are classical inactivated or subunit adjuvanted vaccines. With the aim to reduce the incidence of injection site reactions, a non-adjuvanted canarypox virus vectored vaccine has been developed where the recombinant canarypox virus vector expresses envelope glycoproteins (p15E and gp70) and capsid proteins of FeLV A, which have been shown to provide protection against FeLV oro-nasal challenge [21-23]. Efficacy data have been published for the different types of vaccines but few comparative studies are available [20]. In addition, most of the published studies rely on artificial challenge models, using the intra-peritoneal route or high doses of challenge virus with simultaneous administration of glucocorticoids [24]. Although less commonly performed, natural challenge models of infection are generally regarded as the most valuable method of assessing FeLV vaccine efficacy, mimicking natural infection as much as possible.

This study was designed to assess the efficacy of a non-adjuvanted canarypox virus vectored vaccine (EURIFEL® FeLV renamed PUREVAX® FeLV, Merial) and a sub-unit vaccine, LEUCOGEN® in a natural challenge model of FeLV infection [25]. LEUCOGEN®is a p45 sub-unit vaccine adjuvanted with aluminium hydroxide and saponin [26].

MATERIALS AND METHODS

Animals and challenge Specific pathogen free (SPF) kittens were used for the study and housed in a confined environment. All kittens were FeLV negative by p27 antigen screening (IDEXX, Westbrook, USA) prior to inclusion in the study. The kittens were divided into four groups:

- Group A comprised 18 kittens which served as the source of natural challenge. They were challenged at 8-9 weeks of age with 1×10^6 focus forming units of Glasgow-1 strain of FeLV-A with 0.25 ml administered into each nostril and 0.5 ml orally to induce persistent viraemia.
- Groups B and C comprised 24 kittens in each and received one of the two vaccines being tested
- Group D comprised 23 kittens given placebo to serve as controls.
- Cats from groups B, C and D were also shown to be free of antibodies against gp70 at the time of inclusion. Allocation to these groups B, C and D was performed using a computerized randomization program based on age, sex, parentage and weight in descending order of priority.

Vaccination

Kittens in Groups B and C were vaccinated according to the manufacturer's recommendations. Kittens in group B were vaccinated at 8-9 weeks of age and four weeks later with EURIFEL® FeLV (renamed PUREVAX® FeLV), a non-adjuvanted recombinant canarypox virus expressing the env and gag/pro genes of FeLV A (vCP97). Kittens in group C were vaccinated at 9-10 weeks of age and again three weeks later at

12-13 weeks of age with LEUCOGEN® purchased from a veterinary drug wholesaler. Group D kittens received subcutaneous injections of sterile phosphate buffered saline at 8-9 weeks of age and at 12-13 weeks of age as a placebo.

The four groups were initially kept in separate rooms. Two weeks after cats in groups B and C received their second vaccination; the kittens from all four groups were mixed and housed in the same room. They shared litter pans, food bowls and water dishes for the remainder of the trial. Kittens in Group A were approximately four weeks older than kittens from Groups B, C and D.

Post-Challenge Follow-Up

Blood samples were collected by jugular venipuncture from all kittens every two weeks for the first 14 weeks and then every three weeks until the end of the trial, 27 weeks after mixing. The blood samples were tested using both a standard commercial ELISA for FeLV p27 antigen (Inochem, Carnforth, UK or IDEXX, Westbrook, USA) and virus isolation on QN10S cells based on the method of Jarrett et al. (1982) [27]. Persistent viraemia was defined as positive viraemia and/or antigenemia for the final three blood samples of the study or, for the cats which were euthanized before the end of the trial, for the three samples prior to death. Vaccine efficacy was calculated as the preventable fraction (Table 2).

STATISTICAL ANALYSIS

The proportion of persistently viraemic cats in each group was compared by 2 test or Fisher's exact test (comparison between vaccinated groups). The Kaplan-Meier Product-Limit method was used to plot the "survival" curves defining the time to viraemia or antigenaemia, and to compare the median time to viraemia or antigenaemia (Log-rank test). The analyses were two-tailed and conducted with SAS 9.2 (SAS Institute Inc, Cary, NC) or Statgraphics Plus 5.1 (StatPoints Technologies Inc., Warrenton, VA). The type I error was set to α=5%.

RESULTS

Eleven out of 18 kittens in Group A became antigenaemic/viraemic within four weeks of challenge and 14 were antigenaemic/viraemic by the time of mixing (six weeks after challenge). Three of the remaining kittens became antigenaemic/viraemic before the end of the trial and the final kitten remained negative throughout. Four of the viraemic kittens from Group A were euthanized during the trial-two due to severe anaemia at 28 and 32 weeks after challenge, one due to an abdominal mass at 23 weeks after challenge, and one due to paraparesis one week before the trial terminated.

Results of p27 ELISA and virus isolation were highly consistent overall, although viral isolation was slightly more sensitive than p27 ELISA (Table 1). Eighteen of 23 (78%) kittens from Group D became persistently viraemic - one died of unrelated causes during the trial but was persistently viraemic.

Four of the remaining 5 cats in this group became antigen and/or virus isolation positive during the last three weeks of the trial but did not fulfil the criteria for persistent viraemia. Four kittens from Group B became persistently viraemic (time to onset of viraemia was respectively 6, 10, 12 and 18 weeks, Figure 1). Only one other kitten in this group tested positive (on virus isolation), at the end of the trial. Six kittens from Group C became persistently viraemic (time to onset of viraemia was 6 weeks for one cat and 18 weeks for the remainder) and one other kitten became antigenaemic/viraemic on the two final two tests of the trial.

Table 1: Antigenaemia and viraemia status of the cats aier mixing with Group A on week 0

Week	Criteria	Canarypox-FeLV #/24	LEUCOGEN #/24	Control #/23
	Neg	24	24	23
	p27	0	0	0
1	VI	0	0	0
	Neg	24	24	20
	p27	0	0	2
4	VI	0	0	3
	Neg	23	23	19
	p27	0	1	3
6	VI	1	1	4
	Neg	23	23	18
	p27	1	1	5
8	VI	1	1	5
	Neg	22	23	17
	p27	2	1	6
10	VI	1	1	6
	Neg	21	23	12
	p27	2	1	7
12	VI	3	1	11
	Neg	21	23	9
	p27	3	1	13
14	VI	3	1	13
	Neg	20	18	5

	p27	4	6	17
18	VI	4	6	18
	Neg	20	18	5
	p27	4	6	17
21	VI	4	6	18
	Neg	20	17	1
	p27	4	6	20
25	VI	4	7	21
	Neg	19	17	1
	p27	4	7	21
27	VI	5	7	22

neg: neither antigenaemic nor viraemic
p27: antigenaemic; VI: viraemic; #: number of cats

The proportions of persistently viraemic kittens for each group and the preventable fractions achieved by the two vaccines are shown in Table 2.

Table 2: Preventable fraction in vaccinated groups (PF=(Pv-Pc)/(1-Pc) where Pv is the proportion of vaccinated cats which became persistently viraemic and Pc the proportion of controls which became viraemic)

Group	Total number	Number persistently viraemic	Proportion persistently viraemic	Preventable fraction
Canarypox-FeLV	24	4	17%	79%
Leucogen	24	6	25%	68%
Controls	23	18	78%	-

There was a significant difference in the proportion of persistently viraemic kittens between the different groups ($\chi 2$ test; $p<0.0001$) but no significant difference between the two vaccine groups (Fisher's exact test; p=0.5).

The time to positive viraemia or antigenemia was significantly reduced in vaccinated groups (Log-rank test; $p<0.001$), and the difference between vaccinated groups was not statistically significant (Log-rank test; p=0.58).

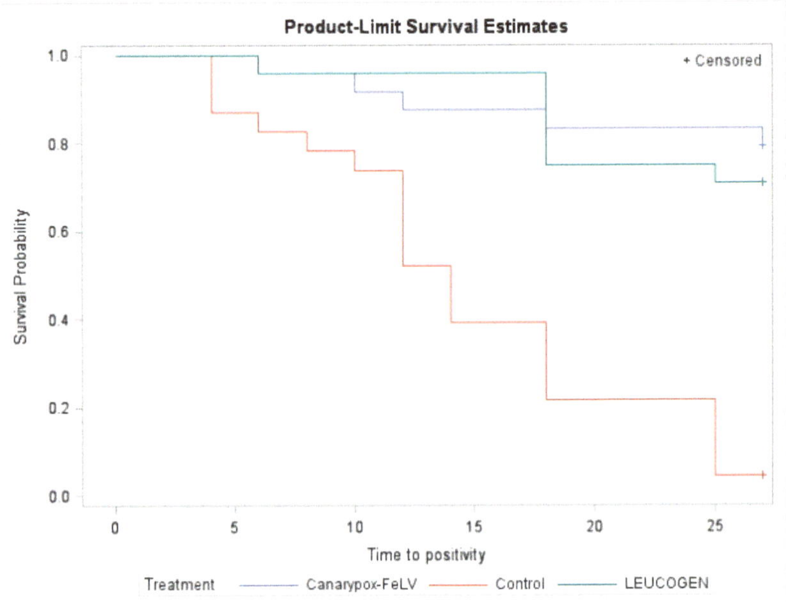

Figure 1: Evolution of the rate of negative cats per group (expressed as survival probability on y-axis in %) aier mixing with Group A on week 0 (x-axis in weeks). A negative cat does not have detectable p27 antigenaemia nor viraemia.

DISCUSSION

In the absence of identified correlate of protection, vaccine efficacy has traditionally been evaluated using experimental challenge with a virulent FeLV strain. The best practice should be to use a challenge model as close as possible to the natural conditions of infection. Using other routes of infection than the oro-nasal route or the concurrent administration of corticosteroids may introduce a bias in the assessment of vaccine efficacy. Although an oro-nasal challenge with a virulent FeLV strain is feasible as shown in our study, the intraperitoneal route or the simultaneous administration of glucocorticoids has frequently been used to increase the efficiency of FeLV challenge [20,24,28]. However, the route of infection may have an impact on the outcome of an infectious challenge and consequently on the efficacy of a vaccine candidate. As an example, Dunham and coll. showed that a vaccine against FIV was able to provide some protection against an intra-peritoneal challenge but not against an intra-muscular one [29]. Similarly, corticosteroids-induced immunosuppression may introduce a bias in the evaluation of vaccine efficacy. Indeed, glucocorticoids suppress cellular (Th1) immunity and promote humoral (Th2) immunity [30]. As a consequence, the impact of corticosteroids on vaccine efficacy may be different depending on the mode of action of the vaccine. Furthermore, administration of a single high dose of challenge virus to ensure a high rate of infection in controls (as required by FeLV vaccine monograph) is not representative of natural conditions and may be an unnecessary difficulty in the development of an efficacious vaccine. The natural transmission is usually the result of prolonged or repeated contacts between cats. In an attempt to address this concern, we used an experimental model which simulates natural transmission of infection and may enable a more reliable determination of the efficacy of protection that can be expected under field conditions.

In the FeLV vaccine monograph of the European Pharmacopeia, the efficacy test for FeLV vaccines is stringent and requires that 80% of the control cats become persistently viraemic. This is one of the reasons why natural transmission contact challenge studies are not routinely used to demonstrate the efficacy of FeLV vaccines, despite the fact that using natural routes of infection for such studies may produce results that are more likely to reflect the true efficacy of vaccines. In our study, the rate of persistent viraemia in controls cats (78%) approached what is often obtained in classical oro-nasal or intra-peritoneal challenges [20]. In addition, three of the four kittens in the control group that did not become persistently viraemic showed evidence of infection by the end of the trial and it is likely that most, if not all, of these would have become persistently viraemic if the follow-up period had been extended. This demonstrates that our challenge model was rigorous compared with previous natural models, which displayed lower infection rates [31-37]. The origin of the cats, housing conditions and/or the FeLV challenge strain may explain some of these differences. The strong virulence of Glasgow-1 strain was indeed illustrated by the appearance of clinical signs strongly suggestive of FeLV infection in kittens from group A (anaemia, abdominal mass, paraparesis).

The overall rate of antigenaemic cats observed in our study is much higher than what is usually reported in the field. In some high-risk environments the proportion of antigenaemic cats can reach 10-20% [38,39], far lower than in the current study. However, those populations included cats of varying ages and it is well recognized that susceptibility to FeLV infection is higher in young kittens than in adult cats [32,40], and the cats in our study were actually all young. Our study confirmed that transmission of FeLV is very efficient in young cats living in close contact and in confinement in a restricted environment.

Results of p27 antigenemia and virus isolation on blood samples were comparable in this study. Virus isolation appeared to be slightly more sensitive than antigenaemia, although the ease of detecting antigenaemia generally makes this the method of choice to assess the FeLV status of cats in many clinical studies. In the European Pharmacopeia, persistent antigenaemia or viraemia is defined by three consecutive positive results or five positive results at any time during the follow-up period. However, the results at the end of the trial may be more relevant indicators of FeLV status and potential persistent viraemia. This is particularly true for a natural challenge model where it generally takes longer for persistent viraemia to become established. In our study, comparable to previous reports [35], the time between mixing the groups and the first detection of viraemia varied from 4 to 27 weeks and it took more than 21 weeks to get close to 80% of the control cats persistently infected. This is likely to be the result of the overall infectious pressure increasing as new cats became persistently viraemic.

In recombinant canarypox-FeLV and LEUCOGEN® vaccinated cats, only 4 and 6 cats out of 24 in each group became persistently viraemic respectively. In both groups, one additional cat was positive by the end of the study. Overall, both vaccines significantly reduced the risk of persistent viraemia with preventable fractions of 79% and 68% respectively. While we cannot rule out the possibility that those figures would have changed if the cats had been kept in contact for a longer period [32], we believe that contact for more than 6 months can be considered as a good challenge model, especially given the infection rate seen in the control cats. A contact challenge over a 6 month period is likely to be a mix of immediate, late and repeated infections via the natural route of transmission. This suggests that the canarypoxvectored FeLV vaccine-induced immunity against FeLV was early and sustained over the 6-month follow-up period. These results are consistent with previous data demonstrating the efficacy of the nonadjuvanted canarypox-vectored FeLV vaccine against classical challenges performed 2-3 weeks or one year after vaccination [19,21,22]. Of note, the canarypox-FeLV vaccine protected more than 80% of the cats against persistent viraemia as requested by the FeLV monograph of the European Pharmacopeia.

In this study, infectious pressure increased with time while new cats became persistently viraemic and thereby additional shedders of FeLV. In that respect, the challenge model was likely more severe than in the usual field conditions where prophylaxis against FeLV relies also on the detection and isolation of FeLV positive cats to reduce the risk of exposure for non-infected animals.

CONCLUSION

The natural challenge model to assess FeLV vaccines in this study proved to be a potent method to reproduce FeLV challenge, confirming that under appropriate conditions FeLV is efficiently transmitted. Despite the severity of the challenge, both vaccines provided a comparable and good protection against persistent viraemia over a 6- month contact period which led to persistent viraemia in most of the controls. This study confirmed the efficacy of a non-adjuvanted canarypox-vectored FeLV vaccine against a contact challenge mimicking the natural conditions of infection.

ACKNOWLEDGEMENTS

The authors want to thank Franz Oberly for the statistical analyses.

REFERENCES

1. Hartmann K (2012) Clinical aspects of feline retroviruses: a review. Viruses 4: 2684-2710.
2. Willett BJ, Hosie MJ (2013) Feline leukaemia virus: half a century since its discovery. Vet J 195: 16-23.
3. Loar AS (1993) Feline leukemia virus. Immunization and prevention. Vet Clin North America 23: 193-211.

4. McClelland AJ, Hardy WD Jr, Zuckermann EE (1980) Prognosis of healthy feline leukemia virus infected cats. Dev Cancer Res 4: 121.

5. Hoover EA, Mullins JI (1991) Feline leukemia virus infection and diseases. J Am Vet Med Assoc 199: 1287-1297.

6. Helfer-Hungerbuehler AK, Widmer S, Kessler Y, Riond B, Boretti FS et al. (2014) Long-term follow up of feline leukemia virus infection and characterization of viral RNA loads using molecular methods in tissues of cats with different infection outcomes. Virus Res 197: 137-150.

7. Bandecchi P, Dell'Omodarme M, Magi M, Palamidessi A, Prati MC (2006) Feline leukaemia virus (FeLV) and feline immunodeficiency virus infections in cats in the Pisa district of Tuscany, and attempts to control FeLV infection in a colony of domestic cats by vaccination. Vet Rec 158: 555-557.

8. Gleich SE, Krieger S, Hartmann K (2009) Prevalence of feline immunodeficiency virus and feline leukaemia virus among client-owned cats and risk factors for infection in Germany. J Feline Med Surg 11: 985-992.

9. Lee IT, Levy JK, Gorman SP, Crawford PC, Slater MR (2002) Prevalence of feline leukemia virus infection and serum antibodies against feline immunodeficiency virus in unowned free-roaming cats. J Am Vet Med Assoc 220: 620-622.

10. Little S (2011) A review of feline leukemia virus and feline immunodeficiency virus seroprevalence in cats in Canada. Vet ImmunolImmunopathol 143: 243-245.

11. Rypuła K, Płoneczka-Janeczko K, Bierowiec K, Kumala A, Sapikowski G (2014) Prevalence of viral infections in cats in southwestern Poland in the years 2006 to 2010. Berl Munch TierarztlWochenschr 127: 163-165.

12. Duarte A, Fernandes M, Santos N, Tavares L (2012) Virological Survey in free-ranging wildcats (Felissilvestris) and feral domestic cats in Portugal. Vet Microbiol 158:400-404.

13. Arjona A, Escolar E, Soto I, Barquero N, Martin D, Gomez-Lucia E (2000) Seroepidemiological survey of infection by feline leukemia virus and immunodeficiency virus in Madrid and correlation with some clinical aspects. J ClinMicrobiol 38: 3448-3449.

14. Ortega-Pacheco A, Aguilar-Caballero AJ, Colin-Flores RF, Acosta-Viana KY, Guzman-Marin E, et al. (2014) Seroprevalence of feline leukemia virus, feline immunodeficiency virus and heartworm infection among owned cats in tropical Mexico. J Feline Med Surg 16: 460-464.

15. Cong W, Meng QF, Blaga R, Villena I, Zhu XQ, et al. (2015) Toxoplasma gondii, Dirofilariaimmitis, feline immunodeficiency virus (FIV), and feline leukemia virus (FeLV) infections in stray and pet cats (Feliscatus) in northwest China: co-infections and risk factors. Parasitol Res.

16. Major A, Cattori V, Boenzli E, Riond B, Ossent P, et al. (2010) Exposure of cats to low doses of FeLV: seroconversion as the sole parameter of infection. Vet Res 41: 17.

17. Suntz M, Failing K, Hecht W, Schwartz D, Reinacher M (2010) High prevalence of non-productive FeLV infection in necropsied cats and significant association with pathological findings. Vet ImmunolImmunopathol 136: 71-80.
18. Hofmann-Lehmann R, Cattori V, Tandon R, Boretti FS, Meli ML, et al. (2007) Vaccination against the feline leukaemia virus: outcome and response categories and long-term follow-up. Vaccine 25: 5531-5539.
19. Hofmann-Lehmann R, Cattori V, Tandon R, Boretti FS, Meli ML, et al. (2008) How molecular methods change our views of FeLV infection and vaccination. Vet ImmunolImmunopathol 123: 119-123.
20. Sparkes AH (1997) Feline leukaemia virus: a review of immunity and vaccination. J Small AnimPract 38: 187-194.
21. Tartaglia J, Jarrett O, Neil JC, Desmettre P, Paoletti E (1993) Protection of cats against feline leukemia virus by vaccination with a canarypox virus recombinant, ALVAC-FL. J Virol 67: 2370-2375.
22. Poulet H, Brunet S, Boularand C, Guiot AL, Leroy V, et al. (2003) Efficacy of a canarypox virus-vectored vaccine against feline leukaemia. Vet Rec 153: 141-145.
23. Schlecht-Louf G, Mangeney M, El-Garch H, Lacombe V, Poulet H, et al. (2014) A targeted mutation within the feline leukemia virus (FeLV) envelope protein immunosuppressive domain to improve a canarypox virus-vectored FeLV vaccine. J Virol 88: 992-1001
24. Patel M, Carritt K, Lane J, Jayappa H, Stahl M, Bourgeois M (2015) Comparative Efficacy of Feline Leukemia Virus (FeLV) Inactivated Whole-Virus Vaccine and Canarypox Virus-Vectored Vaccine during Virulent FeLV Challenge and Immunosuppression. Clin Vaccine Immunol 22: 798-805.
25. Jarrett O, Ganière JP (1996) Comparative studies of the efficacy of a recombinant feline leukaemia virus vaccine. Vet Rec 138: 7-11.
26. Kensil CR, Barrett C, Kushner N, Beltz G, Storey J, et al. (1991) Development of a genetically engineered vaccine against feline leukemia virus infection. J Am Vet Med Assoc 199: 1423-1427.
27. Jarrett O, Golder MC, Weijer K (1982) A comparison of three methods of feline leukaemia virus diagnosis. Vet Rec 110: 325.
28. Stuke K, King V, Southwick K, Stoeva MI, Thomas A, et al. (2014) Efficacy of an inactivated FeLV vaccine compared to a recombinant FeLV vaccine in minimum age cats following virulent FeLV challenge. Vaccine 32:2599-2603.
29. Dunham S, Bruce J, MacKay S, Golder M, Jarrett O, et al. (2004) Efficacy of Feline Immunodeficiency Virus vaccines FEL-O-VAX and FIVGL8ΔIN DNA vaccine: effect of the route of challenge on the outcome. Abstract of 7th International Feline Retrovirus Research Symposium, Pisa, Italy.
30. Franchimont D (2004) Overview of the actions of glucocorticoids on the immune response: a good model to characterize new pathways of immunosuppression for new treatment strategies. Ann N Y AcadSci 1024: 124-137.

31. Pedersen NC, Theilen G, Keane MA, Fairbanks L, Mason T, et al. (1977) Studies of naturally transmitted feline leukemia virus infection. Am J Vet Res 38: 1523-1531.
32. Grant CK, Essex M, Gardner MB, Hardy WD Jr (1980) Natural Feline leukemia virus infection and the immune response of cats of different ages. Cancer Res 40: 823-829.
33. Lafrado W (1994) Evaluation of a feline leukemia virus vaccine in a controlled natural transmission study. J Am Vet Med Assoc 204: 914-917.
34. Legendre AM, Mitchener KL, Potgieler LND (1990) Efficacy of a feline leukemia virus vaccine in a natural exposure challenge. J Vet Intern Med 4: 92-98.
35. Legendre AM, Hawks DM, Sebring R, Rohrbach B, Chavez L, et al. (1991) Comparison of the efficacy of three commercial feline leukemia virus vaccines in a natural challenge exposure. J Am Vet Med Assoc 199: 1456-1462.
36. Scarlett JM, Pollock RV (1991) Year two of follow-up evaluation of a randomized, blind field trial of a commercial feline leukemia virus vaccine. J Am Vet Med Assoc 199: 1431-1432.
37. Sebring RW, Chu HJ, Chavez LG, Sandblom DS, Hustead DR, et al. (1991) Feline leukemia virus vaccine development. J Am Vet Med Assoc 199: 1413-1419.
38. Addie DD, Dennis JM, Toth S, Callanan JJ, Reid S, et al. (2000) Long-term impact on a closed household of pet cats of natural infection with feline coronavirus, feline leukaemia virus and feline immunodeficiency virus. Vet Rec 146: 419-424.
39. Bande F, Arshad SS, Hassan L, Zakaria Z, Sapian NA, et al. (2012) Prevalence and risk factors of feline leukaemia virus and feline immunodeficiency virus in peninsular Malaysia. BMC Vet Res 8: 33.
40. Wilson S, Greenslade J, Saunders G, Holcroft C, Bruce L, et al. (2012) Difficulties in demonstrating long term immunity in FeLV vaccinated cats due to increasing age-related resistance to infection. BMC Vet Res 8:125.

6

CHAPTER

UNDERSTANDING THE OSTEOSARCOMA PATHOBIOLOGY: A COMPARATIVE ONCOLOGY APPROACH

Jyotika Varshney, Milcah C. Scott , David A. Largaespada and Subbaya Subramanian

Keywords: *Osteosarcoma*, comparative oncology, microRNAs, prognosis, canine osteosarcoma

INTRODUCTION

Osteosarcoma is an aggressive primary bone tumor most prevalent in human patients. It mostly occurs during adolescence, with a second peak at middle age (older than 40) [1,2]. The tumor is characterized by increased production of osteoid (abnormal bone matrix) and by exceptionally complex karyotypes [3,4]. While the target cell for malignant transformation in the formation of osteosarcoma is not known with certainty, it is thought to be a mesenchymal stem cell (MSC) or a cell committed to the osteoblast lineage [5]. Evidence from mouse models indicates that any of several cell stages could serve as target cells for osteosarcoma development [6]. There are three common histologic types of osteosarcoma: osteoblastic, where tumor cells produce large amounts of tumor osteoid; chondroblastic, where tumor cells produce chondroid (cartilage) in addition to some amount of tumor osteoid; and fibroblastic, where tumor cells are predominantly fibroblasts and can produce both collagen and tumor osteoid [7]. The disease is highly metastatic, with distant spread mostly to lungs and other sites in bone, but osteosarcoma can also metastasize to lymph nodes and intra-abdominal organs [8,9]. The metastatic pattern (lungs, bones, lymph nodes) is similar for dogs and humans [10]. Osteosarcoma may present with macroscopic metastatic disease or

Citation: Jyotika Varshney, Milcah C. Scott, David A. Largaespada and Subbaya Subramanian, Understanding the Osteosarcoma Pathobiology: A Comparative Oncology Approach, doi:10.3390/vetsci3010003.

metastatic disease can occur after therapy. In either case, prognosis is significantly worse once metastasis has been detected [11,12].

In canine patients, osteosarcoma is a disease primarily of adult dogs; the median age at diagnosis is approximately eight years, with a small peak of incidence in young animals (younger than 3 years) [10,13]. This differs from the situation in human patients where the peak age of incidence is in adolescence. Nevertheless, the natural history of the disease is similar in canine and human osteosarcoma patients [14]. Moreover, we have observed that genome wide expression profiles of canine osteosarcoma are indistinguishable from human pediatric osteosarcoma and more like human osteosarcoma than any other human cancer [14,15]. In dogs, there is generally a strong breed preference in the risk for cancer, such as osteosarcoma [16,17]. Many large breed dogs have an increased risk for osteosarcoma compared to other breeds [4,18,19]. The genetic determinants of osteosarcoma susceptibility in dogs are not fully elucidated, and it is possible that these factors will also be important in human osteosarcoma susceptibility. The development of treatment strategies in dogs and people has proven mutually beneficial for both species [20]. In fact, current treatment options are similar in both species.

Osteosarcoma is treated using surgery, radiation and chemotherapy. Surgical techniques have greatly improved with time, and in many cases limb salvage is feasible with low rates of local recurrence in humans [21]. Combination chemotherapies are vital for effective treatment of osteosarcoma [22]. However, despite decades of effort, nothing better than the most often used combination of three chemotherapeutic agents (*i.e.*, methotrexate, doxorubicin and cisplatin) has been found [22].The adjuvant chemotherapy is generally administered prior to surgery and, according to many studies, the extent of necrosis observed in the primary tumor after surgical removal is correlated with the outcome. [21]. The goal of the adjuvant chemotherapy is to eliminate the micrometastases that are thought to be present in >80% of all patients at the time of diagnosis, thus preventing relapse [1]. New research is underway to define specific molecular targets that could be utilized to treat this disease, but their elucidation has been proven difficult. It is possible that osteosarcoma may also be treated using recently developed immunotherapies, such as immune checkpoint blockade or chimeric antigen receptor-engineered T cells [21].

Osteosarcoma is characterized by aneuploidy and extensive genetic instability [23]. Due to this extreme genetic instability, common causes of osteosarcoma development have largely been limited to implicating loss of *RB* and *TP53* regulated cellular activities and upregulation of *MYC* transcriptional activity reviewed by Morrow *et al.* [24]. Beyond these, few alterations are common or well accepted as osteosarcoma drivers. Gene amplification and protein overexpression of the*RUNX2* transcription factor, which is a regulator of bone renewal, has been proposed to drive osteosarcoma [25]. Conflicting data on activation of beta-catenin dependent transcription in osteosarcoma has been reported [26]. In addition, TGF-β signaling has been proposed to promote the acquisition of metastatic disease [27]. Notable, expression of Ezrin at high levels has been found in metastatic human and canine osteosarcoma and functionally validated in model systems as a driver of osteosarcoma metastasis [28]. Recently, a large scale *Sleeping Beauty* (SB) transposon-based forward genetic screen was carried out for osteosarcoma in mice [29]. From this screen, a large number of new candidate osteosarcoma proto-oncogene and tumor suppressors were reported. These included the candidate oncogenes *SEMA4D* and *SEMA6D*, which were partially functionally validated as well as tumor suppressors like *NF1*, *NF2* and *PTEN* [29]. Beyond protein encoding genes, several micro RNAs (miRNAs) and miRNA clusters have been suggested as drivers or suppressors of osteosarcoma development and progression [30]. What remains unclear is which common oncogenic drivers for osteosarcoma should be targeted and how they would be targeted. Unlike the case for other malignancies, osteosarcoma is genetically heterogeneous and common molecular targets may not be present.

Osteosarcoma is much more common in dogs than in people (greater than 15 times) and can be experimentally induced in mice via transgenesis. Perceivably, the opportunity to study osteosarcoma in three different species may make it possible to identify core genes and pathways, whose alterations are central to the osteosarcoma phenotype and that would make good targets for therapy. In the past, the main challenges were the development of improved surgical techniques for limb salvage, prevention of local recurrence and the identification of effective combination chemotherapies. Currently, a major pressing need is the development of new therapies to prevent the outgrowth of metastatic disease and to treat it once it has occurred. It is possible that germline or somatic mutations or tumor gene expression signatures identified through multi-species approaches could help predict which patients will respond well to current treatment regimes and which need to be referred for more intensive therapy or follow-up screening. However, much remains to be learned about what allows microscopic osteosarcoma lesions to resist chemotherapy and to suddenly break tumor dormancy and form a macroscopic mass. Until these questions are answered, we are not fully capable to help many human and canine osteosarcoma patients.

This review is an attempt to address many of the unanswered questions pertaining to osteosarcoma by focusing on recently acquired knowledge from a multi-species approach.

HUMAN OSTEOSARCOMA

Osteosarcoma in human patients is a rare tumor with a peak incidence in the second decade of life. The incidence is roughly 25 cases per 10 million per year in the United States [31]. A second wave of osteosarcoma is diagnosed in individuals between 70 and 80 years of age, often in association with Paget's disease. Paget's disease is an abnormality of bone homeostasis in which excessive bone reabsorption and reformation occur. Genetic and viral origins of Paget's disease have been suggested. While osteosarcoma is a rare manifestation of the disease, risk for osteosarcoma is increased. Osteosarcoma can occur in nearly any part of the skeleton, but commonly affects one of the long bones. As it occurs during a period of intense bone growth, there may be an association between this growth and sensitivity to osteoblast transformation [31]. Indeed, children with osteosarcoma are on average tall for their age [32]. Genetic studies also have suggested an association between the inheritance of certain forms of growth control genes and risk for osteosarcoma [33]. Other risk factors for human osteosarcoma include prior radiation therapy, male gender, and possibly African ancestry [34,35]. A genome-wide association study (GWAS) revealed possible risk alleles in the glutamate receptor, metaotropic 4 (*GRM4*) gene and a gene desert at chromosome 2p25.2 [36]. A recent GWAS also identified a potential high-risk allele for osteosarcoma metastasis at presentation within the transcriptional activator *NFIB* [37], a gene that was also identified as a potential tumor/metastasis suppressor in a transposon-based genetic screen in mice [29].

Some rare inherited cancer predisposition syndromes increase the risk for osteosarcoma. These rare cancers include Li-Fraumeni syndrome, hereditary retinoblastoma and Rothman-Thompson syndrome caused by germline mutations in *TP53, RB1*, and *RECQL4*, respectively [38]. Certain other cancer predisposition syndromes also seem to increase the risk of osteosarcoma development including Neurofibromatosis Type 1 syndrome, Werner's syndrome and Diamond-Blackfan anemia [24]. Patients with hereditary multiple osteochondromas, due to inheritance of mutations in the *EXT1* or *EXT2*genes, are predisposed to development of osteosarcoma also [24].

Human osteosarcoma is typically diagnosed due to swelling and pain often in the limbs. This can cause a limp if the involved limb is a leg or immobility of a joint. Pain may be constant or associated with exertion. In rare cases osteosarcoma will trigger a bone fracture. Diagnosis is made following a complete medical exam and imaging studies. Often an X-ray is done, followed by positron emission tomography or a bone scan. As osteosarcoma can often metastasize to the lungs, lung X-rays are utilized. A definitive diagnosis requires a biopsy. Staging of osteosarcoma is controversial. Most believe that all osteosarcoma should be considered high grade and treated as such although low grade osteosarcoma seems to be a distinct entity [38]. The only commonly accepted staging is localized *versus* metastatic disease.

Human osteosarcoma is commonly treated using surgery and chemotherapy [38]. Chemotherapy for roughly ten weeks that precedes surgery and the extent of necrosis in the surgically removed primary tumor has been suggested to be associated with long term risk for disease recurrence [38]. Chemotherapy is also given after surgery for a period of up to a year. Usually two or three chemotherapeutic agents are given for osteosarcoma treatment. Common combinations include high-dose methotrexate, doxorubicin and cisplatin (sometimes with ifosfamide); doxorubicin and cisplatin; ifosfamide and etoposide; ifosfamide, cisplatin (or carboplatin) and epirubicin [38]. Radiation therapy is used in some cases for non-resectable tumors [38].

The prognosis of human osteosarcoma is affected largely by the presence or absence of metastases. The 5-year survival rate for localized osteosarcoma is estimated to be between 50% and 60%. For metastatic disease the 5-year survival rate is 15% to 30% [39]. There is a better prognosis if metastatic osteosarcoma is present only in the lungs and is all metastatic lesions can be removed surgically [39]. That said, there is a dire need to develop therapies that can be used to treat patients who present with extensive metastatic disease or who recur with metastatic disease. At present, palliative care is often used in such cases or referral for clinical trials [38].

CANINE OSTEOSARCOMA

Canine osteosarcoma accounts for 80%–90% of canine primary bone tumors [40]. Dogs often present with a history of lameness or in some cases with a pathologic fracture of the affected bone. Diagnosis is based on clinical signs, imaging and biopsy. The metaphyseal region of long bones is the most common primary site with front limbs affected twice as often as rear limbs and the distal radius and proximal humerus being the two most common locations [41,42].

It is believed that external factors such as chemical carcinogens, ionization radiation, metallic implants to fix fractures and precedent skeletal disorders such as osteomyelitis and microscopic fractures can lead to canine osteosarcoma [10]. There are implications of genetic factors such as *TP53* and RB1 aberrations, as well as certain viruses and growth factor alterations [43]. Osteosarcoma can affect any breed of dog, but it is more commonly found in the larger breeds. Some breeds, such as the Scottish Deerhound, Great Dane, St. Bernard and Greyhound, are at high risk for developing primary bone tumors suggesting a genetic predilection [40]. In fact, the CDKN2A locus has been recently linked to osteosarcoma risk in dogs, and the risk allele is fixed in certain breeds like Rottweilers and Irish Wolfhounds [4].

Without treatment, the estimated survival for a dog with osteosarcoma is less than 3 months. On the other hand, survival times of approximately 1 year (or about 10% of a dog's lifetime) are achievable for 20%–50% of dogs with osteosarcoma treated using the current standard of care, and a small percentage of dogs can survive up to 5–6 years after diagnosis [44]. Standard of care for dogs is surgery (amputation of limb sparing surgery) with adjuvant chemotherapy [45]. The choice of chemotherapy drugs does not seem to influence survival, thus, toxicity, quality of life and cost tend to be the factors that guide treatment decisions [44]. Chemotherapy is only recommended when the primary tumor is removed and as of current, the drug of choice is carboplatin.

Many well-controlled studies show that a clinical response for osteosarcoma is only achievable with accepted standard of care. In very rare cases, dogs with osteosarcoma that receive palliative care may have prolonged (>1 year) survival, even in face of metastatic disease. Anecdotal benefits reported from herbal or "alternative" treatments, have not been reproducible, and no alternative therapies have been shown to have efficacy or provide consistent clinical benefit in controlled trials.

Metastatic bone cancer is the common cause of death or euthanasia, in 90% of dogs by 1 year [46]. Reducing the primary tumor's ability to metastasize and enhancing the antitumor activity of chemotherapy drugs and yet having minimal negative side effects is still a challenge for veterinary practitioners [10]. Treatment options for canine patients with metastases include pulmonary metastasectomy, but treatment for metastatic disease is only recommended if the primary tumor remains in complete remission [47]. The median survival after pulmonary metastasectomy can be up to 6 months; but without standard surgical procedure, survival outcome is usually less than 2 months [46].

MOUSE MODELS OF OSTEOSARCOMA

The number of genetically engineered or other mouse models of osteosarcoma are fairly restricted. However, these have been useful for studies on the cell of origin for osteosarcoma development and gaining insight into new genes and pathways that influence osteosarcoma initiation, progression and the process of metastasis. Most of the reported models utilize Cre/LoxP mediated deletion of *Trp53* and/or *Rb1* (reviewed in [48]). A few other models have been created by transgenic overexpression of various oncogenes including *Fos* and SV40 large T antigen [49], or co-deletion of one copy of *Twist* and mutation of *Apc* [50]. Osteosarcoma can be induced with high efficiency in mice by osteoblast lineage specific deletion of the*Trp53* gene, although the latency and penetrance is greatly enhanced by co-deletion of both copies of the *Rb1* gene [51].These data are consistent with the centrality of *TP53* and *RB1* loss of function alterations in human osteosarcoma [23]. Mouse osteosarcoma induced by deletion of *Trp53* is genomically unstable, as is seen in human osteosarcoma [52].

Others have created mouse cell lines from spontaneously occurring osteosarcoma. In cases in which these osteosarcoma were induced on a uniform strain background, the osteosarcoma cells can be grown in syngeneic hosts by intravenous, subcutaneous, or orthotopic injections into the tibia (reviewed in [53]). Examples include the K12 and K7M2 derivative that is highly metastatic, and the Dunn along with its metastatic derivative LM8. These cell lines have been useful for testing the role of various components of the immune system on primary osteosarcoma tumor growth and osteosarcoma metastasis [54]. Such cell lines have also been used to create matched pairs of poorly and highly metastatic cell lines for study [53]. These have been useful for developing candidate genes and pathways that may regulate the process of metastasis, such as high-level expression of ezrin [28].

Quist *et al.* reported that osteosarcoma could be induced in mice via homozygous Cre/LoxP-mediated deletion of *Trp53*and *Rb1* in undifferentiated mesenchyme, pre-osteoblasts or infrequently cycling mature osteoblasts [6]. These data suggest that a variety of cell types could be targets for osteosarcoma development. This plasticity may also be the basis for the ready acquisition of new osteosarcoma phenotypes in patients, including chemo/radiotherapy resistance and the ability to readily colonize the lung.

From osteosarcoma mouse models, we have learned that osteosarcoma cells have a predilection to metastatic colonization of the lung, but, interestedly, have observed a metastatic potential spectrum across various cell lines. Intriguingly, in mouse models of Li-Fraumeni, the rate of lung metastasis is influenced by the nature of the p53 mutant allele used and when in the lifetime of the mouse Cre is used to induce mutation of the p53 gene [51]. The rate of spontaneous development of osteosarcoma and the frequency of lung metastasis is higher in mice heterozygous for the $Trp53^{R272H}$ allele than in mice heterozygous for the carry $Trp53^{R270H}$ allele [55].

Recently, a new mouse model of osteosarcoma was developed which utilizes the *Sleeping Beauty* (SB) transposon mutagenesis system [29]. In this project, a SB transposon vector designed to activate proto-oncogenes or inactivate tumor suppressor genes by insertional mutagenesis, was mobilized specifically in *Osx1+* cells using a tissue-specific mutagenesis approach. Mutagenesis by SB was able to induce osteosarcoma in otherwise wild type mice or accelerate osteosarcoma in mice with tissue-specific induction of the $Trp53^{R270H}$ allele. Transposon insertion mutations in specific regions of the genome are found recurrently in SB induced tumors and these regions are called "common insertion sites" or CIS [29]. CIS result from selection for insertions that occur within or near a cancer gene in the right position and the right orientation so as to give the cell a selective advantage and drive the development of a tumor. Thus, the identification of genes at or near CIS defines new candidate drivers of cancer development.

CONSERVED DRIVERS OF OSTEOSARCOMA

Genomic Alterations

It has been reported that genomic alterations are necessary for development of osteosarcoma in mouse models (*TP53*) and are accepted as being commonly shared in humans and dogs [13,29,56].

Highly chaotic karyotypes encompass a key feature that characterizes some mouse models used for osteosarcoma studies, and naturally occurring osteosarcoma in dogs, as well as in human patients. The average human osteosarcoma harbors roughly 30 coding alterations [23,57] while in dog osteosarcoma and mouse models, this figure is not known with certainty. Many of the candidate genes implicated in the pathogenesis and progression of osteosarcoma in people have also been characterized in the canine disease. Notable examples of these genes are *PTEN* (phosphatase and tensin homolog), *RB1*(retinoblastoma), and *TP53* (tumor protein 53), and *MET* (mesenchymal-epithelial transition factor).

Genetic alterations of the retinoblastoma susceptibility (*RB1*) gene have been implicated in the development and progression of osteosarcoma. In people, almost 70% of osteosarcomas have at least one *RB1* gene alteration and the percentage is similar in dog osteosarcomas [13]. We recently reported that an aberrant RB-E2F1 regulatory pathway is predictive of biological behavior [58]. Since our work, another group has reported that RB1 alterations may serve as a prognostic marker for the management of osteosarcoma patients [59].

Approximately 50% of human osteosarcomas have been reported to have somatic *TP53* deletions or point mutations detected using exon sequencing strategies [23]. However, a recent study that used whole genome sequencing of human osteosarcomas suggests that nearly all osteosarcoma tumors have p53 pathways lesions, which in many cases are translocations that break in the first intron of *TP53* gene [57]. Thus, it would appear that p53 pathway loss might be a requirement for osteosarcoma development in people. Clearly, germline *TP53* mutations, which cause Li-Fraumeni syndrome, predispose to osteosarcoma. However, it is unclear whether *TP53* mutations act as initiating mutations or progression mutations in sporadic osteosarcoma. In any case, p53 pathway alterations are common in genetically engineered mouse models as well as spontaneous canine and human osteosarcoma. Therefore, mouse models could be used to develop therapies that exploit p53 pathway alterations in patient osteosarcoma.

In humans and dogs, several oncogenes have been identified as possibly playing a role in osteosarcoma including *MET,FOS*, *IGF1R* (Insulin-Like Growth Factor 1 Receptor), *PVT1/MYC*, *RUNX2*, and *HER2*. Some of these changes involve copy number alterations. Consistent genome and chromosome copy number changes have been reported in canine and human osteosarcoma [17]. For instance, a high copy number gain of the *RUNX2* locus has been reported in both human and dog osteosarcoma [56].

Some of these genes, or the pathways they regulate, including the *PVT1/MYC* locus, *MET* signaling, and *IGF1R* have been implicated in genetically engineered mouse models of osteosarcoma [29,52].

Recurrent point mutations have been observed in osteosarcoma, but there are few beyond *RB1* and *TP53* that reach statistical significance. This is in part because too few samples have been sequenced. However, point mutations or deletions of several tumor suppressor genes, likely to be drivers of osteosarcomagenesis, were observed in a recent report of human osteosarcoma including *NF1*, *NF2* and *PTEN*, all of which were also recovered in a transposon-based screen for osteosarcoma in mice [29]. Overlap exists between other reported candidate human osteosarcoma genes after genome-wide copy number and whole exome sequencing were done [23], and also after transposon based screening in a mouse model including activation of *PI3KCA*, and *AKT1*, and inactivation of *ARID1A* [29].

Deregulation of Micrornas in Canine and Human Osteosarcoma

microRNAs (miRNAs) are small non coding RNAs that regulate more than 60% of the genome post transcriptionally. Several studies have identified deregulated miRNAs in osteosarcoma [60,61,62,63,64,65,66]. One of the earliest studies reported four differentially expressed miRNAs in a handful of osteosarcoma samples compared to controls [67]. Since these initial studies, additional research has shown that miRNA deregulation is potentially central to osteosarcoma development and progression [68]. Indeed, our group generated a Sarcoma MicroRNA Expression Database (S-MED) that represents 22 different sarcoma types, including osteosarcoma [69]. Through S-MED we found that osteosarcoma clustered separately from all other sarcoma types indicating the presence of potentially biologically important miRNAs. One of the unique miRNA signatures we found revealed the significant downregulation of around 50 miRNAs in the human 14q32 locus compared to the controls [65]. Most importantly, we have also shown a comparable decrease in expression of orthologous 14q32 miRNAs in canine osteosarcoma samples [65]. Interestingly we did not observe any copy number changes at the 14q32 locus, suggesting epigenetic changes at the locus. We confirmed that subset of these 50 miRNAs (miR-382, miR-369-5p, miR-544 and miR-134) could target the 3′ UTR of cMYC transcript. Additionally, overexpression of these miRNAs in osteosarcoma cells decreased the cMYC levels and induced apoptosis [65,70]. Also cMYC has been shown to transactivate a commonly known miRNA cluster, miR-17-92 [71]. We showed that restoration of the 14q32 miRNAs not only did decrease the cMYC levels but also significantly reduced the levels of mir-17-92 [70].

It was observed in other studies that miR-135b, -150, -370, -542-5p, -652, and -654 were highly expressed compared to osteoblasts [72,73,74]. Many of them play crucial roles in bone differentiation and key signaling pathways (miR-206 and -286) [75]. Additionally, miRNAs target *TP53*, which is an important tumor suppressor gene, was mutated in more than 60% osteosarcoma tumors [76]. One of the key miRNAs in the *TP53* pathway is miR-34, which is significantly downregulated in many osteosarcoma tumors that affects the cell cycle and proliferation [77,78,79].

The role of miRNAs in canine osteosarcoma remains to be fully elucidated. Since the discovery of miRNAs, there have been few studies that show a correlation between deregulation of miRNAs and canine osteosarcoma. A recent study investigated the role of miR-196a and its target Annexin V in human (143B, MG63) and canine (DAN) osteosarcoma cell lines to identify potential targets for new therapeutic agents in both the species [80]. They observed that miR-196a is downregulated in many of the canine osteosarcoma tumors compared to the normal bone, which is in contradiction with some earlier studies [66,81]. Further studies need to be performed on a larger cohort to establish that miR-196a is a potential therapeutic target and can impact multiple downstream targets in canine osteosarcoma.

A study led by Fenger *et al.*, sought to characterize miRNA expression in canine primary tumors among the major large breeds (greyhounds, rottweilers, golden retrievers and some mixed breeds) [43,82]. Using Nanominer software, they determined 189 miRNAs that were differentially expressed. Of these, miR-494 was highly expressed in all the breeds compared to normal canine osteoblasts.

As mentioned earlier, our group was among the first groups to observe a significant downregulation of around 50 miRNAs in the human 14q32 chromosomal region, which was highly conserved in the dog genome. Out of the 50 miRNAs, 2 miRNAs, miR-134 and mir-544, shared 100% conservation with the canine genome and mapped to the predicted synteny in canine osteosarcoma [14]. We have comprised a table of key miRNAs that play an important role in survival outcome and chemoresponse that can potentially lead to osteosarcoma diagnosis, subtyping and therapeutics in human and canine osteosarcoma (Table 1).

Table 1: miRNAs as potential markers for survival outcome and/ or chemosensitivity

miRNAs Deregulated in OS	Expression Levels Compared to the Controls	Overall Function	References
miR-382	Down-regulated	Poor survival outcome and metastasis marker	[70,83]
miR-154	Down-regulated	Poor survival outcome	[70]
miR-33a	Up-regulated	Chemoresistance	[84]
miR-34c	Down-regulated	Chemoresistance	[85]

Epigenetic Changes in Osteosarcoma

Most forms of human cancer have changes in the epigenome compared to the normal cellular counterparts from which they are derived. Indeed, changes to the epigenome seem to be a ubiquitous feature of cancer. Epigenetic changes are revealed in alterations to the pattern of DNA methylation, histone modifications and nucleosome remodeling (reviewed in [24]). Osteosarcoma, like other forms of human cancer, seems to have many such epigenome changes compared to normal osteoblasts, the presumptive target cell for transformation. Several studies have analyzed the epigenome in a genome-wide manner, albeit with low numbers of cases [86,87]. These studies confirm that specific methylation events are heterogeneous among different cases of human osteosarcoma and that these differences may help explain differences in the clinical behavior of different osteosarcomas. These genome wide studies in human osteosarcoma have been restricted to the study of DNA methylation. Work on other chromatin modification remains to be done. The study of genome wide epigenetic changes has not been undertaken on a large scale in genetically engineered mouse models or canine osteosarcoma samples.

Many studies in osteosarcoma have focused on methylation of specific genes or gene regions. These studies suggest that certain genes and genetic pathways are subject to control by DNA methylation and attendant modifications to the histone code. Among these are alterations to the RB and p53 pathways. While these specific genes are not frequent targets of methylation based gene silencing, genes in these pathways have been reported as targets for pathogenic methylation. Specifically the *CDKN2A* locus, encoding the cyclin dependent kinase inhibitor $p16^{INK4a}$ and the Mdm2 inhibitor $p14^{Arf}$, has been reported [88,89]. Several genes that are targets of p53, or modulate p53 activity, have been shown to be methylated and silenced in osteosarcoma cell lines or xenograft tumors including *CDKN1A*, *HIC1* and *GADD45* [90,91,92]. Many other tumor suppressor genes are silenced by promoter hypermethylation in osteosarcoma cell lines including *RASSF1A*, *TIMP3*, DAPK1 and others (review in Morrow and Khanna, Critical Reviews in Oncogenesis, 2015). Methylation and silencing of tumor suppressive miRNA genes has also been observed as specific events in human osteosarcoma cell lines and primary tumors. Promoter hypomethyation, and probable overexpression, of oncogenes is less well studied in osteosarcoma, but several reports have been made suggesting such a mechanism, notably for the metastasis promoting gene *IRX1* and the growth factor gene *IGF2* [93,94]. Several candidate osteosarcoma oncogenes found in a transposon-based forward genetic screen in mice are also hypomethylated and overexpressed in human osteosarcoma compared to normal osteoblasts, including *SEMA4D*, *RAF1* and *PAK1* [29]. Some of these epigenetic changes, including aberrant repression and activation, are associated with loss of imprinting control at specific loci in osteosarcoma cells [95,96,97].

Genome wide studies of epigenetic alterations in human osteosarcoma need to incorporate many more samples before we learn to what extent they may explain molecular subtypes and clinical behavior of different cases. No such studies have been reported for canine osteosarcomas or mouse models either. When they are, they will allow cross-species comparisons that could help reveal the most meaningful alterations. Despite these limitations, it is apparent that osteosarcoma development is accompanied by changes to the epigenome that drive progression and confer specific cancer phenotypes. Published data does suggest that epigenome targeted therapies, including histone deacetylase inhibitors and DNA demethylating agents, can alter gene expression and inhibit osteosarcoma growth and/or metastasis [93,98]. Indeed, one study suggests that osteosarcoma cell lines can be reprogrammed using induced pluripotency genes and that the accompanying epigenetic changes reduce tumorigenic potential [99]. Taken together, these data suggest that modification of osteosarcoma epigenomes will be a useful therapeutic approach.

ADVANTAGES OF A MULTI-SPECIES, COMPARATIVE OSTEOSARCOMA STUDY APPROACH

Using comparative genetic studies in multiple organisms, it is possible to understand more about the inherited and somatically acquired genetic alterations that are informative of osteosarcoma risk and clinical behavior, especially metastasis. It is reasonable that genetic alterations that are present in human, dog, and mouse osteosarcomas represent the most likely true drivers of osteosarcoma progression, based on the concept of convergent evolution. Singly, mouse models offer opportunities to discover new genes and pathways important in disease initiation and progression. Dogs bring many other advantages to the table. Notably, since they show remarkable intra-breed homogeneity, which, together with noticeable interbreed heterogeneity, the dog offers distinctive opportunities to understand the genetics underlying osteosarcoma. Taken all together, an interspecies approach offers a possibly broader view and understanding of osteosarcoma since, for example, what is found to be altered at the genetic level in one species may be epigenetically silenced altered in another, but would be hard to pick out based on changes to gene expression alone.

Findings from mouse models and naturally occurring osteosarcoma in dogs need to be translated into therapeutic approaches in a clinically relevant model. Advantages of clinical trials in dogs are numerous and include that there are many more cases of canine osteosarcoma than human osteosarcoma [100,101]. In addition, disease progression in dogs, even with standard of care, is rapid so that assessments of improvement can be made in comparatively short periods of time [102].

It has been shown that histological response is not a good predictor (St. Jude, CTOS 20th Annual Meeting) in human osteosarcoma patients, and so there is an urgent need for informative biomarkers. The 14q32 locus is a new and promising marker, which was discovered by our group through a comparative species approach [65].

CONCLUSIONS

In more than 70% of osteosarcoma patients, current standard-of-care therapies ultimately fail to prevent relapse and metastasis. This dismal outcome has not improved over the past three decades, indicating a desperate need for novel drugs and treatment strategies. As osteosarcoma is genetically heterogeneous, successful therapies will need to target conserved pathobiology. In this review, we discussed the presence of multiple conserved signaling mechanisms as well as some of the approaches for understanding osteosarcoma pathobiology. Recent studies highlight the role of microRNAs in regulation of these conserved signaling pathways. In addition, we have just begun to understand the roles of the regulatory small RNAs and long-noncoding RNAs (lncRNAs). Further, intricacy in gene regulations does not end with identification of regulatory RNAs and its interacting partners. Molecular intricacy is also heavily dependent on our understanding of the implications of other layers of gene regulation such as role for competing endogenous RNAs along with pseudogenes, circular RNAs and lncRNAs. Acquiring such breadth and depth of knowledge is critical for developing therapies that will prevent bypass mechanisms of resistance to therapies. Moreover, cell non-autonomous functions of secreted factors such as exosomes are currently being investigated. In addition, emerging concepts of immune regulation by cancer and recent advancements in immunotherapy hold promise for treating and better outcomes in osteosarcoma.

ACKNOWLEDGMENTS

We thank Jaime Modiano and Aaron Sarver for helpful discussions and Anne Sarver for assisting in manuscript preparation. Due to the space restrictions we could not cite many other significant contributions made by numerous researchers and laboratories in this potentially important and rapidly progressing field. Subbaya Subramanian and David A. Largaespada are supported by research grants funded by American Cancer Society Grant (RSG 13-381-01-RMC), the Sobiech osteosarcoma fund, Children's cancer research funds, the Wyckoff Rein in Sarcoma Foundation.

AUTHOR CONTRIBUTIONS

Jyotika Varshney and Subbaya Subramanian developed the concept for the review. Milcah C. Scott and David A. Largaespada provided input in the canine osteosarcoma and epigenetics of osteosarcoma.

REFERENCES

1. Moore, D.D.; Luu, H.H. Osteosarcoma. *Cancer Treat Res.* 2014, *162*, 65–92.
2. Ottaviani, G.; Jaffe, N. The epidemiology of osteosarcoma. *Cancer Treat Res.* 2009, *152*, 3–13.
3. Letson, G.D.; Muro-Cacho, C.A. Genetic and molecular abnormalities in tumors of the bone and soft tissues. *Cancer Control* 2001, *8*, 239–251.
4. Karlsson, E.K.; Sigurdsson, S.; Ivansson, E.; Thomas, R.; Elvers, I.; Wright, J.; Howald, C.; Tonomura, N.; Perloski, M.; Swofford, R.; *et al.* Genome-wide analyses implicate 33 loci in heritable dog osteosarcoma, including regulatory variants near CDKN2A/B. *Genome Biol.* 2013, *14*, R132.
5. Mutsaers, A.J.; Walkley, C.R. Cells of origin in osteosarcoma: Mesenchymal stem cells or osteoblast committed cells?*Bone* 2014, *62*, 56–63.
6. Quist, T.; Jin, H.; Zhu, J.F.; Smith-Fry, K.; Capecchi, M.R.; Jones, K.B. The impact of osteoblastic differentiation on osteosarcomagenesis in the mouse. *Oncogene* 2015, *34*, 4278–4284.
7. Yoshida, H.; Adachi, H.; Hamada, Y.; Aki, T.; Yumoto, T.; Morimoto, K.; Orido, T. Osteosarcoma. Ultrastructural and immunohistochemical studies on alkaline

phosphatase-positive tumor cells constituting a variety of histologic types.*Acta Pathol. Jpn.* 1988, *38*, 325–338.

8. Dirik, Y.; Cinar, A.; Yumrukcal, F.; Eralp, L. Popliteal lymph node metastasis of tibial osteoblastic osteosarcoma. *Int. J. Surg. Case Rep.* 2014, *5*, 840–844.
9. Jeffree, G.M.; Price, C.H.; Sissons, H.A. The metastatic patterns of osteosarcoma. *Brit. J. Cancer* 1975, *32*, 87–107.
10. Morello, E.; Martano, M.; Buracco, P. Biology, diagnosis and treatment of canine appendicular osteosarcoma: Similarities and differences with human osteosarcoma. *Vet. J.* 2011, *189*, 268–277.
11. Gill, J.; Ahluwalia, M.K.; Geller, D.; Gorlick, R. New targets and approaches in osteosarcoma. *Pharmacol. Ther.* 2013,*137*, 89–99.
12. Jaffe, N. Osteosarcoma: Review of the past, impact on the future. The American experience. *Cancer Treat Res.* 2009,*152*, 239–262.
13. Modiano, J.F.; Breen, M.; Lana, S.E.; Ehrhart, N.; Fosmire, S.P.; Thomas, R.; Jubala, C.M.; Lamerato-Kozicki, A.R.; Ehrhart, E.J.; Schaack, J.; *et al.* Naturally occurring translational models for development of cancer therapy. *Gene Ther. Mol. Biol.* 2006, *10*, 31–40. [Google Scholar]
14. Scott, M.C.; Sarver, A.L.; Gavin, K.J.; Thayanithy, V.; Getzy, D.M.; Newman, R.A.; Cutter, G.R.; Lindblad-Toh, K.; Kisseberth, W.C.; Hunter, L.E.; *et al.* Molecular subtypes of osteosarcoma identified by reducing tumor heterogeneity through an interspecies comparative approach. *Bone* 2011, *49*, 356–367.
15. Paoloni, M.; Davis, S.; Lana, S.; Withrow, S.; Sangiorgi, L.; Picci, P.; Hewitt, S.; Triche, T.; Meltzer, P.; Khanna, C. Canine tumor cross-species genomics uncovers targets linked to osteosarcoma progression. *BMC Genom.* 2009, *10*, 625.
16. Schiffman, J.D.; Breen, M. Comparative oncology: What dogs and other species can teach us about humans with cancer. *Philos. Trans. R. Soc. Lond. B Biol. Sci.* 2015, *370*.
17. Thomas, R.; Wang, H.J.; Tsai, P.C.; Langford, C.F.; Fosmire, S.P.; Jubala, C.M.; Getzy, D.M.; Cutter, G.R.; Modiano, J.F.; Breen, M. Influence of genetic background on tumor karyotypes: Evidence for breed-associated cytogenetic aberrations in canine appendicular osteosarcoma. *Chromosome Res.* 2009, *17*, 365–377.
18. McNeill, C.J.; Overley, B.; Shofer, F.S.; Kent, M.S.; Clifford, C.A.; Samluk, M.; Haney, S.; van Winkle, T.J.; Sorenmo, K.U. Characterization of the biological behaviour of appendicular osteosarcoma in Rottweilers and a comparison with other breeds: A review of 258 dogs. *Vet. Comp. Oncol.* 2007, *5*, 90–98.
19. Dobson, J.M. Breed-predispositions to cancer in pedigree dogs. *ISRN Vet. Sci.* 2013, *2013*, 941275.
20. Paoloni, M.; Khanna, C. Translation of new cancer treatments from pet dogs to humans. *Nat. Rev. Cancer* 2008, *8*, 147–156.

21. Isakoff, M.S.; Bielack, S.S.; Meltzer, P.; Gorlick, R. Osteosarcoma: Current treatment and a collaborative pathway to success. *J. Clin. Oncol.* 2015, *33*, 3029–3035.

22. Ferrari, S.; Serra, M. An update on chemotherapy for osteosarcoma. *Expert Opin. Pharmacother.* 2015, *16*, 2727–2736.

23. Perry, J.A.; Kiezun, A.; Tonzi, P.; van Allen, E.M.; Carter, S.L.; Baca, S.C.; Cowley, G.S.; Bhatt, A.S.; Rheinbay, E.; Pedamallu, C.S.; *et al.* Complementary genomic approaches highlight the PI3K/mTOR pathway as a common vulnerability in osteosarcoma. *Proc. Natl. Acad. Sci. USA* 2014, *111*, 5564–5573.

24. Morrow, J.J.; Khanna, C. Osteosarcoma genetics and epigenetics: Emerging biology and candidate therapies. *Crit. Rev. Oncog.* 2015, *20*, 173–197.

25. Li, N.; Luo, D.; Hu, X.; Luo, W.; Lei, G.; Wang, Q.; Zhu, T.; Gu, J.; Lu, Y.; Zheng, Q. RUNX2 and osteosarcoma.*Anticancer Agents Med. Chem.* 2015, *15*, 881–887.

26. Tian, J.; He, H.; Lei, G. Wnt/beta-catenin pathway in bone cancers. *Tumour Biol.* 2014, *35*, 9439–9445.

27. Lamora, A.; Talbot, J.; Bougras, G.; Amiaud, J.; Leduc, M.; Chesneau, J.; Taurelle, J.; Stresing, V.; Le Deley, M.C.; Heymann, M.F.; *et al.* Overexpression of smad7 blocks primary tumor growth and lung metastasis development in osteosarcoma. *Clin. Cancer Res.* 2014, *20*, 5097–5112.

28. Khanna, C.; Wan, X.; Bose, S.; Cassaday, R.; Olomu, O.; Mendoza, A.; Yeung, C.; Gorlick, R.; Hewitt, S.M.; Helman, L.J. The membrane-cytoskeleton linker ezrin is necessary for osteosarcoma metastasis. *Nat. Med.* 2004, *10*, 182–186.

29. Moriarity, B.S.; Otto, G.M.; Rahrmann, E.P.; Rathe, S.K.; Wolf, N.K.; Weg, M.T.; Manlove, L.A.; LaRue, R.S.; Temiz, N.A. A Sleeping Beauty forward genetic screen identifies new genes and pathways driving osteosarcoma development and metastasis. 2015, *47*, 615–624.

30. Chang, L.; Shrestha, S.; LaChaud, G.; Scott, M.A.; James, A.W. Review of microRNA in osteosarcoma and chondrosarcoma. *Med. Oncol.* 2015, *32*, 613.

31. Geller, D.S.; Gorlick, R. Osteosarcoma: A review of diagnosis, management, and treatment strategies. *Clin. Adv. Hematol. Oncol.* 2010, *8*, 705–718.

32. Mirabello, L.; Pfeiffer, R.; Murphy, G.; Daw, N.C.; Patino-Garcia, A.; Troisi, R.J.; Hoover, R.N.; Douglass, C.; Schuz, J.; Craft, A.W.; *et al.* Height at diagnosis and birth-weight as risk factors for osteosarcoma. *Cancer Causes Control* 2011, *22*, 899–908.

33. Savage, S.A.; Woodson, K.; Walk, E.; Modi, W.; Liao, J.; Douglass, C.; Hoover, R.N.; Chanock, S.J. Analysis of genes critical for growth regulation identifies Insulin-like Growth Factor 2 Receptor variations with possible functional significance as risk factors for osteosarcoma. *Cancer Epidemiol. Biomark. Prev.* 2007, *16*, 1667–1674.

34. Miller, R.W. Contrasting epidemiology of childhood osteosarcoma, Ewing's tumor, and rhabdomyosarcoma. *Natl. Cancer Inst. Monogr.* 1981, *56*, 9–15.

35. Jawad, M.U.; Cheung, M.C.; Min, E.S.; Schneiderbauer, M.M.; Koniaris, L.G.; Scully, S.P. Ewing sarcoma demonstrates racial disparities in incidence-related and sex-related differences in outcome: An analysis of 1631 cases from the SEER database, 1973–2005. *Cancer* 2009, *115*, 3526–3536.

36. Savage, S.A.; Mirabello, L.; Wang, Z.; Gastier-Foster, J.M.; Gorlick, R.; Khanna, C.; Flanagan, A.M.; Tirabosco, R.; Andrulis, I.L.; Wunder, J.S.; *et al.* Genome-wide association study identifies two susceptibility loci for osteosarcoma.*Nat. Genet.* 2013, *45*, 799–803.

37. Mirabello, L.; Koster, R.; Moriarity, B.S.; Spector, L.G.; Meltzer, P.S.; Gary, J.; Machiela, M.J.; Pankratz, N.; Panagiotou, O.A.; Largaespada, D.; *et al.* A Genome-wide scan identifies variants in NFIB associated with metastasis in patients with osteosarcoma. *Cancer Discov.* 2015, *5*, 920–931.

38. Gorlick, R.; Khanna, C. Osteosarcoma. *J. Bone Miner. Res.* 2010, *25*, 683–691.

39. Hameed, M.; Dorfman, H. Primary malignant bone tumors—Recent developments. *Semin. Diagn. Pathol.* 2011, *28*, 86–101.

40. Anfinsen, K.P.; Grotmol, T.; Bruland, O.S.; Jonasdottir, T.J. Breed-specific incidence rates of canine primary bone tumors—A population based survey of dogs in Norway. *Can. J. Vet. Res.* 2011, *75*, 209–215.

41. Liptak, J.M.; Dernell, W.S.; Straw, R.C.; Rizzo, S.A.; Lafferty, M.H.; Withrow, S.J. Proximal radial and distal humeral osteosarcoma in 12 dogs. *J. Am. Anim. Hosp. Assoc.* 2004, *40*, 461–467.

42. Boerman, I.; Selvarajah, G.T.; Nielen, M.; Kirpensteijn, J. Prognostic factors in canine appendicular osteosarcoma—A meta-analysis. *BMC Vet. Res.* 2012, *8*, 56–56.

43. Fenger, J.M.; London, C.A.; Kisseberth, W.C. Canine osteosarcoma: A naturally occurring disease to inform pediatric oncology. *ILAR J.* 2014, *55*, 69–85.

44. Szewczyk, M.; Lechowski, R.; Zabielska, K. What do we know about canine osteosarcoma treatment? Review. *Vet. Res. Commun.* 2015, *39*, 61–67.

45. Berg, J. Canine osteosarcoma: Amputation and chemotherapy. *Vet. Clin. N. Am. Small Anim. Pract.* 1996, *26*, 111–121.

46. Straw, R.C.; Withrow, S.J.; Powers, B.E. Management of canine appendicular osteosarcoma. *Vet. Clin. North Am. Small Anim. Pract.* 1990, *20*, 1141–1161.

47. Gilson, S.D. Principles of surgery for cancer palliation and treatment of metastases. *Clin. Tech. Small Anim. Pract.* 1998,*13*, 65–69.

48. Guijarro, M.V.; Ghivizzani, S.C.; Gibbs, C.P. Animal models in osteosarcoma. *Front. Oncol.* 2014, *4*, 189.

49. Ruther, U.; Komitowski, D.; Schubert, F.R.; Wagner, E.F. c-fos expression induces bone tumors in transgenic mice.*Oncogene* 1989, *4*, 861–865.

50. Entz-Werle, N.; Choquet, P.; Neuville, A.; Kuchler-Bopp, S.; Clauss, F.; Danse, J.M.; Simo-Noumbissie, P.; Guerin, E.; Gaub, M.P.; Freund, J.N.; *et al.* Targeted apc;twist double-mutant mice: A new model of spontaneous osteosarcoma that mimics the human disease. *Transl. Oncol.* 2010, *3*, 344–353.

51. Walkley, C.R.; Qudsi, R.; Sankaran, V.G.; Perry, J.A.; Gostissa, M.; Roth, S.I.; Rodda, S.J.; Snay, E.; Dunning, P.; Fahey, F.H.; *et al.* Conditional mouse osteosarcoma, dependent on p53 loss and potentiated by loss of Rb, mimics the human disease. *Genes Dev* 2008, *22*, 1662–1676.

52. Rao, P.H.; Zhao, S.; Zhao, Y.J.; Yu, A.; Rainusso, N.; Trucco, M.; Allen-Rhoades, W.; Satterfield, L.; Fuja, D.; Borra, V.J.;*et al.* Coamplification of Myc/Pvt1 and homozygous deletion of Nlrp1 locus are frequent genetics changes in mouse osteosarcoma. *Genes Chromosomes Cancer* 2015, *54*, 796–808.

53. Mohseny, A.B.; Hogendoorn, P.C.; Cleton-Jansen, A.M. Osteosarcoma models: From cell lines to zebrafish. *Sarcoma*2012, *2012*, 417271.

54. Merchant, M.S.; Melchionda, F.; Sinha, M.; Khanna, C.; Helman, L.; Mackall, C.L. Immune reconstitution prevents metastatic recurrence of murine osteosarcoma. *Cancer Immunol. Immunother.* 2007, *56*, 1037–1046.

55. Olive, K.P.; Tuveson, D.A.; Ruhe, Z.C.; Yin, B.; Willis, N.A.; Bronson, R.T.; Crowley, D.; Jacks, T. Mutant p53 gain of function in two mouse models of Li-Fraumeni syndrome. *Cell* 2004, *119*, 847–860.

56. Angstadt, A.Y.; Thayanithy, V.; Subramanian, S.; Modiano, J.F.; Breen, M. A genome-wide approach to comparative oncology: High-resolution oligonucleotide aCGH of canine and human osteosarcoma pinpoints shared microaberrations. *Cancer Genet.* 2012, *205*, 572–587.

57. Chen, X.; Bahrami, A.; Pappo, A.; Easton, J.; Dalton, J.; Hedlund, E.; Ellison, D.; Shurtleff, S.; Wu, G.; Wei, L.; *et al.* Recurrent somatic structural variations contribute to tumorigenesis in pediatric osteosarcoma. *Cell Rep.* 2014, *7*, 104–112.

58. Scott, M.C.; Sarver, A.L.; Tomiyasu, H.; Cornax, I.; van Etten, J.; Varshney, J.; O'Sullivan, M.G.; Subramanian, S.; Modiano, J.F. Aberrant RB-E2F transcriptional regulation defines molecular phenotypes of osteosarcoma. *J. Biol. Chem.* 2015.

59. Ren, W.; Gu, G. Prognostic implications of RB1 tumour suppressor gene alterations in the clinical outcome of human osteosarcoma: A meta-analysis. *Eur. J. Cancer Care* 2015.

60. Sampson, V.B.; Yoo, S.; Kumar, A.; Vetter, N.S.; Kolb, E.A. MicroRNAs and potential targets in osteosarcoma: Review.*Front. Pediatr.* 2015, *3*, 69.

61. Zhang, J.; Yan, Y.G.; Wang, C.; Zhang, S.J.; Yu, X.H.; Wang, W.J. MicroRNAs in osteosarcoma. *Clin. Chim. Acta* 2015,*444*, 9–17.

62. Miao, J.; Wu, S.; Peng, Z.; Tania, M.; and Zhang, C. MicroRNAs in osteosarcoma: Diagnostic and therapeutic aspects.*Tumour Biol.* 2013, *34*, 2093–2098.

63. Zhou, G.; Shi, X.; Zhang, J.; Wu, S.; Zhao, J. MicroRNAs in osteosarcoma: From biological players to clinical contributors, a review. *J. Int. Med. Res.* 2013, *41*, 1–12.

64. Li, Y.; Zhang, J.; Zhang, L.; Si, M.; Yin, H.; Li, J. Diallyl trisulfide inhibits proliferation, invasion and angiogenesis of osteosarcoma cells

by switching on suppressor microRNAs and inactivating of Notch-1 signaling. *Carcinogenesis* 2013,*34*, 1601–1610.

65. Sarver, A.L.; Thayanithy, V.; Scott, M.C.; Cleton-Jansen, A.M.; Hogendoorn, P.C.; Modiano, J.F.; Subramanian, S. MicroRNAs at the human 14q32 locus have prognostic significance in osteosarcoma. *Orphanet J. Rare Dis.* 2013, *8*, 7.
66. Namlos, H.M.; Meza-Zepeda, L.A.; Baroy, T.; Ostensen, I.H.; Kresse, S.H.; Kuijjer, M.L.; Serra, M.; Burger, H.; Cleton-Jansen, A.M.; Myklebost, O. Modulation of the osteosarcoma expression phenotype by microRNAs. *PloS ONE* 2012, *7*, e48086.
67. Lulla, R.R.; Costa, F.F.; Bischof, J.M.; Chou, P.M.; de, F.B.M.; Vanin, E.F.; Soares, M.B. Identification of differentially expressed MicroRNAs in osteosarcoma. *Sarcoma* 2011, *2011*, 732690.
68. Varshney, J.; Subramanian, S. MicroRNAs as potential target in human bone and soft tissue sarcoma therapeutics.*Front. Mol. Biosci.* 2015, *2*, 31.
69. Sarver, A.L.; Phalak, R.; Thayanithy, V.; Subramanian, S. S-MED: Sarcoma microRNA expression database. *Lab. Investig. J. Tech. Methods Pathol.* 2010, *90*, 753–761.
70. Thayanithy, V.; Sarver, A.L.; Kartha, R.V.; Li, L.; Angstadt, A.Y.; Breen, M.; Steer, C.J.; Modiano, J.F.; Subramanian, S. Perturbation of 14q32 miRNAs-cMYC gene network in osteosarcoma. *Bone* 2012, *50*, 171–181.
71. Li, Y.; Choi, P.S.; Casey, S.C.; Dill, D.L.; Felsher, D.W. MYC through miR-17–92 suppresses specific target genes to maintain survival, autonomous proliferation, and a neoplastic state. *Cancer Cell* 2014, *26*, 262–272.
72. Schaap-Oziemlak, A.M.; Raymakers, R.A.; Bergevoet, S.M.; Gilissen, C.; Jansen, B.J.; Adema, G.J.; Kogler, G.; le Sage, C.; Agami, R.; van der Reijden, B.A.; *et al.* MicroRNA hsa-miR-135b regulates mineralization in osteogenic differentiation of human unrestricted somatic stem cells. *Stem. Cells Dev.* 2010, *19*, 877–885.
73. Wei, J.Q.; Chen, H.; Zheng, X.F.; Zhang, B.X.; Wang, Y.; Tang, P.F.; She, F.; Song, Q.; Li, T.S. Hsa-miR-654–5p regulates osteogenic differentiation of human bone marrow mesenchymal stem cells by repressing bone morphogenetic protein 2. *J. Southern Med. Univ.* 2012, *32*, 291–295. [Google Scholar]
74. Fang, S.; Deng, Y.; Gu, P.; Fan, X. MicroRNAs regulate bone development and regeneration. *Int. J. Mol. Sci.* 2015, *16*, 8227–8253.
75. Inose, H.; Ochi, H.; Kimura, A.; Fujita, K.; Xu, R.; Sato, S.; Iwasaki, M.; Sunamura, S.; Takeuchi, Y.; Fukumoto, S.; *et al.* A microRNA regulatory mechanism of osteoblast differentiation. *Proc. Natl. Acad. Sci. USA* 2009, *106*, 20794–20799.
76. Feng, Z.; Zhang, C.; Wu, R.; Hu, W. Tumor suppressor p53 meets microRNAs. *J. Mol. Cell Biol.* 2011, *3*, 44–50.
77. Wang, Y.; Jia, L.S.; Yuan, W.; Wu, Z.; Wang, H.B.; Xu, T.; Sun, J.C.; Cheng, K.F.; Shi, J.G. Low miR-34a and miR-192 are associated with unfavorable prognosis in patients suffering from osteosarcoma. *Am. J. Transl. Res.* 2015, *7*, 111–119.
78. Zhao, H.; Ma, B.; Wang, Y.; Han, T.; Zheng, L.; Sun, C.; Liu, T.; Zhang, Y.; Qiu,

X.; Fan, Q. miR-34a inhibits the metastasis of osteosarcoma cells by repressing the expression of CD44. *Oncol. Rep.* 2013, *29*, 1027–1036.

79. He, C.; Xiong, J.; Xu, X.; Lu, W.; Liu, L.; Xiao, D.; Wang, D. Functional elucidation of MiR-34 in osteosarcoma cells and primary tumor samples. *Biochem. Biophys. Res. Commun.* 2009, *388*, 35–40.
80. Pazzaglia, L.; Leonardi, L.; Conti, A.; Novello, C.; Quattrini, I.; Montanini, L.; Roperto, F.; del Piero, F.; di Guardo, G.; Piro, F.; *et al.* miR-196a expression in human and canine osteosarcomas: A comparative study. *Res. Vet. Sci.* 2015, *99*, 112–119.
81. Zhang, W.; Zhang, C.; Chen, H.; Li, L.; Tu, Y.; Liu, C.; Shi, S.; Zen, K.; Liu, Z. Evaluation of microRNAs miR-196a, miR-30a-5P, and miR-490 as biomarkers of disease activity among patients with FSGS. *Clin. J. Am. Soc. Nephrol.* 2014,*9*, 1545–1552.
82. Gardner, H.L.; Fenger, J.M.; London, C.A. Dogs as a model for cancer. *Annu. Rev. Anim. Biosci.* 2015. in print.
83. Xu, M.; Jin, H.; Xu, C.X.; Sun, B.; Song, Z.G.; Bi, W.Z.; Wang, Y. miR-382 inhibits osteosarcoma metastasis and relapse by targeting Y box-binding protein 1. *Mol. Ther.* 2015, *23*, 89–98.
84. Zhou, Y.; Huang, Z.; Wu, S.; Zang, X.; Liu, M.; Shi, J. miR-33a is up-regulated in chemoresistant osteosarcoma and promotes osteosarcoma cell resistance to cisplatin by down-regulating TWIST. *J. Exp. Clin. Cancer Res.* 2014, *33*, 12.
85. Xu, M.; Jin, H.; Xu, C.X.; Bi, W.Z.; Wang, Y. MiR-34c inhibits osteosarcoma metastasis and chemoresistance. *Med. Oncol.* 2014, *31*, 972.
86. Rosenblum, J.M.; Wijetunga, N.A.; Fazzari, M.J.; Krailo, M.; Barkauskas, D.A.; Gorlick, R.; Greally, J.M. Predictive properties of DNA methylation patterns in primary tumor samples for osteosarcoma relapse status. *Epigenetics* 2015,*10*, 31–39.
87. Kresse, S.H.; Rydbeck, H.; Skarn, M.; Namlos, H.M.; Barragan-Polania, A.H.; Cleton-Jansen, A.M.; Serra, M.; Liestol, K.; Hogendoorn, P.C.; Hovig, E.; *et al.* Integrative analysis reveals relationships of genetic and epigenetic alterations in osteosarcoma. *PLoS ONE* 2012, *7*, e48262.
88. Oh, J.H.; Kim, H.S.; Kim, H.H.; Kim, W.H.; Lee, S.H. Aberrant methylation of p14ARF gene correlates with poor survival in osteosarcoma. *Clin. Orthop. Relat. Res.* 2006, *442*, 216–222.
89. Park, Y.B.; Park, M.J.; Kimura, K.; Shimizu, K.; Lee, S.H.; Yokota, J. Alterations in the INK4a/ARF locus and their effects on the growth of human osteosarcoma cell lines. *Cancer Genet. Cytogenet.* 2002, *133*, 105–111.
90. Al-Romaih, K.; Sadikovic, B.; Yoshimoto, M.; Wang, Y.; Zielenska, M.; Squire, J.A. Decitabine-induced demethylation of 5′ CpG island in GADD45A leads to apoptosis in osteosarcoma cells. *Neoplasia* 2008, *10*, 471–480.
91. Badal, V.; Menendez, S.; Coomber, D.; Lane, D.P. Regulation of the p14ARF promoter by DNA methylation. *Cell Cycle*2008, *7*, 112–119.

92. Chen, W.; Cooper, T.K.; Zahnow, C.A.; Overholtzer, M.; Zhao, Z.; Ladanyi, M.; Karp, J.E.; Gokgoz, N.; Wunder, J.S.; Andrulis, I.L.; *et al.* Epigenetic and genetic loss of Hic1 function accentuates the role of p53 in tumorigenesis. *Cancer Cell* 2004, *6*, 387–398.

93. Lu, J.; Song, G.; Tang, Q.; Zou, C.; Han, F.; Zhao, Z.; Yong, B.; Yin, J.; Xu, H.; Xie, X.; *et al.* IRX1 hypomethylation promotes osteosarcoma metastasis via induction of CXCL14/NF-kappaB signaling. *J. Clin. Investig.* 2015, *125*, 1839–1856.

94. Li, Y.; Meng, G.; Huang, L.; Guo, Q.N. Hypomethylation of the P3 promoter is associated with up-regulation of IGF2 expression in human osteosarcoma. *Hum. Pathol.* 2009, *40*, 1441–1447.

95. Ulaner, G.A.; Vu, T.H.; Li, T.; Hu, J.F.; Yao, X.M.; Yang, Y.; Gorlick, R.; Meyers, P.; Healey, J.; Ladanyi, M.; *et al.* Loss of imprinting of IGF2 and H19 in osteosarcoma is accompanied by reciprocal methylation changes of a CTCF-binding site. *Hum. Mol. Genet.* 2003, *12*, 535–549.

96. Li, Y.; Meng, G.; Guo, Q.N. Changes in genomic imprinting and gene expression associated with transformation in a model of human osteosarcoma. *Exp. Mol. Pathol.* 2008, *84*, 234–239.

97. Lee, D.F.; Su, J.; Kim, H.S.; Chang, B.; Papatsenko, D.; Zhao, R.; Yuan, Y.; Gingold, J.; Xia, W.; Darr, H.; *et al.* Modeling familial cancer with induced pluripotent stem cells. *Cell* 2015, *161*, 240–254.

98. Thayanithy, V.; Park, C.; Sarver, A.L.; Kartha, R.V.; Korpela, D.M.; Graef, A.J.; Steer, C.J.; Modiano, J.F.; Subramanian, S. Combinatorial treatment of DNA and chromatin-modifying drugs cause cell death in human and canine osteosarcoma cell lines. *PLoS ONE* 2012, *7*, e43720.

99. Zhang, X.; Cruz, F.D.; Terry, M.; Remotti, F.; Matushansky, I. Terminal differentiation and loss of tumorigenicity of human cancers via pluripotency-based reprogramming. *Oncogene* 2013, *32*, 2249–2260.

100. Maniscalco, L. Canine osteosarcoma: Understanding its variability to improve treatment. *Vet. J.* 2015, *203*, 135–136.

101. Rodriguez, C.O., Jr. Using canine osteosarcoma as a model to assess efficacy of novel therapies: Can old dogs teach us new tricks? *Adv. Exp. Med. Biol.* 2014, *804*, 237–256.

102. Modiano, J.F.; Bellgrau, D.; Cutter, G.R.; Lana, S.E.; Ehrhart, N.P.; Ehrhart, E.; Wilke, V.L.; Charles, J.B.; Munson, S.; Scott, M.C.; *et al.* Inflammation, apoptosis, and necrosis induced by neoadjuvant fas ligand gene therapy improves survival of dogs with spontaneous bone cancer. *Mol. Ther.* 2012, *20*, 2234–2243.

7

CHAPTER

CHARACTERISTICS OF DOGS HAVING DIABETES MELLITUS; ANALYSIS OF DATA FROM PRIVATE JAPANESE VETERINARY CLINICS

Shiho Usui, Hidemi Yasuda and Yuzo Koketsu

Keywords: Canine, characteristics, diabetes mellitus, descriptive epidemiology

INTRODUCTION

Diabetes mellitus (DM) is one of the most frequently diagnosed endocrine diseases in dogs, accounting for 0.32-0.64% of dogs receiving veterinary care in U.K. and U.S.A. [1-3]. Dogs with DM have been diagnosed by polydipsia, polyuria, polyphagia and weight loss [4]. The cause of canine DM is considered multifactorial, i.e., autoimmune destruction of insulin producing β cells, pancreatitis, chronic hyperglycemia or hormonal disturbances [4]. Also, middle aged to older dogs and intact female dogs have been associated with dog DM [2]. Additionally, excessive overweight in dogs causes hyperinsulinemia and glucose intolerance [2]. Other studies have shown that Miniature Schnauzers and Toy Poodles are high risk breeds for DM [5], whereas Shetland Sheepdogs and Golden Retrievers have reduced risk of DM [1].

No studies in Japan have quantified the characteristic factors (age, sex, neuter status, body condition and breeds) associated with DM in dogs, nor the interactions between these factors in the same model, using medical records. Also, dogs' veterinary medical records are in a multi-level structure because health related checks, guidance and treatments on an individual dog are all performed in a clinic, i.e., dogs are not independent of the clinic. The clinic is a variable that includes some unique information,

Citation: Shiho Usui, Hidemi Yasuda and Yuzo Koketsu, Characteristics of dogs having diabetes mellitus; analysis of data from private Japanese veterinary clinics, DOI : http://dx.doi.org/10.7243/2054-3425-3-5.

such as a clinic's location, the average social and economic status of all owners coming with their dogs to the clinic and veterinary health guidance. Therefore, the objective of the present study was to characterize DM in dogs by using a mixed-effects modelling approach to identify characteristic factors and estimate their effects.

MATERIALS AND METHODS

Database and Body Condition Score (BCS)

A dog database has been created at Meiji University (Kawasaki, Japan) by cooperating with a veterinary service (Spectrum Lab Japan, Tokyo, Japan). The veterinary service recorded information about individual dog's characteristics (age, sex, neuter status, BCS and breed) when they received serum samples for lipoprotein analysis from veterinarians in private clinics throughout Japan. The veterinarians who submitted the samples were not informed about the specific purposes of the present study. The serum samples were collected from clinically-non-diseased dogs that received a health check and from dogs that were being assessed for suspected dyslipidemia or DM. Dogs' health condition was diagnosed by their veterinarians when the serum samples were taken. The diagnosis of DM was determined by the veterinarians on the basis of DM criteria such as polydipsia and polyuria with blood glucose and urine glycosuria [4]. However, the veterinarians did not record separately whether the dogs had insulin deficiency DM or insulin resistance DM. The BCS for each dog was evaluated by the dog's veterinarian using a five-point scale system (1: thin, 2: underweight, 3: ideal, 4: overweight and 5: obese). In addition to the five-point BCS scale used in our study, there is also a nine-point scale system [6] that has been commonly used in the EU and the U.S.A. However, we used the five-point scale system [7] because the website information and brochures about the five-point BCS scale system are widely available to veterinary clinics across Japan, provided by Pet Food Institute (Washington D.C., U.S.A.) and a nutrition company (Hill's-Colgate JAPAN Ltd., Tokyo, Japan). At the time of the study, three most popular types of dogs in Japan were Toy Poodle, Chihuahua and Miniature Dachshund [8].

Data and Exclusion Criteria

The database comprised data of 7,982 dogs from 109 breeds, collected from 1,198 veterinary clinics across Japan between January 2006 and January 2013. Of the 11,032 small animal clinics in Japan [9], 10.9% were included in our project. Records of second visits or more were not used in the present study (1,886 records). Records of dogs having hypothyroidism or hyperadrenocorticism health problems, which would influence body condition, were excluded from the dataset (753 records). The diagnoses of these endocrine diseases were made by the dogs' veterinarians on the basis of symptoms such as polydipsia and polyuria with blood and urinary tests. Thus, the dataset included the records of 5,343 diabetic or non-diabetic dogs in 102 breeds from 1,131 clinics.

The proportions of the 6,096 samples included in East Japan (including Tokyo) and West Japan were 61.7 and 38.3%, respectively. The samples were submitted from all the

47 prefecture regions in Japan. Additionally, the proportions of the samples submitted in January to March, April to June, July to September and October to December were 22.9, 28.3, 24.5 and 24.3%, respectively.

Categories and Definitions

Dog ages were calculated in years that have passed since their time of birth. Dogs classed as 0 years old were puppies between 5 and 11 months old. Dogs were categorized into four BCS groups; thin dogs (15 records) were included in the underweight dog group. Additionally, dogs were classified into two sex groups (male dogs or female dogs) and also two neuter status groups (intact dogs or neutered dogs). Preliminary analysis identified two breeds, Toy Poodles and Miniature Schnauzers, as having the highest percentages of dogs with DM; they also had relatively large sample size (450 dogs or more). In contrast, Shetland Sheepdogs have less propensity of dog DM [1], and they also had a relatively large sample size in our study (over 500 dogs). Therefore, these three breeds, Toy Poodles, Miniature Schnauzers and Shetland Sheepdogs, were used as breed groups in our study, along with a fourth group called Other breeds that comprised all the remaining 3,611 dogs. This simple grouping is done to test the hypothesis that dog breed affects dogs having DM.

Statistical Analysis

Two-level analysis was applied, using a clinic at level 2 and an individual dog at level 1, to take account of the hierarchical structure of the individual dogs within a clinic. This design was used to account for the fact that an individual dog received a health check and possible treatments at an individual clinic, and that the clinic represents information similar for its average clients but not collected otherwise; such as a dog's approximate location, the dog owner's social status and the specific health guidance taken by a clinc. A two-level mixed-effects logistic regression model using the GLIMMIX procedure with logit link function was fit to the data to determine characteristics for DM in dogs. The GLIMMIX procedure with the ILINK (Inverse link function) was used to convert the logit to a probability [10]. Pairwise multiple comparisons were performed using the Tukey-Kramer test [11]. Based on an assumption of normality, figures were also generated from the estimates in the final model. All statistical analyses were performed using SAS software (SAS Int. Inc., Cary, U.S.A.).

Age, sex, neuter status, BCS group and breed group were included in the model as possible characteristics (explanatory variables). Quadratic expressions of age and all possible twoway interactions between the explanatory variables were also examined, and then removed from the model if they were not significant. A significance level of $\alpha=0.05$ was applied. The sampled year was taken as a block in the model. Additionally, the model included the clinic as a random intercept. The adequacy of the model assumptions was evaluated by visual inspection of normal probability plots [10]. To assess the variations in the probability of dogs having DM that could be explained by the clinic, intraclass correlation coefficients (ICC) were calculated by the ICC equation in Dohoo et al. [12] :

$$\rho = \frac{\sigma^2_{Clinic}}{\sigma^2_{Clinic} + (\pi^2/3)}$$

where ρ represents the intraclass correlation coefficient σ^2_{Clinic}, is the between-clinic variance and $\pi^2/3$ is the assumed variance at the individual dog level.

Finally it was assessed which breeds in the studied population had the highest propensity for DM, and whether the proportion of dogs with DM differed between breeds. Only breeds with at least 60 dogs in the same population were selected, resulting in 10 breeds that were examined. A chi-squared test was also used to examine whether the percentage of DM dogs differed between the 10 breeds with the highest proportions of DM dogs (only breeds with sample size at least 60 dogs).

RESULTS

The mean age in all the studied dogs was 8.6±0.05 years old ranging from 0 to 17 years. Of 2,372 male dogs and 2,585 female dogs, 62.2% and 74.2% were neutered, respectively. Relative frequencies (%) of BCS 1, 2, 3, 4 and 5 were 0.3, 4.2, 41.4, 39.7 and 14.4%, respectively (Table 1). Prevalence (±SEM) of dogs having DM was 3.6±0.01% in this studied population.

Table 1: Relative frequency of 5,343 dogs categorized on the basis of body condition score groups

Measurements	N	%
Body condition score group*	--	--
1: Thin	15	0.3
2: Underweight	207	4.2
3: Ideal	2,052	41.4
4: Overweight	1,967	39.7
5: Obese	714	14.4

*The remaining records (5,343-N) were treated as missing values.

Table 2 shows the final model for dogs having DM. Dogs having DM was associated with age, BCS and breed groups ($P<0.05$), whereas was not associated with ($P=0.41$) and neuter status ($P=0.68$). Increased age was non-linearly associated with a higher probability of dogs having DM ($P<0.05$), with the probability peaking at 9 years of age, and then declining (Figure 1). The odds ratio of dogs having DM was 5.6 for underweight and thin dogs compared with ideal dogs ($P<0.05$).

Table 2: Estimates of fixed effects and random effect variance included the final binary logistic regression model (including breed groups) of the probability of a dog having diabetes mellitus (DM)

Fixed effects and variance	Estimate (±SE)	P-value
Intercept	-3.378 (0.293)	<0.01
Age	0.092 (0.104)	0.11
Age squared	-0.042 (0.010)	<0.01
Body condition score group	--	<0.01
Obese dogs	0	--
Overweight dogs	-0.316 (0.333)	--
Ideal dogs	0.044 (0.303)	--
Underweight and thin dogs	1.816 (0.372)	--
Breed group	--	<0.01
Toy Poodles	1.218 (0.274)	--
Miniature Schnauzers	0.580 (0.248)	--
Shetland Sheepdogs	-2.719 (1.164)	--
Others	0	--
AgexBody condition score group	--	0.01
AgexObese dogs	0	--
AgexOverweight dogs	0.093 (0.124)	--
AgexIdeal dogs	-0.052 (0.118)	--
AgexUnderweight and thin dogs	-0.258 (0.131)	--
AgexBreed group	--	0.02
AgexToy Poodles	0.288 (0.092)	--
AgexMiniature Schnauzers	0.125 (0.096)	--
AgexShetland Sheepdogs	0.150 (0.417)	--
AgexOthers	0	--
Clinic variance	0.46	--
Intraclass correlation coefficient, %	12.2	--

*Year effect was not shown because it was not relevant to the study objectives.

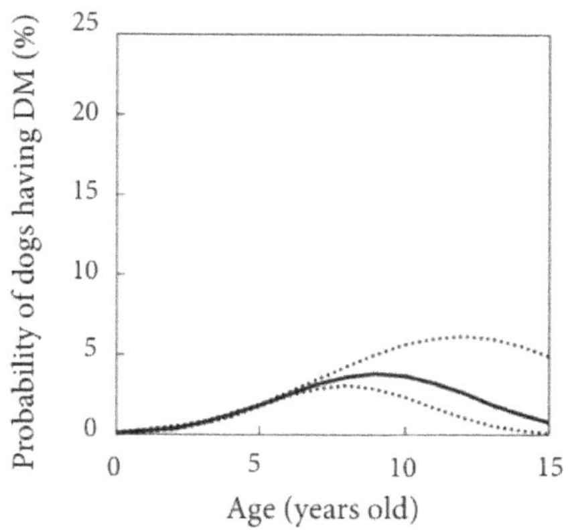

Figure 1: Estimated probability (%) of dogs having diabetes mellitus (DM) at different age (dotted lines represent 95% confidence intervals).

Additionally, underweight and thin dogs had 9.4-10.1% higher probability of having DM than dogs in the other BCS groups (P<0.05; Table 3). The odds ratios of Toy Poodles and Miniature Schnauzers were 3.1 and 1.6, respectively (P<0.05) compared to Other breeds. Also, Toy Poodles and Miniature Schnauzers had 4.9-9.3% higher probabilities of having DM than Shetland Sheepdogs (P<0.05).

Table 3: Comparisons between explanatory variables (risk factors) for the probability of dogs having diabetes mellitus (DM) and the odds ratios from the final model for the DM

Risk factors*	**Probability of dogs having DM, %**		**Odds ratio (95% confidence interval)**	**P-value**
	N**	**Mean±SE†**		
Body condition score group				
Obese dogs	714	1.6±0.50[b]	0.7 (0.4-1.2)	0.19
Overweight dogs	1,967	1.7±0.43[b]	0.7 (0.5-1.1)	0.17
Ideal dogs	2,052	2.3±0.53[b]	Reference	--
Underweight and thin dogs	222	11.7±3.11[a]	5.6 (3.3-9.8)	<0.01
Breed group§				
Toy Poodles	453	9.8±2.10[a]	3.1 (1.9-5.0)	<0.01
Miniature Schnauzers	766	5.4±1.15[b]	1.6 (1.0-2.6)	0.04
Shetland Sheep-dogs	513	0.5±0.38[d]	0.1 (0.0-0.7)	0.01
Others	3,611	3.4±0.46[c]	Reference	--

[a-d]Means within a column with different letters differ (P<0.05).
*Year effect was not shown because it was not a research purpose.
**The remaining records (5,343-N) were treated as missing values.
†Mean and SE were estimated by a mixed-effects multivariable model.

There were two two-way interactions between the dog age and BCS (P=0.01) or breed groups (P=0.02), respectively, for dogs having DM (Table 2). In underweight and thin dogs, the probability of dogs having DM increased from 4.5% to a peak of 21.2% as dog age rose from 1 to 7 years old (P<0.05; Figure 2), whereas in obese and overweight dogs the probabilities increased from 0.14 to 2.3%, and from 0.07 to 2.2%, respectively, over the same age range. There was only a low overall probability of dogs of ideal weight having DM, but the probability still rose from 0.2% at 1 years old to a peak of 4.3% at 9 years old.

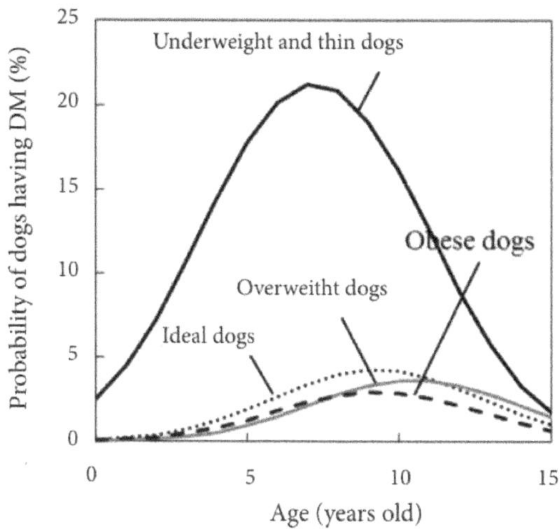

Figure 2: Estimated probability (%) of dogs in four body condition score groups having diabetes mellitus (DM) at different age..

Figure 3 shows that the probability of Toy Poodles and Miniature Schnauzers having DM increased non-linearly from 2.2 to 18.6% and from 2.0 to 6.6%, respectively, as dog age rose from 5 to 12 years old ($P<0.05$), whereas over the same age range DM in Shetland Sheepdogs increased non-linearly from 0.2 to only 0.6%.

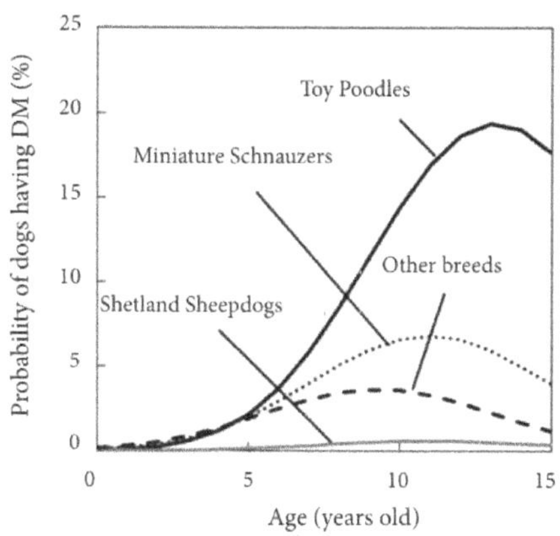

Figure 3: Estimated probability (%) of dogs in four breed groups having diabetes mellitus (DM) at different age.

Toy Poodles had the highest percentage of dogs having DM out of 102 breeds (Table 4). A chi-squared test also showed that the percentages of DM dogs differed between the 10 selected breeds ($P<0.05$). Finally, with regard to the ICC, the clinic effect explained 11.0-13.4% of the total variation for the probability of dogs having DM.

Table 4: Top 10 breeds with the highest percentages of dogs having diabetes mellitus (DM) out of 102 breeds studied*

Rank	Breed	Body size	Number of dogs	Number DM dogs	Percentage of DM dogs, %
1	Toy Poodle	Toy	453	37	8.2
2	Miniature Schnauzer	Small	766	48	6.3
3	Pomeranian	Toy	237	13	5.5
4	Maltese	Toy	187	10	5.3
5	Labrador Retriever	Large	61	3	4.9
6	Yorkshire Terrier	Toy	250	12	4.8
7	Mongrel	Unknown	372	17	4.6
8	Welsh Corgi	Medium	100	4	4.0
9	Beagle	Medium	88	2	2.3
10	Shiba Inu	Small	146	3	2.1

*The Table includes only 10 breeds with more than 60 dogs.

DISCUSSION

The present study quantified the associations between increased age and the probability of dogs having DM, and showed that the probability peaked at middle age. Also, in our study most dogs (65.1%) were found to have had DM between 5 and 11 years of age. These results confirm findings from a previous study [4], indicating that DM develops over months or years through several pathophysiological stages before dogs are diagnosed as DM dogs.

Our study also showed that dogs evaluated as underweight or thin have a higher odds ratio of being diagnosed for DM as compared to dogs in the other BCS groups. Weight loss is one of the clinical signs for DM, and therefore DM dogs are likely to become underweight and thin [4]. The results in the present study and those in a previous study [4] imply that the owners are more likely to recognize that their dogs have a disease problem due to the dogs being underweight, thin or suffering weight loss. In our study obesity was not associated with DM, but obesity may be a factor because it is associated with an increased risk of pancreatitis and glucose intolerance, both of which are a common cause of DM [3,4].

There was also an interaction between age and breed, which indicates that the probability of dogs having DM in middle age or older varies greatly between breed groups. The higher likelihood of Toy Poodles and Miniature Schnauzers having DM is consistent with previous studies [1,13]. Overall, the differences in the percentages of DM dogs between the top 10 breeds (Table 3) indicate that breeds have an important predictor for dogs having DM. Such differences in breed susceptibility to DM are associated with multiple genes, which increase the risk of DM, and differences in the haplotype between breeds [2,14].

The lack of any effects of sex or neuter status on the probability of dog DM may be explained by the fact that our data included many neutered dogs. Approximately 74% of the female dogs (1,919/2,585 female dogs) were neutered, and it is likely that many or most of these dogs would have been neutered at an early age, although the records did not include the timing of neutering. Previous studies have shown that female dogs were more likely to have DM compared to male dogs [1], and that intact female dogs had a higher percentage of DM than neutered female dogs [2]. Neutering reduces synthesis of progesterone [2], and this is likely to reduce the risk of DM in neutered dogs [4]. Therefore, neutering at an early stage is recommended in the U.K. [2] and also it has been shown that neuter status is not a factor for DM [1].

CONCLUSIONS

Characteristics of dogs having DM were high age, low BCS and specific breeds. This finding could help veterinarians to identify subclinical DM dogs, by taking these characteristics into account. Our study also shows that there are some difference between clinics in terms of DM dogs, as indicated by the ICCs of 11.0-13.4% for clinic variance. This suggests that some clinic related factors could be related to dog DM, such as clinic location, a neighborhood and social economic status of the average owner in that area and veterinarians' guidance for dogs.

Finally, it should be noted that there are some limitations to this present study. Dogs were not randomly selected because it was a cross-sectional study to examine possible risk factors using veterinarian-submitted samples. The proportion of DM (3.6%) in our study was relatively high. It is possible that samples from clinics with a high prevalence of DM dogs are overpresented. Also, the veterinarians did not record separately the type of diabetes that each dog had. Additionally, there is still possibility that we have had samples from certain clinics which may be highly related to high or low risk DM breeds. Furthermore, neither the dogs' rearing environments nor their nutrition were taken into account in the analyses. The level of agreement between the BCS evaluations conducted by the participating veterinarians was not evaluated. However, our statistical models included the clinic as a random effect in order to adjust some clinic or veterinarian effects. Even with such limitations, this research provides valuable information for veterinarians about the characteristics related to dog DM.

AUTHORS' CONTRIBUTIONS

Authors' contributions	SU	HY	YK
Research concept and design	√	--	√
Collection and/or assembly of data	√	√	--
Data analysis and interpretation	√	--	√
Writing the article	√	--	√
Critical revision of the article	--	√	√
Final approval of article	√	√	√
Statistical analysis	√	--	√

ACKNOWLEDGEMENT

The authors gratefully thank the cooperating veterinarians for providing their data for use in the present study. We also thank Dr. I. McTaggart for his critical review of this manuscript.

REFERENCES

1. Guptill L, Glickman L and Glickman N. **Time trends and risk factors for diabetes mellitus in dogs: analysis of veterinary medical data base records (1970-1999).** *Vet J.* 2003; 165:240-7.
2. Catchpole B, Ristic JM, Fleeman LM and Davison LJ. **Canine diabetes mellitus: can old dogs teach us new tricks?** *Diabetologia.* 2005; 48:1948-56.
3. Mattin M, O'Neill D, Church D, McGreevy PD, Thomson PC and Brodbelt D. **An epidemiological study of diabetes mellitus in dogs attending first opinion practice in the UK.** *Vet Rec.* 2014; 174:349.
4. Fleeman L and Rand J. Canine Diabetes Mellitus. In Rand J (Ed), Clinical Endocrinology of Companion Animals. *Wiley-Blackwell, Ames.* 2013; 143-168.
5. Hess RS, Saunders HM, Van Winkle TJ and Ward CR. **Concurrent disorders in dogs with diabetes mellitus: 221 cases (1993-1998).** *J Am Vet Med Assoc.* 2000; 217:1166-73.
6. Edney AT and Smith PM. **Study of obesity in dogs visiting veterinary practices in the United** Kingdom.*Vet Rec.* 1986; 118:391-6.
7. Laflamme D. P. Development and validation of a body condition score system for dogs. Canine Practice. 1997; 22:10-15.
8. JKC (Japan Kennel Club). Popular dog breeds in Japan. 2009.
9. MAFF (Ministry of Agriculture, Forestry and Fisheries). Statistics 2013 in the number of animal hospitals in Japan.
10. Littell RC, Milliken GA, Stroup WW, Wolfinger RD and Schabenberger O. SAS System for Mixed Models. 2nd edn. SAS Inst. Inc., Cary. 2006; 525-566.
11. SAS/STAT User Guide. The Glimmix Procedure. SAS Institute, Cary. 2013; 3080-3209.
12. Dohoo IR, Martin SW and Stryhn H. Veterinary Epidemiologic Research. 2nd edn. VER Inc., Charlottetown. 2009; 579-606.
13. Hess RS, Kass PH and Van Winkle TJ. **Association between diabetes mellitus, hypothyroidism or** hyperadrenocorticism, and atherosclerosis in dogs. *J Vet Intern Med.* 2003; 17:489-94.
14. Short AD, Saleh NM, Catchpole B, Kennedy LJ, Barnes A, Jones CA, Fretwell N and Ollier WE. **CTLA4 promoter polymorphisms are associated with canine diabetes mellitus.** *Tissue Antigens.* 2010; 75:242-52.

8
CHAPTER

COMPARATIVE PHARMACOTHERAPY OF THYROID DISEASES IN DOGS AND CATS

Marina Mickael, Eric Morris, Mollie M Roush and Inder Sehgal

Keywords: Veterinary pharmacy, Hypothyroid, Hyperthyroid, Levothyroxine, Methimazole, Dog, Cat

INTRODUCTION

Retail pharmacies are receiving an increasing number of prescriptions for pets, primarily dogs and cats, to receive humanapproved medications. Retail pharmacists are not routinely trained by pharmacy schools in veterinary-specific pharmacotherapy, yet they have a duty to provide necessary counselling. They may need to help the pet client with questions regarding signs of therapeutic efficacy, time from initiation of therapy until clinically noticeable improvement, remedies to drug administration difficulties and potential adverse effects. Pharmacist-to-client counselling should take into account differences in pet vs. human behaviors. This article will cover the most common endocrine diseases of dogs and cats—thyroid diseases. While diabetes is by far the most common endocrine disease in people, in dogs and cats, diseases of the thyroid are the most frequent endocrinopathies. For dogs, hypothyroidism is far more frequent than hyperthyroidism, while in cats, the opposite is true. As with people, thyroxine (T4) and triiodothyronine (T3) exist both in bound-to-plasma-protein and in unbound, free states, and only the free molecules have biological effects and can be readily metabolized.

Citation: Mickael M, Morris E, Roush MM, Sehgal I (2015) Comparative Pharmacotherapy of Thyroid Diseases in Dogs and Cats, J Pharma Care Health Sys S3-002. doi:10.4172/2376-0419.S3-002.

HYPOTHYROIDISM

Background

In dogs, hypothyroidism is usually primary, i.e., due to atrophy of the thyroid gland. In the majority of cases, this atrophy is associated with acquired autoimmune lymphocytic thyroiditis, similar to Hashimoto's thyroiditis in humans, as both are characterized by cellular lymphocytic, as well as humoral autoantibodies against thyroglobulin, T4 and T3 in the thyroid gland [1]. The remainders of canine hypothyroid causes are non-inflammatory or of unknown etiology; congenital hypothyroidism is rare [2].

Hypothyroidism is most often diagnosed in middle-aged dogs (approximately 7-8 years old) and is more likely in pure breeds such as Golden and Labrador Retrievers, Doberman Pinschers, and Irish Setters. It is also more common in neutered and spayed dogs [3]. In people, hypothyroidism is more frequent in women; however, female dogs do not appear to be at greater risk.

Hypothyroidism Symptoms and Diagnosis

Signs that the client notices in dogs have usually developed over time and are similar to those observed in people. These dogs have dry and brittle hair with poor growth progressing to symmetrical alopecia. Hypothyroid people also develop dry, thinning hair. Hypothyroid dogs have dry skin, which may have dark pigmentation and, like people with chronic severe hypothyroidism, dogs can progress to dermatologic myxedema. Both hypothyroid people and dogs show fatigue, weight gain and exercise intolerance. However, in dogs, neurologic deficits are uncommon [2]; while in people hypothyroidism is associated with memory deficits [4]. Hypothyroidism is one of the few disease conditions in dogs that can result in hypercholesterolemia and even coronary artery disease.

In people, a rise in thyroid stimulating hormone (TSH) is the first suggestive diagnostic of hypothyroidism, as the free T4 levels remain normal initially [5]. In dogs, TSH is not the initial diagnostic, total T4 is. A low total T4 in a dog is highly suggestive of hypothyroidism. In people, >95% of T4 levels are regulated by TSH, therefore, an elevated TSH strongly suggests hypothyroidism. In dogs however, T4 is only regulated approximately 70% by TSH because growth hormone regulates the remainder; thus, as opposed to human medicine, TSH levels in dogs usually play little or no role in routine diagnosis. In people, diagnosis is often made using TSH in combination with free T4 measurements. In dogs, total and free T4 measurements correlate in >95% of suspected canine hypothyroid cases and therefore, the routine testing of both total and free T4 in dogs provides no significant added benefit in the general diagnostic setting [6]. Only in select circumstances is a free T4 assay useful to differentiate dogs with, for instance, non-thyroidal illness or atypical clinical signs [6]. The common-place diagnosis of canine hypothyroidism is based on a low T4 with clinical symptoms followed by a positive response to therapy.

Hypothyroidism Therapy

Thyroid hormone replacement, levothyroxine, is usually administered once a day and adjusted frequently early in treatment. Dogs may be given levothyroxine as a trial to rule out other non-thyroid illnesses. In this case, levothyroxine is administered over approximately 2 months, and if symptoms resolve, the drug is withdrawn over 4-6 weeks. Re-appearance of symptoms indicates hypothyroidism. Ideally, as with people, thyroid replacement should be administered without food, but in the home setting, clients may need to provide a small meatball of food with the oral tablets so that their dog takes the pill. It is important for the client to be reminded to develop a consistent time and method of administering levothyroxine to their pet so that plasma concentrations and drug effects are also consistent on a daily basis. A Client Information Sheet (CIS) on levothyroxine is available on-line at: https://sites.google.com/site/vetpharmcis/home, and this CIS can be used to assist with client counseling. This CIS is part of a series written by Marshall University School of Pharmacy students taking a veterinary pharmacy elective.

In people, a treatment goal is maintenance of the patient's TSH and free T4 within normal range. This is not the goal with dogs. For dogs, resolution of symptoms and normal total T4 values often suffice. The client can be counseled that successful treatment is demonstrated by the return of normal energy levels and a healthier hair coat. Loss of the extra body weight the dog has gained will follow. These responses can occur over 2 weeks to 2 months, with anticipated resolution of most symptoms in 4 weeks [7]. There are no particular adverse reactions associated with levothyroxine therapy at the recommended dosage levels; however, over dosage will result in the signs of thyrotoxicosis, not dissimilar from people. Symptoms of levothyroxine overdose may include excitability, dizziness and fainting, increased thirst, urination and hunger, and panting [8].

The doses of levothyroxine given to dogs are strikingly higher than those doses typically administered to people, and to an unaccustomed pharmacist, they may appear incorrect. While the dose for an adult person can be 75 to 125 μg a day, a medium-sized (25 kg) dog would begin therapy at ≈500 μg a day (assuming a dose of 20ug/kg/day [8]) and half of dogs may need an upward adjustment of this dose and/ or frequency [7]. Cats rarely develop hypothyroidism; however, in those that do, the levothyroxine dose is one-half the dog dose. Humanlabeled products, such as Synthroid are sold in tablet strengths from 25 micrograms to 300 micrograms; however to accommodate medium and large dogs, veterinary-labeled products such as Soloxine are available in strengths up to 1 mg [8]. Clients should be encouraged not to switch between different brands of levothyroxine due to some reports of bioavailability differences.

The dramatic difference in comparative dosing levels is partially explained by the different plasma levels of thyroid binding globulin (TBG). Dogs have only one-fourth the amount of TBG as people, while cats have no detectable TBG [9]. The lower level of plasma proteinbound T4 leads to T4 half-lives in dogs and cats that is much shorter than in people. The half-life of canine T4 is approximately 12h [7]; feline T4 is approximately 10h, compared with people, who have a T4 half-life of approximately

7 days [5]. In addition, the oral bioavailability of levothyroxine is much lower in dogs than humans [8].

In summary, hypothyroidism is very similar in dogs and humans in its pathophysiology, symptoms and drug therapy. The difference most relevant to pharmacy staff is the large dosing necessary in dogs. Pharmacy staff should readily contact the referring veterinarian regarding answers to questions or concerns they or their clients have about the therapy of hypothyroidism in dogs or cats.

HYPERTHYROIDISM

Background

Hyperthyroidism is the endocrine disease most frequent in cats. Feline thyroid disease is primarily caused by a functional thyroid adenoma (adenomatous hyperplasia). A similar adenomatous condition, toxic adenoma, also occurs in people; however, in people, the most frequent cause of hyperthyroidism is an autoimmune syndrome referred to as Grave's disease, which occurs rarely, if ever, in cats [10]. Hyperthyroid dogs most often have thyroid carcinoma [11]; therefore this article will focus on the treatable disease in the cat. Feline hyperthyroidism occurs primarily in middle-aged and older cats (between 10 and 13 years of age [12] with no gender predisposition [10]; in contrast, Grave's disease usually develops in people under 40 years of age and is diagnosed eight times more commonly in women [5].

Hyperthyroidism Symptoms and Diagnosis

The signs of hyperthyroidism in cats that are most noticed by the owner are weight loss and increased appetite. Owners may also observe their cats to be hyper-excitable, to have polydipsia and polyuria, and to have gastrointestinal signs including vomiting, diarrhea, and increased fecal volume [11]. People with Grave's disease share the signs of weight loss and increased appetite, along with diarrhea and anxiety. They also have an exophthalmos that cats do not [5]. As is the case with free T4 assay in the hypothyroid dog, free T4 analysis in the cat adds little benefit to the accuracy of the total T4 alone; therefore, feline hyperthyroidism is presumptively diagnosed by a high T4 and accompanying clinical signs [10,11]. People suspected of hyperthyroidism are diagnosed through elevated serum free T4, total T3 and low TSH levels [5].

Hyperthyroidism Therapy

Pharmacologic therapy for both cats and people involve the administration of thiourea drugs. Methimazole is most often the drug used to treatment of feline hyperthyroidism. Propylthiouracil, a secondline therapy in people, is rarely used in pets because of its greater adverse effects [8]. Mechanistically, methimazole and propothiouracil inhibit the enzyme thyroid peroxidase. To form natural thyroid hormones, iodide is oxidized by this enzyme and then incorporates onto tyrosine amino acid residues. The thioureas also inhibit other steps in thyroid hormone synthesis [5].

In the cat, therapy begins with 2.5-10mg methimazole total dose per animal, which is administered 2-3 times daily for a trial period of approximately 3 weeks. After this trial period, the veterinarian will likely re-assess total T4 levels and clinical response by improvement in signs. The methimazole dose will then be adjusted with the ultimate goal of reaching just once daily administration. Up to 50% of cats receiving methimazole over 6 months will require a dose reduction due to the production of antinuclear antibodies. In comparison with cats, adult humans receive methimazole in dose ranges from 5mg given three times daily for mild hyperthyroidism to 20mg given three times daily. It terms of dosing equivalency per mg body weight, cats will typically receive about twice the dose level as people. A cat client can expect to see clinical improvement in their pet in approximately three weeks [12], while people with Grave's disease expect to benefit in 4-8 weeks [5]. If severe tachycardia has developed, a beta blocker such as propranolol, may be prescribed as adjunctive therapy as in people to reduce palpitations and anxiety. The cat client should be counseled on the importance of consistently administering the methimazole in order to control symptoms, since the disease is not itself cured [8]. A Client Information Sheet (CIS) on methimazole is available on-line at: https:// sites.google.com/site/vetpharmcis/home.

Administering oral medications to cats can be challenging in general and methimazole presents an additional problem since it has a bitter taste. Because it is critical for the drug to be taken consistently, methimazole is a favorite medication referral by veterinarians to compounding pharmacies where it can be reformulated and dispensed as a transdermal gel [13]. A variety of applicators for dispensing the transdermal methimazole compound are available [14,15]. The typical point of application is inside the inner ear pinna every 12 hours. If applying by hand, the client should be counseled to wear a glove. Reported disadvantages of the transdermal formulation are that it is more expensive, less effective in some cats, and that it has a shorter shelf life (approximately 2 weeks) [8].

As opposed to the treatment of dogs for hypothyroidism, adverse reactions are not uncommon in the cat treated for hyperthyroidism. Any concerns from the client or pharmacist should be referred back to the veterinarian. Most adverse reactions, if they occur, occur early in treatment and may warrant a dosage adjustment to reduce theseverity of adverse symptoms. These are most frequently vomiting, anorexia, lethargy and depression. A rare, yet relevant adverse reaction by some cats, is pruritus and self-induced facial excoriation. In people, methimazole is also associated with pruritic rashes, as well as occasional nausea, vomiting, epigastric distress, and a more common adverse effect, benign transient leukopenia, which occurs in up to 12% of adult people [5]. Agranulocytosis is a less frequent, yet serious effect in people with incidences from 0.5 to 6% [5]. Cats (approximately 15%) also develop transient leukopenia within the first 2 months of therapy, and less frequently, approximately 4% of cats also show the more severe agranulocytosis [8]. Key counseling points to give to clients on adverse effects are to observe for lethargy, vomiting, anorexia or pruritus and to contact their veterinarian if adverse reactions occur. Reasons to consider a switch to transdermal methimazole are difficulty in administering the oral drug to defiant cats and/or frequent vomiting with the tablet form [8].

In summary, feline hyperthyroidism arises through a different etiology than the most frequent cause of human hyperthyroidism, Grave's disease; yet both are treated pharmacologically with methimazole. The relative dose is much higher in cats, yet consistent, chronic administration is essential in both cats and people to ensure effective reduction in thyroid hormone levels and signs of clinical pathology. Drug-related adverse effects are similar, but their relative frequencies differ between the two species with vomiting more common in cats. A pet-owner can often administer a pill by hand to a dog if the dog does not take the pill with food; however, cats are difficult for most clients to pill by hand, especially if it must be done daily. Therefore, in consultation with the referring veterinarian, a transdermal delivery option should be considered for cats that do not take oral methimazole well.

REFERENCES

1. Miller J, Popiel J, Chelmonska-Soyta A (2015) Humoral and Cellular Immune Response in Canine Hypothyroidism. J Comp Pathol 153: 28-37.
2. Mooney CT (2011) Canine hypothyroidism: a review of aetiology and diagnosis. N Z Vet J 59: 105-114.
3. http://www.dog-health-guide.org/hypothyroidismcanine.html
4. He XS, Ma N, Pan ZL, Wang ZX, Li N, et al. (2011) Functional magnetic resource imaging assessment of altered brain function in hypothyroidism during working memory processing. Eur J Endocrinol 164: 951-959.
5. Jonklass J, Talbert RL (2014) Chapter 58 Thyroid disorders. In: J DiPiro, RL Talbert, G Yee, G Matzke, B Wells, ML Posey (Eds.), Pharmacotherapy A Pathophysiologic Approach. (9thEdn), McGraw Hill Education, New York.
6. Rasmussen SH, Anderson HH, Kjelgaard-Hansen M (2014) Combined assessment of serum free and total T4 in a general clinical setting seemingly has limited potential in improving diagnostic accuracy of thyroid dysfunction in dogs and cats. Veterinary Clinical Pathology 43: 1-3
7. Van Dijl IC, Le Traon G, Van de Meulengraaf BD, Burgaud S, Horspool LJ, et al. (2014) Pharmacokinetics of total thyroxine after repeated oral administration of levothyroxine solution and its clinical efficacy in hypothyroid dogs. J Vet Intern Med 28: 1229-1234.
8. Plumb DC (2015) Plumb's Veterinary Drug Handbook (8th edn). John Wiley & Sons, Inc, Stockholm, WI.
9. Larsson M, Pettersson T, Carlström A (1985) Thyroid hormone binding in serum of 15 vertebrate species: isolation of thyroxine-binding globulin and prealbumin analogs. Gen Comp Endocrinol 58: 360-375.
10. Taylor JA, Jacobs RM, Lumsden JH, Bonnett BN (1989) Perspectives on the diagnosis of feline hyperthyroidism. Can Vet J 30: 477-481.
11. http://www.merckvetmanual.com/
12. http://www.aspca.org/pet-care/cat-care/hyperthyroidism

13. Lécuyer M, Prini S, Dunn ME, Doucet MY (2006) Clinical efficacy and safety of transdermal methimazole in the treatment of feline hyperthyroidism. Can Vet J 47: 131-135.

14. http://www.wedgewoodpetrx.com/learning-center/professional-monographs/efficacy-and-safety-of-methimazole-for-once-daily-transdermal-treatment-of-cats-with-hyperthyroidism.html

15. http://www.vetrxdirect.com/product/view/methimazole-transdermal-gel-compounded-for-cats

9
CHAPTER

IN VITRO CHARACTERIZATION OF THE PERCUTANEOUS ABSORPTION OF TRAMADOL INTO INNER EAR DOMESTIC FELINE SKIN USING THE FRANZ SKIN FINITE DOSE MODEL

August S. Bassani, Daniel Banov, Chris Simmons and Ha Phan

Keywords: Domestic feline(s), pain, pharmaceutical compounding, percutaneous absorption, tramadol, Lipoderm, PLO, Franz skin finite dose model

INTRODUCTION

Companion animals such as cats and dogs are popular pets in many countries around the world. In the United States, the estimated percentages of households owning pets are 30.4% for cats and 36.5% for dogs [1]. Though both domestic animals are cherished by their caregivers, cats are often under-treated for pain in comparison to dogs. Domestic cats, also referred to as domestic felines, belong to the larger family of felines, which also includes tigers, lions, jaguars, and wild cats. Only 56% of domestic felines receive adequate analgesia due to the increased difficulty for caregivers to recognize and assess pain in these animals [2].

The types of pain experienced by domestic felines can be divided into two categories: acute pain and chronic pain. Acute pain is often a result of trauma or surgery, while chronic pain is usually associated with Degenerative Joint Disease (DJD), a condition that involves deterioration of tissues surrounding the joints. Opioids such as morphine or fentanyl are commonly used for acute pain, while Nonsteroidal Anti-Inflammatory Drugs (NSAIDs) such as meloxicam or ketoprofen are commonly used for chronic pain [3]. Though opioids and NSAIDs are common treatment options, there

Citation: August S. Bassani, Daniel Banov, Chris Simmons and Ha Phan, In vitro characterization of the percutaneous absorption of tramadol into inner ear domestic feline skin using the Franz skin finite dose model, DOI: http://dx.doi.org/10.7243/2054-3425-3-3.

are disadvantages with the use of these medications in domestic felines. As obligated carnivores, the feline family has low capacity for the metabolism of drugs via hepatic glucuronidation, a pathway that develops as a result of exposure to phytoalexins in plants. Deficiency in this pathway can lead to decreased efficacy with morphine, as the glucuronidation pathway is required to convert morphine to its active metabolite, Morphine-6-Glucuronide (M-6-G) [2,3]. Although NSAIDs do not require the glucuronidation pathway for activation, long-term exposure to this medication class can lead to gastrointestinal toxicity (e.g., bleeding, ulcerations) and renal damage, which limits the chronic use of NSAIDs [3]. Due to the limitations of current therapies, pain management in domestic felines has become increasingly challenging for practitioners and pharmacists.

In recent years, tramadol has been researched for the treatment of domestic feline pain. Tramadol is a synthetic opioid that exerts analgesic effects by binding to μ-opioid receptors as well as inhibiting neuronal reuptake of norepinephrine and serotonin [4]. Previous studies have shown that tramadol can be used alone or in combination with NSAIDs for the treatment of mild to moderate pain in domestic felines [5,6]. The conventional routes of administration for tramadol include oral, Intravenous (IV), and Subcutaneous (SC) administration [5]. Both IV and SC administration are invasive and, therefore, it may be challenging for caregivers to successfully administer tramadol in a home environment. Although oral administration of tramadol is non-invasive, this route of administration requires physical restraint of the animal by its owner to administer each dose, which can lead to non-compliance and treatment failure [3].

The Food and Drug Administration (FDA) has recognized the need for pharmaceutical compounding in veterinary medicine. Particularly with regards to domestic felines, pharmaceutical compounding can be utilized to overcome the limitations of conventional therapies [7]. Pharmaceutical compounding involves the preparation of customized medications to meet the individual patient needs [8]. When compounded, tramadol can be incorporated into transdermal bases such as Pluronic Lecithin Organogel (PLO) or Lipoderm for transdermal delivery. In comparison to oral, IV, and SC administration, transdermal delivery is a non-invasive route of administration that allows for the percutaneous absorption of drugs. Following application, the medication is intended to be directly absorbed into systemic circulation over a period of time, bypassing first-pass metabolism [9].

PLO is a first generation transdermal base that contains Pluronic F-127, soya lecithin, and IPP (Isopropyl Palmitate)/IPM (Isopropyl Myristate). PLO is composed of two phases, an aqueous phase (pluronic phase) and an oil phase (lecithin phase), continuously mixed with one another until a homogenous gel is formed. The gel is intended to dissolve both hydrophobic and hydrophilic drugs, with hydrophobic drugs dissolving in the oil phase and hydrophilic drugs dissolving in the aqueous phase [10]. Lipoderm, on the other hand, is a transdermal base that consists of a proprietary liposomal component shown to successfully facilitate the penetration of drugs into and through ex vivo human skin under *In vitro* conditions [11]. Although transdermal delivery of tramadol in PLO or Lipoderm is advantageous in comparison to conventional routes, there is limited data to support the efficacy of compounded tramadol for transdermal delivery in domestic felines. The purpose of this study is to characterize the percutaneous absorption of two tramadol formulations (Tramadol 100 mg/g in PLO and Tramadol 100 mg/g in Lipoderm), when applied to the inner ear of domestic feline skin, *In vitro*, using the Franz skin finite dose model. In domestic felines, transdermal delivery usually involves the rubbing of medication to the animal's inner ear skin surface, a location that cannot be licked and is usually hairless [12]. The Franz skin finite dose model has proven to be a valuable tool in predicting *in vivo* percutaneous absorption of topically applied drugs [11,13]. Therefore, this model was selected to characterize the percutaneous absorption of tramadol into and through the ex vivo inner ear skin of domestic feline donors.

MATERIALS AND METHODS

Materials

Details relating to the composition of the samples used for testing are shown in Table 1.

Table 1: Composition of the samples used for testing

Tramadol 100 mg/g in PLO			
Ingredients	**Quantity**	**Lot number**	**Source**
Tramadol HCl	10 g	C129073	PCCA
Propylene glycol	8 g	C129628	PCCA
Lecithin isopropyl palmitate base	22 g	2007156	PCCA
Poloxamer 407 20% gel	q.s. to 100 g	1722672	PCCA
Tramadol 100 mg/g in Lipoderm			
Tramadol HCl	10 g	C129073	PCCA
Propylene glycol	8 g	C129628	PCCA
Lipoderm	q.s. to 100 g	2039478	PCCA

Tramadol 100 mg/g in PLO

Tramadol hydrochloride (HCl), in an amount necessary to result in a concentration of 100 mg/g, was added to Lecithin Isopropyl Palmitate solution base along with 10% Propylene Glycol as a wetting agent. Poloxamer 407 20% gel was then added in sufficient quantity to reach the final weight. The formulation was mixed using an electronic mortar and pestle (EMP) for 3 min on a setting of 7, sheared twice using an ointment mill at a setting of 1, and remixed for 1 min on a setting of 5. The specific gravity of the final formulation was 1.002 g/mL.

Tramadol 100 mg/g in Lipoderm

Tramadol HCl, in an amount necessary to result in a concentration of 100 mg/g, was added to Lipoderm along with 10% Propylene Glycol as a wetting agent. The formulation was mixed with the aid of an EMP for 3 min at a setting of 7, sheared twice using an ointment mill on a setting of 1, and remixed with an EMP for 1 min at a setting of 5 to achieve accurate content uniformity. The density of the final formulation was 0.726 g/mL, thus the final tramadol HCl concentration in weight per volume was 72.6 mg/mL.

Skin preparation

The percutaneous absorption of two tramadol formulations were evaluated using normal feline ventral inner ear skin obtained from two different donors, a domestic short hair feline female (donor 1) and male (donor 2). Prior to use, the skin was thawed in water at approximately 37°C and rinsed with tap water to remove blood and other material from the surface. The ventral (inner) surface of the skin was then separated from the dorsal layer. The skin from the two donors were cut into multiple sections to fit nominal 0.8 cm^2 Franz diffusion cells, a chamber that cultures the skin cells and allows for the condition of the skin to be maintained at a temperature and humidity that matches *in vivo* conditions [13]. Seven skin cross-sections were obtained from the two donors. Each skin section was assigned to one chamber, with four chambers for donor 1 and three for donor 2 (Table 2). Within the chambers, the cells were mounted on a diffusion apparatus so that the epidermal surface is exposed to the laboratory environment via the chimney (Figure 1). The receptor compartment of the chamber was filled to capacity with isotonic Phosphate- Buffered Saline (PBS), pH 7.4±0.1, stirred magnetically at approximately 600 rpm. The skin surface was maintained at a temperature of 32°C±1°C.

Table 2: Dosing details for the seven chambers

	Donor 1				Donor 2		
Skin chamber	1	2	3	4	5	6	7
Tramadol in PLO	X	X	--	--	X	--	--
Tramadol in Lipoderm	--	--	X	X	--	X	X

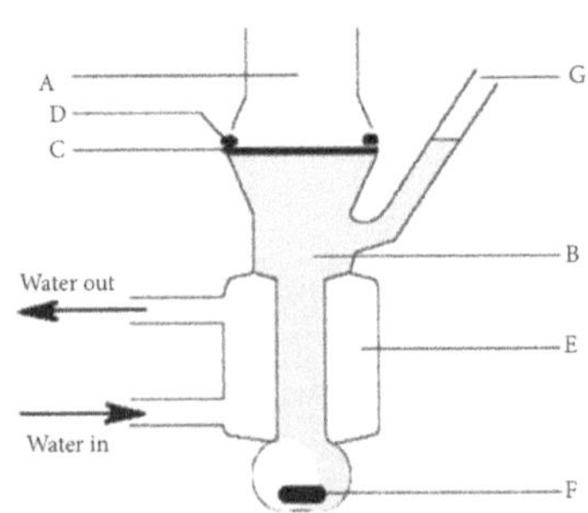

A. Chamber chimney (open to environment)
B. Receptor solution compartment (4.5-6.5 ML)
C. O-ring seal
D. Skin (1.0cm²)
E. Heated water jacket
F. Magnetic stir bar
G. Sampling port

Figure 1: Franz diffusion cell.

Dosing and Sample Collection

Prior to dosing, the receptor solution was removed and replaced with fresh solution containing 0.1xPBS with 0.1% Volpo. The chimney was next removed to allow for access to the epidermal surface for dose application. The two formulations were tested on duplicate sections from two different donors for percutaneous absorption of tramadol over a 48 hr dosing period. Due to the odd number of skin sections available from the two donors, tramadol in PLO was applied to three skin sections (two from donor 1 and one from donor 2) while tramadol in Lipoderm was applied to four skin sections (two from each donor) (Table 2). Using the finite dose technique, a variable finite dose (e.g., 25 μg/cm^2) of each formulation was applied to the outer surface of each skin section using a positive displacement pipette set to deliver 5 μL formulation/cm^2 [11]. The dose was then spread across the surface with a glass rod and the chimney was replaced five to ten minutes after dose application. At 2, 4, 8, 12, 24, 32, and 48 hr following dose application, the receptor solution was removed, replaced with fresh receptor solution, and a predetermined volume of aliquot was saved for subsequent High-Performance Liquid Chromatography (HPLC) analysis. Samples that were not assayed on the day of collection were stored at or below -20°C.

Following collection of the last receptor solution sample at 48 hr, surfaces of the skin were washed twice (0.5 mL each time) with 80:20 Ethanol:Water to remove unabsorbed formulation from skin surfaces. The intact skin was then removed from the chamber and extracted in 80:20 Ethanol:Water overnight at room temperature. Tramadol skin content was determined via HPLC analysis of the extractant sample.

Analytical Testing

Tramadol contents within the skin, in the surface wash, and in each receptor solution sample collected at the predetermined time intervals were quantified using HPLC/UV (Ultraviolet). HPLC was conducted on a Hewlett-Packard 1100 Series HPLC system with a diode array detector at a wavelength of 220 ηm (4 ηm) to 500 ηm (50 ηm). A solvent system consisting of 70% Water (pH 9.5) with 10 mM Ammonium Formate and 30% Methanol was run through a Phenomenex Gemini C18 column (3 μ, 50x3 mm) at a flow rate of 0.4 mL/min. The column temperature was maintained at 25°C.

RESULTS

To characterize the percutaneous absorption of tramadol, a total of 4 parameters were determined for each of the 7 chambers, as follows: total absorption, rate of absorption, surface wash, and skin content. Since each chamber had corresponding values for the 4 parameters, mean values and standard deviation were calculated for each parameter across the 2 donors. Mean values were expressed as percentages of the applied dose to further compare the abilities of PLO and Lipoderm in facilitating the percutaneous absorption of tramadol. Summary of results across the two donors can be found in Tables 3 and 4 and Figure 2.

Table 3: Across donor summary: mean total absorption, surface wash and skin content (mean±SE (standard error) as percent applied dose, n=2)

	Total absorption (μg)	Total absorption (%)	Surface wash (μg)	Surface wash (%)	Skin content (μg)	Skin content (%)
Tramadol in Lipoderm	277.10±11.39	100.40±3.24	9.86±0.15	3.65±0.14	2.97±0.28	1.09±0.07
Tramadol in PLO	333.70±43.09	90.28±14.70	39.66±54.79	10.45±14.42	<LOD	<LOD

Table 4: Across donor summary: mean flux (μg/cm²/hr) (mean±SE, n=2 donors).

Time (hr)	Tramadol in PLO	Tramadol in Lipoderm
1	17.91±19.00	13.57±3.19
3	15.40±16.28	15.40±0.71
6	10.32±8.70	13.80±0.54
10	10.31±6.68	14.21±1.73
18	12.55±2.78	9.80±1.02
28	6.48±3.93	4.36±1.05
40	4.09±5.01	1.50±0.21

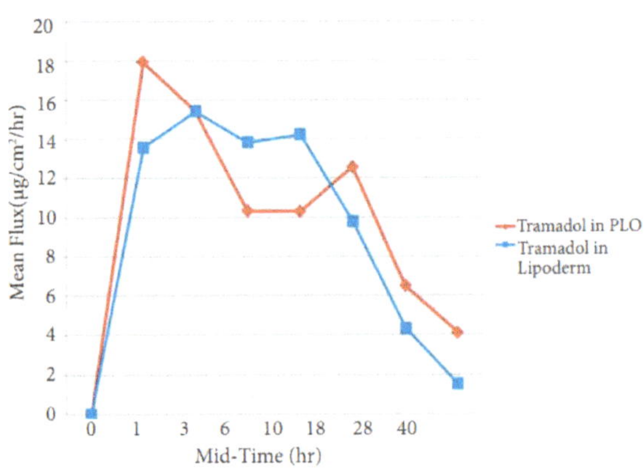

Figure 2: Across donor summary: mean flux (μg/cm²/hr) for two compounded transdermal formulations.

Total absorption (μg) was calculated as the sum of tramadol content (μg) within the 7 samples collected over 48 hr. Mean total absorption (μg) was the average of total absorptions for all chambers from the 2 donors. The mean total absorption of tramadol in PLO was 333.70 μg±43.09, corresponding to 90.28%±14.70 absorption of the applied dose. For tramadol in Lipoderm, mean total absorption was 277.10 μg±11.39, corresponding to 100.40%±3.24 absorption of the applied dose.

Rate of absorption, presented as flux (μg/cm²/hr) of tramadol into receptor solution, was determined by dividing the amount of tramadol absorbed during a time interval and the length of that interval. Flux is a value reported at midpoint of sample collection for a sampling period. For instance, if samples are collected at 4 and 8 hr, the flux of tramadol during that time interval is equal to the amount of tramadol in the receptor solution between 4 and 8 hr, divided by the time span of 4 hr. Flux is then plotted at 6 hr, midpoint of 4 and 8 hr. Mean flux (μg/cm^2/hr), shown inTable 4, was calculated across donors for each sampling interval. Figure 2 illustrates mean flux data plotted as the amount of tramadol absorbed through the skin against time.

Surface wash (μg) refers to the amount of tramadol remaining on the surface of the skin after 48 hr of dose application. Surface wash was 39.66 μg±54.79 for tramadol in PLO and 9.86 μg±0.15 for tramadol in Lipoderm, corresponding to 10.45%±14.42 and 3.65%±0.14 of the applied dose, respectively.

Skin content (μg) refers to the amount of tramadol found within the skin after 48 hr. Mean skin content was calculated as the average tramadol content in the skin sections across 2 donors. Mean tramadol skin content was less than the Lower Limit of Detection (LOD) for tramadol in PLO. For tramadol in Lipoderm, mean skin content was 2.97 μg±0.28, which is equivalent to a mean of 1.09%±0.07 of the applied dose.

DISCUSSION

Results of this study show that both PLO and Lipoderm were capable of facilitating the percutaneous absorption of tramadol across ex-vivo feline inner ear skin using the Franz skin finite dose model. For both transdermal formulations (tramadol in PLO and tramadol in Lipoderm), the majority of the applied dose penetrated the skin as more than 90% was found in the receptor solution after 48 hr. However, the mean total absorption of tramadol when in Lipoderm (100.40%±3.24) was higher than when in PLO (90.28%±14.70). The higher mean percent total absorption of tramadol seen with Lipoderm potentially indicates that this transdermal base has greater penetration potentials in comparison to PLO. If the tramadol in PLO and tramadol in Lipoderm are both applied to domestic feline inner ear skin, tramadol plasma concentrations may be higher in domestic felines receiving the Lipoderm formulation.

When examining rate of absorption, mean flux profile reveal similar time course of tramadol absorption for PLO and Lipoderm, with a rapid rise to a peak flux within 2.5 hr of dose application for both transdermal formulations. Though tramadol, when in Lipoderm, had a lower peak flux, the decline in rate was more steady, forming a more predictable and reliable absorption profile in comparison to the rapid decline and fluctuations in rate for tramadol in PLO (Figure 2). The steadier decline in flux seen with tramadol in Lipoderm may be helpful when managing domestic feline pain as the analgesic effects of tramadol can slowly taper off overtime rather than having a rapid reduction followed by erratic fluctuations of analgesic effects with PLO.

As for surface wash, tramadol content in the surface wash was lower when in Lipoderm than when in PLO. This difference indicates that more tramadol was absorbed when in Lipoderm. Such results then show that Lipoderm may be more efficient at facilitating the percutaneous absorption of tramadol in comparison to PLO as less tramadol remained on the surface following application of the tramadol in Lipoderm formulation. Surface wash results potentially correlate to the higher total absorption of tramadol seen with Lipoderm.

While very minute amounts of the applied dose were found within the skin, tramadol content in the skin was higher for the Lipoderm than the PLO formulation. The higher tramadol skin content may be due to the ability of Lipoderm to partition into various layers of the skin to a greater extent than PLO. Having higher skin content potentially correlates to a slow and steadier decline in flux as tramadol is slowly released from the skin into receptor solution overtime.

The higher mean total absorption, steadier decline in flux, lower surface wash, and higher skin content seen with the tramadol in Lipoderm formulation show that Lipoderm may be a more appropriate transdermal base for the transdermal delivery of tramadol in comparison to PLO. However, since the study was conducted *In vitro*, future studies need to be conducted *in vivo* to fully inform practitioners and pharmacists on the efficacy of tramadol in Lipoderm compared to tramadol in PLO for domestic feline pain.

CONCLUSIONS

Knowledge of this study's results can be used to predict the *in vivo* rate and extent of percutaneous absorption of tramadol in domestic felines. The data collected can augment the limited efficacy data relating to compounded tramadol for transdermal delivery in domestic felines. Based on the *In vitro* results of this study, one may likely hypothesize that tramadol, when in Lipoderm, may potentially have a higher total absorption and a steadier decline in rate of absorption in comparison to when in PLO. The prediction can guide practitioners and pharmacists, when prescribing and compounding with tramadol for feline use, to select a transdermal base with the best and most predictable percutaneous absorption potential.

AUTHORS' CONTRIBUTIONS

Authors' contributions	ASB	DB	CS	HP
Research concept and design	√	√	--	--
Data analysis and interpretation	√	√	--	√
Writing the article	√	√	--	√
Critical revision of the article	√	√	√	√
Final approval of article	√	√	√	√

Acknowledgement

The authors would like to thank Paul A. Lehman, MSc (Cetero Research, Fargo, ND, USA) for conducting the Franz finite dose model experiments, which were funded by PCCA.

REFERENCES

1. American Veterinary Medical Association. *U.S. Pet Ownership Statistics 2012.* 2015.

2. Robertson SA. Assessment and management of acute pain in cats. *J Vet Emerg Crit Care.* 2005; 15:261-72.

3. Robertson SA. Chapter 24: cat-specific considerations. In J. Gaynor & W. Muir III (Eds.), *Handbook of Veterinary Pain Management.* St. Louis, Missouri: Mosby. 2015; 493-516.

4. Takasuga S, Yamamoto R, Mafune S, Sutoh C, Kominami K, Yoshida Y, Ito M and Kinoshita M. In-vitro and in-vivo transdermal iontophoretic delivery of tramadol, a centrally acting analgesic. *J Pharm Pharmacol.* 2011; 63:1437-45.

5. Ray J, Jordan D, Pinelli C, Fackler B, Boggess D and Clark J. Case studies of compounded Tramadol use in cats. *Int J Pharm Compd.* 2012; 16:44-9.

6. Gaynor J and Muir III W. Chapter 14: Alternative drugs and novel therapies used to treat pain. In J. Gaynor & W. Muir III (Eds.), *Handbook of Veterinary Pain Management.* St. Louis, Missouri: Mosby. 2015; 283-284.

7. U.S. Food and Drug Administration. *Animal drugs.* 2015.

8. U.S. Pharmacopeial Convention. *Pharmaceutical Compounding-Nonsterile Preparations*, in: U.S.P. Convention (Ed.) 795, U.S. Pharmacopeial Convention, US, 2014.

9. Muir III W. Chapter 15: Factors influencing analgesic drug selection, dose, and routes of drug administration. In J. Gaynor & W. Muir III (Eds.), *Handbook of Veterinary Pain Management.* St. Louis, Missouri: Mosby. 2015; 329-330.

10. Belgamwar V, Chauk D, Pandey M and Surana S. Pluronic lecithin organogel. *Asian Journal of Pharmaceutics.* 2008; 2:134.

11. Bassani AS, Banov D and Lehman PA. Evaluation of the Percutaneous Absorption of Promethazine Hydrochloride, In Vitro, Using the Human Ex Vivo Skin Model. *Int J Pharm Compd.* 2008; 12:270-273.

12. Papich MG. Drug compounding for veterinary patients. *AAPS J.* 2005; 7:E281-7.

13. Franz TJ, Lehman PA and Raney SG. Use of excised human skin to assess the bioequivalence of topical products. *Skin Pharmacol Physiol.* 2009; 22:276-86.

10
CHAPTER

EFFICACY OF GLUCOCORTICOID MONOTHERAPY FOR TREATMENT OF CANINE MENINGOENCEPHALOMYELITIS OF UNKNOWN ETIOLOGY: A PROSPECTIVE STUDY IN 16 DOGS

Miyu Mercier and Heidi L. Barnes Heller

INTRODUCTION

Canine meningoencephalomyelitis is a heterogeneous collection of inflammatory and infectious diseases of the central nervous system (CNS). In the majority of dogs, meningoencephalomyelitis has an inflammatory non-infectious etiology. There are several non-infectious inflammatory forms of meningoencephalomyelitis, including granulomatous meningoencephalitis (GME), necrotizing meningoencephalitis (NME), necrotizing leukoencephalitis (NLE) and eosinophilic meningoencephalitis (EME). Due to the distinctive high eosinophil presence in CSF and on histopathology, EME can be readily distinguished from GME, NME, and NLE. Dogs with GME, NME, and NLE may be any age, breed, or sex. Many dogs diagnosed with GME, NME, or NLE are small-breed dogs, but the presence of the disease is not restricted to this population. (Granger *et al.* 2010) Diagnostic imaging for GME, NME, or NLE often involves magnetic resonance imaging (MRI) and may be normal or show focal or multifocal changes. Mononuclear pleocytosis is often present but this varies widely, and cerebrospinal (CSF) analysis may be normal in 12–22% of cases. (Granger *et al.* 2010) In the absence of histopathologic examination, GME, NME, and NLE are indistinguishable on the basis of clinical presentation, breed, sex, age, advanced imaging, and CSF analysis. When histopathologic examination is not available for a given dog, the term meningoencephalomyelitis of unknown etiology (MUE) is used to describe suspected GME, NME, or NLE. (Zarfoss *et al.* 2006; Granger *et al.* 2010; Talarico & Schatzberg 2010)

Citation: Miyu Mercier and Heidi L. Barnes Heller, Efficacy of glucocorticoid monotherapy for treatment of canine meningoencephalomyelitis of unknown etiology: a prospective study in 16 dogs, DOI: 10.1002/vms3.4.

Following a diagnosis of MUE, initial therapy consists of glucocorticoid (GC) drugs, with or without the addition of other immunosuppressant medications. (Adamo *et al.* 2007; Coates*et al.* 2007; Menaut *et al.* 2008; Pakozdy *et al.* 2009; Talarico & Schatzberg 2010; Wong *et al.* 2010; Flegel *et al.* 2011; Lowrie *et al.* 2013) Glucocorticoid monotherapy has been considered the standard therapy (Zarfoss *et al.* 2006; Adamo *et al.* 2007; Jung*et al.* 2007; Pakozdy *et al.* 2009; Talarico & Schatzberg 2010; Wong *et al.* 2010; Flegel*et al.* 2011); however, its efficacy without adjunct immunosuppression in the treatment of MUE has been evaluated in only a limited number of studies. (Munana & Luttgen 1998; Jung*et al.* 2007; Pakozdy *et al.* 2009; Flegel *et al.* 2011) Use of GC drugs, with variable dosing within each study, has been reported in 59 dogs. The doses have ranged from 5–30 mg/kg per day (Pakozdy *et al.* 2009), 0.17–2.5 mg/kg per day (Flegel *et al.* 2011), 1 mg/kg per day (Jung *et al.* 2007), and 0.5–4 mg/kg per day. (Munana & Luttgen 1998) Therefore, the aims of the current study were compare the CSF analysis at diagnosis and after treatment with a standard GC dose in dogs with MUE. The second aim was to determine the survival time in dogs with MUE treated with GC monotherapy. We hypothesized that abnormal CSF findings would normalize in dogs with MUE, and survival time would be longer than in previous studies utilizing variable GC protocols.

MATERIALS AND METHODS

Study Population and Inclusion Criteria

In this prospective study, client-owned dogs were accrued continuously between September 2006 and May 2009. All clients signed informed consent forms prior to enrollment. Complete physical and neurologic examinations were performed by 1 of the authors. Dogs were included in the study if the following inclusion criteria were met: (1) normal minimum database; (2) GC was not administered within 5 days prior to presentation; (3) MRI consistent with meningoencephalitis/myelitis; (4) negative infectious disease titres, including, tick-borne agents (*Borrelia bergdorferi*, *Rickettsia rickettsii*, and *Ehrlichia canis*), protozoa (*Neospora caninum*), fungi (*Histoplasma, Blastomyces, Aspergillus, Coccidioidomyces*, and *Cryptococcus*) and paired serum and CSF distemper virus titers; and (5) abnormal CSF findings without evidence of neoplastic or infectious etiology. A minimum database was defined as a complete blood count, serum biochemical panel, urinalysis, and three-view thoracic radiographs. Large breed dogs with cervical hyperpathia only were excluded from the study.

Diagnostic Testing

Magnetic resonance imaging (GE Horizon 1.0 Tesla magnet, Pittsburg, PA, USA) was performed under general anesthesia in all dogs based on lesion localization from the neurologic examination. Dogs were pre-medicated with hydromorphone (Baxter Pharmaceutical, Deerfield, IL, USA) at 0.1 mg/kg IV and diazepam (Valium; Hospira, Lake Forest, IL, USA) at 0.25 mg/kg IV and induced with propofol (PropoFlo; Abbott Animal Health, Abbott Park, IL, USA) at 4 mg/kg IV to effect. Anesthesia was maintained with isoflurane (IsoFlo®; Abbott Animal Health). The standard MRI protocol for this study included T1- and T2- weighted images in sagittal and transverse planes, fluid attenuated inversion recovery images in the transverse planes, and T1-weighted images after administration of Gadolinium (MultiHance; Bracco Diagnostics, Monroe Township, NJ, USA) in transverse and sagittal planes. Magnetic resonance imaging findings were classified as normal, focal or multifocal for this study.

Cerebrospinal fluid (CSF) was collected from the cerebellomedullary or lumbar cisterns during the same anesthetic episode as neuroimaging. Normal CSF analysis was defined as nucleated cell count (TNCC) <5 cells/μL and protein concentration <25 mg/dL for cerebellomedullary cistern puncture and <40 mg/dL for lumbar puncture. (Platt & Olby 2004) After collection, the CSF sample was divided into two aliquots for transportation; in 1 sample, a 1:10 dilution of CSF to autologous serum was made to improve cell stabilization for transportation, and the other sample was CSF only. (Cellio 2001) All samples were transported in additive-free sterile glass tubes. Analysis was performed by an affiliated laboratory (Antech Diagnostic Laboratory, Oakbrook, IL, USA) within 12 h of collection and analysed according to standard procedure. Correction factors were not applied to the data, and all reported values were uncorrected. (Summers *et al.* 1995) Approximately 1 month after initial CSF analysis, a second CSF sample was collected from the same cistern, using the same anesthetic protocol, and analysed as detailed above.

Treatment Protocol

Immediately upon recovery from anesthesia all dogs received intravenous methylprednisolone (Solu-Medrol; Pfizer, New York, NY, USA) at 30 mg/kg IV followed by 15 mg/kg IV 3 h after the initial dose and 10 mg/kg IV 3 h after the second dose was administered. Following treatment with methylprednisone, prednisone (West-Ward Pharmaceutical, Eatontown, NJ, USA) or prednisolone (Lloyd, Inc., Shenandoah, IA, USA) at 1 mg/kg PO q12 h, sulfadimathoxine/ormetoprim (Primor® tablets; Pfizer) at 15 mg/kg PO q12 h, doxycycline (Doxycycline tablets; West Ward Pharmaceutical) at 5–10 mg/kg PO q24 h, and famotidine (Famotidine tablets; Wockhardt, Ltd, Morton Grove, IL, USA) at 1 mg/kg PO q24 h were initiated. After obtaining negative results for infectious disease testing, sulfadimathoxine/ormetoprim and doxycycline were discontinued.

If the second CSF results were within reference intervals, the dog was classified as a CSF responder and a gradually decreasing dose of prednisone or prednisolone was administered as follows: 1 mg/kg *per os* q24 h × 30 days, then 1 mg/kg *per os* q48 h × 30 days and then discontinued. If the second CSF results were abnormal, the dog was classified as a CSF non-responder and the same dose of prednisone or prednisolone was continued for an additional 30 days. If dogs did not improve at 60 days or greater following the above treatment, or worsened during treatment, additional immunosuppressive agents were recommended.

Referring veterinarians were contacted by telephone within 48 months after diagnosis of MUE and questioned about the survival of each dog. If the dog had died, the reason for the death was noted. Referring veterinarians were asked if clinical signs had recurred for CSF responders. Relapse was defined as a reoccurrence of clinical signs in CSF responders, after discontinuing GC therapy.

Statistical Analysis

Descriptive statistics including medians, minimums and maximums were recorded for continuous data. A Kaplan–Meier survival curve was created for survival data. Overall survival time and survival time of CSF responders and CSF non-responders was evaluated with the Mantel-Cox Log-Rank test comparison.

RESULTS

Sixteen dogs met the inclusion criteria. Breeds included Lhasa apso ($n = 2$), Dachshund ($n = 2$), and 1 each of the following breeds: Golden Retriever, Retriever mix, Pug, Welsh Springer Spaniel, Boston Terrier, Pug-Beagle mix, Beagle, Jack Russell Terrier, Rottweiler, Collie, Maltese terrier and mixed breed. The median age was 4.5 years (2–11 years) and the median weight was 12.0 kg (5.2–38.4 kg). Neuroanatomical lesion localization, based on the neurologic examination, was prosencephalon (5/16 dogs), brainstem (3/16 dogs), T3-L3 myelopathy (2/16 dogs), L6-S2 radiculopathy (1/16 dogs) and peripheral neuropathy (1/16 dogs) involving the vestibulocochlear nerves. Four of 16 dogs were diagnosed with multifocal lesion localization. Magnetic resonance imaging findings were normal in 2 dogs, focal in 3 dogs and multifocal in 11 dogs. Abnormalities on MRI corresponded with the neuroanatomic lesion localization in all dogs. The median prednisone or prednisolone dose was 1 mg/kg (0.8–1.2 mg/kg) PO q12 h. Sulfadimethoxine/ormetoprim and doxycycline were discontinued by day 7 of treatment in all dogs.

Initial CSF analysis

Initial CSF samples were collected from the cerebellomedullary cistern in 13 dogs and the lumbar cistern in 3 dogs. See Table 1 for median CSF TNCC and protein concentration. Results indicated mixed mononuclear or lymphocytic pleocytosis ($n = 15$) and neutrophilic pleocytosis ($n = 1$); in 3 dogs the TNCC was within the reference interval, but the protein concentration was increased.

Table 1: Median CSF TNCC and protein concentration for dogs diagnosed with MUE

	Median CSF TNCC (cell/μL)		Median CSF protein (mg/dL)	
	Initial	1 month	Initial	1 month
Responder	8.5 (0–1160)	0 (0–1)	40.5 (25–251)	19 (13–24)
Non-responder	59 (0–1400)	15 (0–120)	68.5 (28–293)	38 (17–175)
Combined	39 (0–1400)	49 (25–293)	1 (0–120)	24 (13–175)

CSF, cerebrospinal fluid; TNCC, total nucleated cell count; MUE, meningoencephalomyelitis of unknown etiology. Responders achieved normal CSF results at 1 month; non-responders did not achieve normal CSF results at 1 month. Combined values refer to CSF responders and CSF non-responders together.

Second Evaluation and CSF Analysis

In seven of 16 dogs (44%), CSF analytes were within reference intervals and they were therefore considered CSF responders. One dog did not have sufficient sample to perform CSF protein concentration therefore this dog was considered a CSF responder based on the TNCC. Median TNCC and protein concentration for CSF responders and CSF non-responders are listed in Table 1.

The neurologic examination was normal in 10 of 16 dogs (63%) and abnormal in 6 dogs (38%). In 5 of 10 dogs (50%) with normal neurologic examinations, CSF analysis was also normal. In 2 of 6 dogs (33%) with abnormal neurologic examinations, CSF analysis was normal. All abnormalities on neurologic examination indicated persistent changes; no new abnormalities were detected. Three CSF non-responders started adjunct immunosuppression at a median of 68 days (62–75 days) from diagnosis due to a failure to improve on GC treatment. All 3 dogs received cytosine arabinoside (Generic; Hospira Inc, Lake Forrest, IL, USA) at 50 mg/m^2 *subcutaneous* q 12 h. for 48 h, repeated every 3 weeks as needed.

Survival Time

Follow-up information was obtained within 48 months (45–1100 days) of initial diagnosis in all dogs. One of seven CSF responders (14%) was reported to have clinical signs consistent with relapse and was euthanized without additional diagnostic testing or treatment.

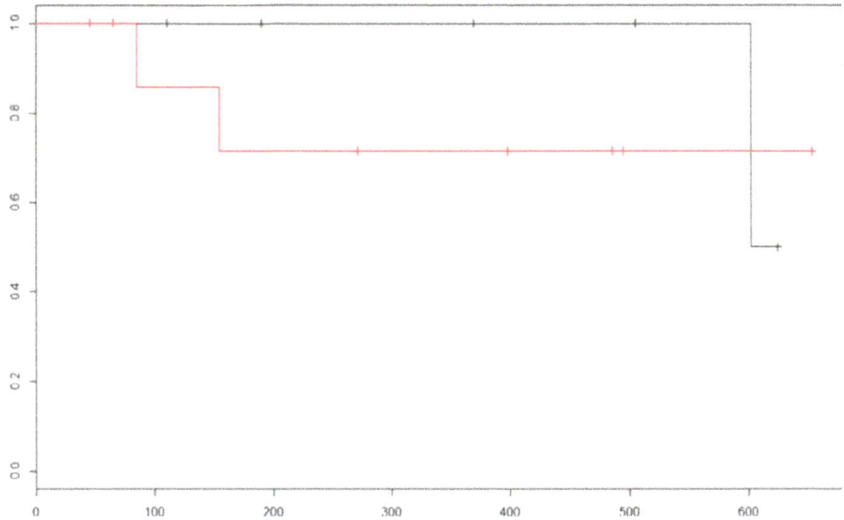

Figure 1: Kaplan-Meier survival curves for 7 responder dogs (black line) and 8 non-responder dogs (red line) with meningoencephalomyelitis of unknown etiology (MUE). Tick marks represent dogs censured for events other than progression of disease.

Two CSF non-responders were euthanized because of progressive disease; two CSF non-responders and one CSF responder were euthanized due to unrelated causes; and two CSF responders and one CSF non-responder were euthanized or died acutely of unknown causes. The remaining three CSF responders and four CSF non-responders dogs were alive at the time of writing (Median 485 days). Median survival for all dogs based on Kaplan–Meier survival analysis was 602 days (45–654 days). Median survival for CSF responders was 602 days and the median was not reached in the CSF non-responders. (Fig. 1) There was no significant difference in survival between the CSF responders and CSF non-responders ($P = 0.85$). Due to the small number of dogs that died due to disease, reporting of survival time between CSF responders and CSF non-responders was not accurate. Additional statistical analysis was not performed due to small sample size.

DISCUSSION

Treatment of dogs with MUE using standardized GC monotherapy resulted in normalization of the CSF analytes in 44% of dogs. None of the previous studies evaluating solo GC therapy has evaluated repeated CSF analysis as a marker for immunosuppression in canine MUE. However, repeated CSF analysis has been evaluated for other immunosuppressant protocols used in treating MUE (Lowrie *et al.* 2013), as well as other inflammatory CNS diseases. (Cizinauskas *et al.* 2000) One study suggested that serial monitoring of CSF TNCC and protein concentrations is a sensitive indicator of successful treatment of inflammatory disease; however, clinical relapse was not evaluated statistically. (Cizinauskas *et al.* 2000) Another study failed to find an association between normal CSF analysis and improved outcome, but did find an association between abnormal CSF analysis and relapse or poor outcome. (Lowrie *et al.* 2013) In the current study, only one CSF responder was reported to have relapsed, suggesting that CSF analysis may be a valid tool for monitoring success or failure of treatment in dogs diagnosed with MUE and treated with GC monotherapy. Larger studies are needed to evaluate this association more fully.

Survival times for dogs in the current study were longer than those in all previous studies of dogs treated with GC monotherapy. Median survival times were reported to be 28 (Pakozdy*et al.* 2009), 91 (Lowrie *et al.* 2013), and 323 (Lowrie *et al.* 2013) days, compared with 602 days in this study. The difference in survival times among studies may reflect different immunosuppression protocols or the prospective nature of the current study. In the current study, we evaluated an immunosuppressive dose of GC that was standardized for all 16 dogs. Methylprednisolone was administered intravenous following the initial diagnosis in all dogs to try to achieve rapid immunosuppression. In studies of treatment protocols using GC in combination with other immunosuppressant agents, median survival times ranged from 26 to 1834 days (Adamo *et al.* 2007; Coates *et al.* 2007; Menaut *et al.* 2008; Pakozdy *et al.* 2009; Talarico & Schatzberg 2010; Wong *et al.* 2010; Flegel *et al.* 2011; Lowrie *et al.* 2013), with a combined median survival time of 375 days. Some of these studies attributed the survival times exclusively to the alternative immunosuppressant. Based on the current study, GC immunosuppression may be a contributing factor to survival times reported for studies, using combination treatments. Furthermore, the long median survival time in this study supports the use of GC monotherapy for dogs diagnosed with MUE.

Lack of a histopathologic diagnosis was a limitation of this study. Although antemortem diagnostic criteria have been established for MUE, inclusion of patients with acute phase infectious disease or neoplasia is an inherent risk in the diagnosis of MUE. (Granger *et al.* 2010) To partially address this possibility, extensive serologic testing was performed at the time of diagnosis for the most common infectious disease in the geographic area as well as paired CSF and serum titres for distemper virus. Serologic testing evaluates immune response to a specific pathogen, therefore it is possible that a dog with acute infectious disease may not yet have mounted an immune response and therefore had negative serology when initially tested. Death or euthanasia due to worsening signs would be expected for dogs with infectious diseases receiving immunosuppressive treatment without concurrent long-term antimicrobial treatment. All dogs included in the study survived for the first 30 days of treatment; therefore it is unlikely that dogs with infectious meningoencephalomyelitis were included. Although neoplastic cells were not identified in CSF, histopathologic examination of the CNS would be expected to be more sensitive than CSF analysis for detection of neoplasia. Brain biopsy was not performed in the dogs in this study due to the risk of complications. Additionally, necropsy was not required and was not obtained in any of the deceased dogs. Requiring diagnosis by either CNS biopsy or necropsy may have resulted in bias towards shorter survival. Therefore, although considered unlikely, occurrence of neoplastic diseases mistakenly diagnosed as meningoencephalomyelitis cannot be excluded. Other limitations of this study included the small size of the study population and limited follow-up time. Larger studies may be able to detect prognostic variables, such normalization differences in CSF protein or TNCC for dogs with MUE that were not evaluated in the current study.

CONCLUSIONS

In dogs with MUE, 44% had normal CSF analysis after 1 month of GC immunosuppression; further studies are needed to determine if a relationship exists between prognosis and results of CSF analysis. Dogs with normal CSF findings at 1 month had longer survival times than dogs with abnormal CSF findings at 1 month. Glucocorticoid therapy in this study, resulted in median survival time longer than previously reported times in studies evaluating combination immunosuppressant protocols; therefore a positive GC effect on survival time in those studies should be considered. Dogs may benefit from the administration of combination immunosuppression protocols if the side effects of GC warrant limited use of GC. In conclusion, this study supports the use of immunosuppression with GC monotherapy in dogs diagnosed with MUE.

ACKNOWLEDGEMENT

This study was supported by VCA-Antech.

REFERENCES

1. Adamo P.F., Rylander H. & Adams W.M. (2007) Ciclosporin use in multi-drug therapy for meningoencephalomyelitis of unknown aetiology in dogs. The Journal of Small Animal Practice 48, 486–496.
2. Cellio B.C. (2001) Collecting, processing, and preparing cerebrospinal fluid in dogs and cats. Compendium Continuing Education for Veterinarians 23, 786–792.
3. Cizinauskas S., Jaggy A. & Tipold A. (2000) Long-term treatment of dogs with steroid-responsive meningitisarteritis: clinical, laboratory and therapeutic results. The Journal of Small Animal Practice 41, 295–301.
4. Coates J.R., Barone G., Dewey C.W., Vitale C.L., Holloway-Azene N.M., Sessions J.K. (2007) Procarbazine as adjunctive therapy for treatment of dogs with presumptive antemortem diagnosis of granulomatous meningoencephalomyelitis: 21 cases (1998–2004). Journal of Veterinary Internal Medicine 2, 100–106.
5. Flegel T., Boettcher I.C., Matiasek K., Oevermann A., Doherr M.G., Oechtering G., Henke D. (2011) Comparison of oral administration of lomustine and prednisolone or prednisolone alone as treatment for granulomatous meningoencephalomyelitis or necrotizing encephalitis in dogs. Journal of the American Veterinary Medical Association 238, 337–345.
6. Granger N., Smith P.M. & Jeffery N.D. (2010) Clinical findings and treatment of non-infectious meningoencephalomyelitis in dogs: a systematic review of 457 pub lished cases from 1962 to 2008. Veterinary Journal 184, 290–297.
7. Jung D.I., Kang B.T., Park C., Yoo J.H., Gu S.H., Jeon H.W., Kim J.W., Heo R.Y., et al. (2007) A comparison of combination therapy (cyclosporine plus prednisolone) with sole prednisolone therapy in 7 dogs with necrotizing meningoencephalitis. Journal of Veterinary Medical Science 69, 1303–1306.
8. Lowrie M., Smith P.M. & Garosi L. (2013) Meningoencephalitis of unknown origin: investigation of prognostic factors and outcome using a standard treatment protocol. The Veterinary Record 172, 527–533.
9. Menaut P., Landart J., Behr S., Lanore D., Trumel C. (2008) Treatment of 11 dogs with meningoencephalomyelitis of unknown origin with a combination of prednisolone and cytosine arabinoside. The Veterinary Record 162, 241–245.
10. Munana K.R. & Luttgen P.J. (1998) Prognostic factors for dogs with granulomatous meningoencephalomyelitis: 42 cases. Journal of the American Veterinary Medical Association 212, 1902–1906.
11. Pakozdy A., Leschnik M., Kneissl S., Gumpenberger M., Gruber A., Tichy A., Thalhammer J.G. (2009) Improved survival time in dogs with suspected GME treated with cyclosporin. The Veterinary Record 164, 89–91.
12. Platt S.R. & Olby N.J. (2004) In BSAVA Manual of Canine and Feline Neurology, 35–53. British Small Animal Veterinary Association: Gloucester.
13. Summers B.A., Cummings J.F., deLahunta A. (1995) Inflammatory diseases of the central nervous system. In: Veterinary Neuropathology, (This is the only edition of this book), pp. 95–162. Mosby: St. Louis.

14. Talarico L.R. & Schatzberg S.J. (2010) Idiopathic granulomatous and necrotizing inflammatory disorders of the canine central nervous system: a review and future perspectives. The Journal of Small Animal Practice 51, 138–149.

15. Wong M.A., Hopkins A.L., Meeks J.C., Clarke J.D. (2010) Evaluation of treatment with a combination of azathioprine and prednisone in dogs with meningoencephalomyelitis of undetermined etiology: 40 cases (2000–2007). Journal of the American Veterinary Medical Association 237, 929–935.

16. Zarfoss M., Schatzberg S., Venator K., Cutter-Schatzberg K., Cuddon P., Pintar J., et al. (2006) Combined cytosine arabinoside and prednisone therapy for meningoencephalitis of unknown aetiology in 10 dogs. The Journal of Small Animal Practice 47, 588–595.

11

CHAPTER

INFLUENCE OF THE DIETARY FIBRE LEVELS ON FAECAL HAIR EXCRETION AFTER 14 DAYS IN SHORT AND LONG-HAIRED DOMESTIC CATS

Mickael Weber, Laura Sams, Alexandre Feugier, Sandrine Michel and Vincent Biourge

INTRODUCTION

A cat can spend 25% to 30% (Benjamin 1976; Panaman 1981) of its time on grooming. Grooming time may be greater than this for cats with limited outdoor access. Grooming behaviour may serve several functions for cats including cooling by coat moistening, removal of shed fur and ectoparasites and stress reduction (Willemse *et al.* 1994; Eckstein & Hart 2000a,b). Since the cat's tongue is covered with keratinous papilla, a large amount of hair is ingested while licking. On average, a short-haired (SH) cat loses approximately 28 g of hair per kg of body weight per year, with two-thirds of this loss being ingested and found in excrement (Hendriks *et al.* 1998). Usually ingested hair is eliminated in faeces however large quantities can accumulate in the digestive tract forming trichobezoars (or hairballs) that can cause digestive problems.

There is no previously published data regarding the incidence of hairballs in pet cats. An epidemiological survey of a large number of cats is necessary to shed more light on the topic. With this aim, a survey of cat owners was recently conducted in order to estimate how common it is for domestic cats to bring up hairballs (Cannon 2013). The survey, based on 48 SH cats, suggested that there was an overall incidence of hairball vomiting of approximately 10% in healthy SH cats. Vomiting, abdominal pain and constipation are the most frequent clinical signs, but hairballs can also result in severe consequences such as anorexia or intestinal obstruction, leading to surgery. This phenomenon is particularly noticeable in long-haired (LH) cats living indoors and during moulting (spring and autumn) but any cat may be affected.

Citation: Mickael Weber, Laura Sams, Alexandre Feugier, Sandrine Michel and Vincent Biourge, Influence of the dietary fibre levels on faecal hair excretion after 14 days in short and long-haired domestic cats, DOI: 10.1002/vms3.6.

For cats that regularly or intermittently suffer from hairballs, preventive treatment is indicated. Common suggestions include regular brushings (Cannon 2013), the use of petroleum-based laxatives or lubricants (Ryan & Wolfer 1978; Barrs *et al.* 1999; Agnello & Kantrowitz2003) or specific dry products (Dann *et al.* 2004; Beynen *et al.* 2011).

Diets formulated to reduce the incidence of hairballs generally contain increased levels of soluble and/or insoluble fibre with the aim of increasing the passage of hair through the gastrointestinal tract and in faeces without causing obstruction or constipation, as well as minimizing formation of hairballs in the digestive tract.

A recent study reported that a diet enriched with insoluble fibre (cellulose) reduced the severity of clinical signs in cats with existing hairballs (Beynen *et al.* 2011). A chew enriched in slippery elm and psyllium husk, a gel-forming and soluble fibre source, has also been shown to reduce the severity of hairball clinical signs in cats by delaying the gastric content (Dann *et al.* 2004). However, the efficacy of these diets has been evaluated from questionnaires or surveys and hairball elimination was subjectively assessed by cat owners. There are no published studies measuring objectively the efficacy of hairball products on faecal hair excretion in cats. This could be due to the difficulty of precisely quantifying faecal hair excretion.

The aim of this study was therefore to assess the impact of psyllium husk and the influence of different levels of total dietary fibre (6% vs. 11% vs. 15% TdF) on faecal hair excretion in short and LH cats by directly measuring hair in their faeces.

MATERIALS AND METHODS

The present study was performed in summer (from July to September).

Animals

Twenty-one healthy adult research cats (4.8 ± 1.1 kg) participated in the study. One panel ($n = 7$) was used to assess fur shedding throughout the study: this panel (called 'shedding panel') was composed of three LH cats (two Birmans and one Maine coon) and four SH cats (four European domestic SH cats). Two collective panels ($n = 7$) were used to evaluate the impact of the diets on faecal hair excretion: a SH panel composed of six Chartreux and one British Short Hair, and an LH panel composed of five European domestic LH cats, one Ragdoll and one Birman.

Ten cats were female and 11 cats were male, and were matched across groups: three females and four males were used in SH and shedding panels and four females and three males in LH panel. All cats were neutered and the median age was 4 years (range 2–11 years). All cats remained healthy throughout the study, based on physical examination. They were treated monthly with a topical flea – tick product (Frontline® Plus; Merial, Dultuh, GA, USA). They were housed in closed indoor (13 m^2) and outdoor (14 m^2) runs with unlimited outdoor access. Every morning, the cattery was cleaned. In order to prevent cats from being disturbed by external noises, music was played inside the cattery during the day. Temperature remained constant at 22–23°C in the cattery and cats were exposed to normal day length and natural lighting throughout the study.

Housing and management protocols adhered to European regulatory guidelines for animal welfare, whilst all experimental protocols complied with European Union guidelines on animal welfare and were approved by the Royal Canin Committee for Animal Ethics and Welfare.

Diet and Food Intake

Three experimental dry, expanded, complete and balanced maintenance diets designed for adult cats were used in the present study (Table 1). The diets varied in TdF and psyllium contents. The control diet (diet 6) contained a low-fibre level (6% TdF) and no psyllium. The first test diet (diet 11) presented moderate fibre content (11% TdF) and 0.5% psyllium husk. The second test diet (diet 15) contained a high fibre level (15% TdF) and 0.5% psyllium husk. The increase in TdF was obtained by supplementation of cellulose: 0% for diet 6, 5.17% for diet 11 and 9.68% for diet 15. During the study, all cats were fed *ad libitum* and the diet was given once a day, in the morning. All food consumptions were measured out using electronic scales (XS4001S; Mettler Toledo, Columbus OH, USA) accurate to within 0.1 g.

Table 1: Dietary composition of the three diets used in the study

	Units	Diet 6	Diet 11	Diet 15
Dry matter	$g\ 100\ g^{-1*}$	94.2	94.7	94.4
Crude protein	$g\ 100\ g^{-1}$	33.8	34.7	34.8
Fat	$g\ 100\ g^{-1}$	14.4	14.1	13.6
Ash	$g\ 100\ g^{-1}$	7.3	7.3	7.3
Crude fibre	$g\ 100\ g^{-1}$	1.2	4.6	7.2
TdF	$g\ 100\ g^{-1}$	6.0	11.2	14.9
Nitrogen free extract	$g\ 100\ g^{-1}$	43.2	39.3	37.1
Metabolizable energy†	$kJ\ kg^{-1}$	16 565	15 963	15 336

Protocol Design

Study #1: Assessment of Shedding Throughout the Study in the Shedding Panel

Three times a week, each cat of the shedding panel received 24 brush strokes: six on the back, four on the neck, the head and the breast and two on the tail and the hind legs. For each cat, the hair collected was weighed carefully to quantify shedding over the study (a total of 8 weeks divided into four 14 day long phases designated phases 1–4).

Study #2: Impact of the Diets on Faecal Hair Excretion in SH and LH Cats

One week before starting the study, SH and LH panels underwent a purge for 3 days to eliminate accumulated hair in the digestive tract (Savorial, MSD Santé animale, Beaucouzé, France). Then they were fed diet 6 for 14 days during phase 1. In phase 2 (14 days), both panels were fed either diet 11 or diet 15. In phase 3, all cats returned to diet 6 for 14 days before crossing over to the other experimental diet (diet 15 or diet 11) in phase 4 (14 days). In order to avoid digestive disorders, 3 days of gradual food transition were made at the beginning of each phase (Fig. 1).

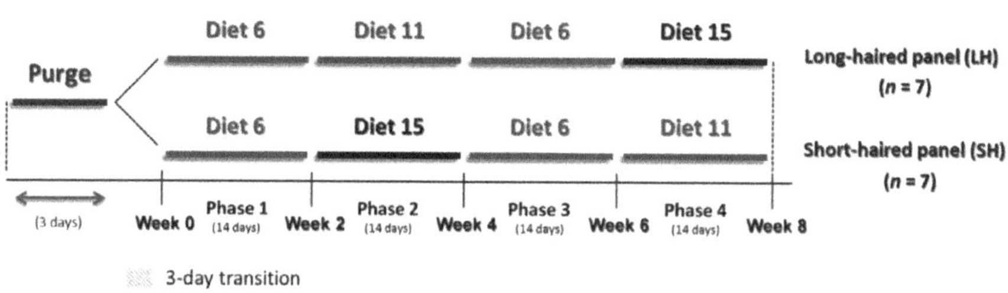

Figure 1: Study design 2: impact of the diets on faecal hair excretion.

Faecal hair excretion was quantified daily for each collective panel fed each diet according to the modified method of Hendriks *et al.* (1998) and Tournier *et al.* (2005). All faeces excreted were collected every morning, pooled and stored at −20°C. Pooled faeces were then dried in an oven (70°C, 24 h) then ground carefully in a blender (GM200; Retsch Grindomix, Haan, Germany) for 12 s at medium speed. Through a sieve (1 mm), hair was then collected and washed using a solution of 20 mL of detergent (IDOS 2000; Elcopharma, Villeneuve s/Yonne, France), and 2 L of boiling water for 30 min. A second stage of sieving and washing (15 min) was then performed. After a third sieving process, hair samples were isolated by vacuum filtration, and then hair moisture was evaporated in an oven (110°C, 15 h). The hair sample obtained was finally weighed by a precision balance (XP504 DR; Mettler Toledo, OH, USA).

Statistical Analysis

Statistical analyses were performed with the SAS version 9.3 software (SAS Institute Inc., Cary, NC, USA). Results were expressed as mean ± SEM.

Study #1

A mixed model was performed to evaluate the impact of the following fixed effects: hair length (long or short), phase (from 1–4) and the interaction hair length × phase on the quantity of hair brushed. The cat was defined as a random term considering that each cat was its own control through weekly measurements. False discovery rate method was used to avoid alpha risk inflation due to multiple comparisons. In this respect, P-values were adjusted to compare phase within hair length and hair length within phase.

Study #2

A generalized linear model was used to assess the effects of panel (SH/LH), diet (diet 6/diet 11/diet 15) and the interaction panel × diet on faecal hair excretion and energy consumption. For faecal hair excretion, food intake was added as covariate to this two-way analysis of variance.

Residuals of each model were checked for fit with normal distribution according to Kolmogorov–Smirnov, Cramer-von Mises and Anderson-Darling tests. Results are expressed as least square means ± SEM. Differences in Least-squares (LS) means were assessed using the Scheffe test to correct for the multiple comparisons. Significance level was set at 5%.

RESULTS

Study #1

The quantity of hair brushed in the shedding panel was impacted by hair length ($P = 0.013$) but not by phase ($P = 0.409$). Significant interaction was found (hair length × phase: $P < 0.001$). The quantities of hair collected were higher in LH cats than in SH cats in the second phase (519.3 ± 20.7 mg vs. 311.2 ± 30.2 mg, $P = 0.0155$), the third phase (552.5 ± 23.0 mg vs. 312.6 ± 33.4 mg, $P = 0.0055$) and the fourth phase (552.9 ± 23.5 mg vs. 316.7 ± 31.6 mg, $P = 0.006$). This effect was not significant during the first phase (338.2 ± 17.8 mg vs. 484.1 ± 65.2 mg, $P = 0.088$). No significant individual effect was observed on the quantity of hair brushed ($P = 0.061$).

Study #2

Energy Consumption

Energy consumption results expressed in kJ day^{-1} are shown in Table 2. Energy consumption was influenced by diet and panel effects (diet effect: $P < 0.001$; panel effect $P < 0.001$; panel × diet: $P < 0.001$). Indeed diet effect depended on the panel considered. For LH panel, energy consumption did not vary between the different diets. For SH panel, no difference was found in energy intake during the phases 2, 3 and 4. However, significantly higher energy consumption was observed when cats were fed diet 6 in phase 1 ($P < 0.001$).

Table 2: Values (mean ± SEM) of the daily energy consumption (in kJ day^{-1}) and faecal hair excretion (in mg day^{-1}) for SH and LH panels

LH panel	Diet 6	Diet 11	Diet 6	Diet 15
Energy consumption (kJ day^{-1})	812.2 ± 91.3	824.4 ± 17.6	862.9 ± 15.1	826.5 ± 14.7
Faecal hair excretion (mg day^{-1})	1512 ± 185^{a}	2735 ± 254^{b}	1610 ± 177^{a}	3435 ± 164^{b}
SH panel	**Diet 6**	**Diet 15**	**Diet 6**	**Diet 11**
Energy consumption (kJ day^{-1})	1062.6 ± 18.0^{a}	916.5 ± 25.1^{b}	897.2 ± 13.4^{b}	903.5 ± 18.8^{b}
Faecal hair excretion (mg day^{-1})	1627 ± 156	1631 ± 105	1084 ± 107	1431 ± 109

LH, long-haired; SH, short-haired. Different superscript letters (a, b) in the same line are significantly different ($P < 0.05$).

Faecal Hair Excretion

On the day after the 3 days of purge, 2.45 and 6.31 g of hair were recovered in faeces of SH and LH panels respectively.

Faecal hair excretion data for LH and SH cats fed different diets are given in Table 2. Faecal hair excretion was influenced by diet only in LH panel (diet effect: $P < 0.001$; panel effect $P < 0.001$; panel × diet: $P < 0.001$). Indeed in LH cats, faecal hair excretion significantly increased by 81% in diet 11 and by 113% in diet 15 compared to diet 6 ($P < 0.001$). The cumulative amounts of hair excreted during the 14-day period were 40.5 and 48.1 g when LH panels were fed diet 11 and diet 15 respectively but only 22 g when fed diet 6. No significant differences in faecal hair excretion were observed between phases 1 and 3 when the cats were fed diet 6, and between diet 11 and 15 fed in phases 2 and 4. In SH cats, no difference was observed in faecal hair excretion when fed diet 6, 11 or 15.

DISCUSSION

The objective of the present study was to assess the influence of psyllium and different levels of TdF (6% vs. 11% vs. 15%) on faecal hair excretion in short and LH cats.

The predisposition of cats to forming hairballs following hair ingestion could be due to their digestive physiological particularities. For example, it has been reported that cats lack interdigestive migrating myoelectric complexes (IMMCs). In other species, these motor complexes begin in the stomach during periods of fasting and result in powerful peristaltic waves which facilitate transportation of indigestible substances such as bone, fibre and hair from the stomach through the small intestine (De Vos 1993). In cats, activity resembling IMMCs has only been identified in the distal small intestine (Roche *et al.* 1982). This slow peristalsis in cats could thus explain both the accumulation of hair in their digestive tract and their slow total gastrointestinal transit time (around 35–40 h) (Fucci *et al.* 1995; Peachey *et al.* 2000) compared to small breed dogs (24 h) (Hernot *et al.* 2005).

Very few studies have been conducted to evaluate the efficacy of diets on the incidence of hairballs in cats (Cannon 2013; German & German 2013). This is likely due to the difficulty of precisely quantifying hairballs. Among existing studies, most used questionnaires or surveys and the frequency of hairball vomiting (Cannon 2013) or clinical signs (vomiting, retching and coughing) (Dann *et al.* 2004; Beynen*et al.* 2011) were evaluated by cat owners, making the results quite subjective.

In the present study, hair was quantified directly in faeces. Faecal hair excretion was measured daily according to the modified method of Hendriks *et al.* (1998) and Tournier *et al.* (2005). Two washing and three sieving steps were needed to separate hair from faeces. Although this method was time consuming, it gave accurate and repeatable measurements (data not shown).

At the beginning of this study, a purge was performed for 3 days in SH and LH cats to eliminate hair accumulated in the digestive tract. Although these cats did not show any clinical signs of hairballs, large quantities of hair were recovered in their faeces within the few days after the purge. As expected, higher faecal hair elimination was observed in LH cats than in SH cats (2.5 times more). Hair accumulated in the digestive tract prior to commencing the study could have altered the results.

Shedding is a natural phenomenon which can have a strong impact on faecal hair excretion. It was therefore assessed throughout the study with a normalized brushing three times a week on all shedding panel cats. The quantity of hair brushed in all cats was not significantly different between 2 phases, indicating that the present study did not occur during a shedding season. The quantity of hair recovered per cat and per brush stroke (63 mg on average) was extremely close to that obtained by Tournier *et al.* (2005) outside the shedding season. This previous study showed that semi-long-haired cats lost on average 70 mg hair per brush stroke and that this quantity increased up to 140 mg during the shedding season.

The shedding panel lived in the same environment as SH and LH cats. It is therefore unlikely that the variations of faecal hair excretion observed in these cats were the consequence of a change in hair losses during the study. Because this study was performed during the summer (from July to September), the shedding period was probably finished.

Different factors such as gender, flea burdens or breed could have affected grooming behaviour and thus impacted on the faecal hair excretion results. To our knowledge, no data are available on the effect of gender on grooming behaviour in cats. However, balanced panels in terms of male and female cats were used in the present study to minimize this possible effect. Flea exposure can strongly increase grooming rate in cats (Eckstein & Hart 2000b). A flea treatment was thus used monthly in all cats and regular observations of hair and skin were made to detect any infestation.

Several pedigree cat breeds were used in SH and LH panels, which may have had an impact on the results. Indeed hair coat length and density, as well as the relative proportions of guard and undercoat hairs may vary with breed and this may have had an impact on the hair excretion. However, the majority of cats present in each panel ($n = 7$/ panel) were of the same breed (six Chartreux in SH panel and five European domestic LH cats in LH panel), thereby limiting this potential effect.

Because food intake affects the quantity of fibre ingested, it was important to ensure that both panels consumed similarly diet 6, 11 and 15. In this study, cats surprisingly ingested similar quantities of energy, despite *ad libitum* access to food and differences in food composition. This supports previous studies demonstrating that cats regulate their energy intake when fed foods containing moderate fibre content (9% cellulose; 8.2% crude fibre) (Prola *et al.* 2006).

Higher energy consumption was only observed in SH cats when fed diet 6 in phase 1. Although not statistically significant, the higher faecal hair excretion observed in SH cats fed diet 6 in phase 1 (1627 ± 156 mg) compared with phase 3 (1084 ± 107 mg) could be explained by this larger consumption (+18%; $P < 0.001$).

The impact of fibre level on faecal hair excretion varied according to hair coat length. In LH panel, consumption of diets 11 and 15 induced significantly higher faecal hair excretion, compared to diet 6 ($P < 0.001$), indicating that the combination of psyllium and cellulose facilitate faecal hair elimination in those cats. This supports previous studies based on cat owner questionnaires showing that the supplementation of cellulose in a diet or of psyllium husks in a treat lowered the incidence of clinical signs of hairballs (Dann *et al.* 2004; Beynen *et al.* 2011).

The mechanism by which the ingestion of cellulose and psyllium depresses the clinical signs of hairballs and stimulates their excretion in faeces is not known. Psyllium husk is a source of gel-forming soluble fibre which has the property of increasing viscosity of the digestive content. Psyllium husk could thus promote the binding of hair to food particles and thereby increase the transfer of gastric hair into the duodenum and enhanced passage through the intestine. Cellulose is a dietary insoluble fibre source which enhances the intestinal transit rate of digesta (Burrows *et al.* 1982) and this may promote the excretion of hair in faeces.

The present study cannot determine which of the two fibre sources (psyllium or cellulose) presents the greatest capacity to stimulate hair excretion in cat faeces. The inclusion of a diet containing 6% fibre and 0.5% psyllium or diets with 11% or 15% fibre without psyllium would have been necessary and their lack is a limitation of this study.

Similar low faecal hair excretions were observed when diet 6 was fed in phases 1 and 3 in LH cats, confirming the weak effect of a low-fibre diet on hair transit. No significant difference was found between diet 11 and 15, suggesting that an 11% fibre level would be sufficient to stimulate faecal hair excretion or that the study was too short to observe significantly higher hair excretion in cats fed diet 15.

In SH cats, similar faecal hair excretions were observed when fed diet 6, 11 and 15. This lack of effect could be explained by insufficient ingestion of hair in this population outside the shedding season. Indeed the quantities of hair excreted by SH animals fed diets 11 and 15 were respectively 40 and 60% lower than those found in LH cats fed the same diets. Moreover, when fed diet 15, the highest daily faecal hair excretion observed was equivalent to the lowest faecal hair excretion in LH cats. The exposure to the diets (14 days) might also have been too short to obtain significant results.

CONCLUSIONS

The results of this study showed that dietary fibre significantly affects faecal hair excretion in LH cats over only 14 days, and outside shedding periods. Results obtained suggest that a diet containing psyllium husk and 11% or 15% TdF facilitates faecal excretion of hair in LH cats. Clinical studies are however required to determine whether such psyllium and TdF levels result in a significant reduction in hairball related clinical signs in cats.

In SH cats, 11% and 15% fibre levels combined with psyllium have no effect on faecal hair excretion. This could be explained by the low quantity of hair ingested by those animals outside the shedding season, by the relatively short duration of the study or by the small number of cats included in the study.

Therefore, future studies would be valuable to evaluate the effect of these diets during the shedding season in both short and LH cats, over a longer period of time and on a larger number of cats.

ACKNOWLEDGEMENT

The authors thank Sophie Clément for assistance in writing this manuscript.

REFERENCES

1. Agnello K.A. & Kantrowitz L. (2003) Esophageal obstruction. *Journal of the American Veterinary Medical Association* 15, 1115–1116.
2. Barrs V.R., Beatty J.A., Tisdall P.L., Hunt G.B. & Gunew M. (1999) Intestinal obstruction by trichobezoars in five cats. *Journal of Feline Medicine and Surgery* 1, 199–207.
3. Benjamin L. (1976) Feline behavior. *Feline Practice* 7, 14–17.
4. Beynen A.C., Middelkoop J. & Saris D.H.J. (2011) Clinical signs of hairballs in cats fed a diet enriched with cellulose. *American Journal of Animal and Veterinary Sciences* 6, 69–72.
5. Burrows C.F., Kronfeld D.S., Banta C.A. & Merritt A.M. (1982) Effects of fibre on digestibility and transit time in dogs. *Journal of Nutrition*112, 1726–1732.
6. Cannon M. (2013) Hair balls in cats, a normal nuisance or a sign that something is wrong. *Journal of Feline Medicine and Surgery* 15,21–29.
7. Dann J.R., Adler M.A., Duffy K.L. & Giffard C.J. (2004) A potential nutritional prophylactic for the reduction of feline hairball symptoms.*Journal of Nutrition* 134, 2124S–2125S.
8. De Vos W.C. (1993) Migrating spike complex in the small intestine of the fasting cat. *American Journal of Physiology* 265,G619–G627.
9. Eckstein R.A. & Hart B.L. (2000a) The organization and control of grooming in cats. *Applied Animal Behaviour Science* 68, 131–140.
10. Eckstein R.A. & Hart B.L. (2000b) Grooming and control of fleas in cats. *Applied Animal Behaviour Science* 68, 141–150.

11. Fucci V., Pechman R.D., Hedlund C.S. & Venugopalan C.S. (1995) Large bowel transit times using radiopaque markers in normal cats. *Journal of the American Animal Hospital Association* 31, 473–477.
12. German A.J. & German A.C. (2013) Bad hair day. *Journal of Feline Medicine and Surgery* 15, 6–7.
13. Hendriks W.H., Tartellin M.F. & Moughan P.J. (1998) Seasonal hair loss in adult domestic cats (*Felis catus*). *Journal of Animal Physiology and Animal Nutrition* 79, 92–101.
14. Hernot D., Biourge V., Martin L., Dumon H. & Nguyen P. (2005) Relationship between total transit time and faecal quality in adult dogs differing in body size. *Journal of Animal Physiology and Animal Nutrition* 89, 189–193.
15. Panaman R. (1981) Behavior and ecology of free-ranging female farm cats (*Felis catus* L). *Zeitschrift für Tierpsychologie* 56, 59–73.
16. Peachey S.E., Dawson J.M. & Harper E.J. (2000) Gastrointestinal transit times in young and old cats. *Comparative Biochemistry and Physiology Part A: Molecular & Integrative Physiology* 126, 85–90.
17. Prola L., Dobenecker B. & Kienzle E. (2006) Interaction between dietary cellulose content and food intake in cats. *Journal of Nutrition*136, 1988S–1990S.
18. Roche M., Bueno L., Vagne M. & Blourde C. (1982) Patterns of electrical activity in the digestive tract of the conscious cat. *British Journal of Nutrition* 48, 129–135.
19. Ryan C.P. & Wolfer J.J. (1978) Recurrent trichophytobezoar in a cat. *Veterinary Medicine Small Animal Clinician* 73, 891–893.
20. Tournier C., Dumon H., Nguyen P., Biourge V. (2005) Dietary fiber stimulates fecal hair excretion in cats. *Proceeding of the 9th European Society of Veterinary and Comparative Nutrition Congress* 112, 27–28.
21. Willemse T., Mudde M., Josephy M. & Spruijt B.M. (1994) The effect of haloperidol and naloxone on excessive grooming behavior of cats. *European Neuropsychopharmacology* 4, 39–45.

12

CHAPTER

GRAPIPRANT: AN EP4 PROSTAGLANDIN RECEPTOR ANTAGONIST AND NOVEL THERAPY FOR PAIN AND INFLAMMATION

Kristin Kirkby Shaw, Lesley C. Rausch-Derra, and Linda Rhodes

INTRODUCTION

Prostanoids are metabolites of arachidonic acid (AA) and have been the target of medicinal therapies for centuries (Appelboom 2002). However, until recently, preparations aimed at inhibiting the action of prostanoids have, with varying degrees of prostanoid specificity, prevented their production and thus impacted both pathologic and homeostatic activity (Curry et al. 2005; KuKanich et al. 2012). The evolution of pain management has entered a new era – that of selectively blocking the single prostanoid receptor that is primarily responsible for pain and inflammation, thereby preserving the production and activity of homeostatic prostanoids (Nakao et al. 2007; Kawabata 2011).

This manuscript reviews the mechanism of action of anti-inflammatory drugs for use in animals and introduce the first-in-class drug for managing pain and inflammation associated with osteoarthritis (OA) in veterinary patients: grapiprant, an EP4 prostaglandin receptor antagonist (PRA).

AA Cascade Revisited

Arachidonic acid is an omega 6 polyunsaturated lipid that is an integral part of cell membranes and is liberated from the cell membrane by the enzyme phospholipase A_2 (PLA_2) as part of normal cellular metabolism and following cell injury (Curry et al. 2005; KuKanich et al.2012). The freed AA molecule is then shuttled into one of three pathways that generate three groups of molecules: prostanoids, leukotrienes

---

Citation: Kristin Kirkby Shaw, Lesley C. Rausch-Derra, andLinda Rhodes, Grapiprant: an EP4 prostaglandin receptor antagonist and novel therapy for pain and inflammation, DOI: 10.1002/vms3.13.

and epoxides (Curry et al. 2005; KuKanich et al. 2012). This manuscript will focus on the prostanoid group.

The enzymes cyclo-oxygenase 1 and 2 (COX-1 and COX-2) convert AA into prostaglandin H_2 (PGH_2), and PGH_2 is subsequently converted, via tissue-specific isomerases and oxidoreductases, to five active prostanoid molecules: thromboxane (TXA), PGD_2, PGI_2(prostacyclin), $PGF_2\alpha$ and PGE_2 (Simmons et al. 2004; Ricciotti & FitzGerald 2011). COX-1 is expressed constitutively in most cells and is the dominant source of prostanoids that are involved in gastric epithelial cytoprotection and homeostasis. COX-2 is constitutively expressed in some tissues, but is also inducible by inflammatory stimuli, and is an important source of prostanoid formation in periods or locations of inflammation. In inflammation, the profile of prostanoid production is determined by the differential expression of these enzymes within cells at the site of inflammation (Ricciotti & FitzGerald 2011). Production of PGE_2 and PGI_2 predominates in sites where COX-2 is activated (Simmons et al. 2004).

In the mid-1990s, prostanoid receptors were identified and continue to be characterized (Woodward et al. 2011). These receptors have varying distributions throughout the body and mediate the activities of each prostanoid. Each prostanoid interacts with at least one distinct receptor to mediate specific physiological effects, and in some cases this includes specific receptor subtypes for a particular prostanoid.

Inhibiting Prostanoid Production: The Good and the Bad

Prostanoids are responsible for a wide range of homeostatic functions in mammals including regulation of renal haemodynamics and ion transport, gastrointestinal cytoprotection and motility, vascular and bronchial smooth muscle activity, immune function and platelet aggregation (Woodward et al. 2011; KuKanich et al. 2012). Pain and inflammation are also mediated by prostanoids, in particular PGE_2, and thus therapeutic drugs are often used to decrease the production and activity of this molecule (Curry et al. 2005; KuKanich et al. 2012). Steroids and cyclo-oxygenase inhibiting drugs have until now been the primary options for treating pain and inflammation, and because of their mechanism of action, these approaches have some drawbacks that are discussed below (Stahn et al. 2007; KuKanich et al. 2012).

Corticosteroids inhibit the enzyme PLA_2, acting up-stream of the COX enzymes in inhibiting the metabolism of AA (Stahn et al. 2007). Corticosteroids prevent the synthesis of prostanoids, leukotrienes and epoxides, and thus have broad anti-inflammatory action, but also inhibit the production of many homeostatic AA metabolites. Short-acting corticosteroids can be important therapeutics in the management of acute allergic reactions, and while they may also provide some degree of pain relief, the untoward side effects make them a poor choice for long-term treatment of pain in veterinary patients.

Salicylic acid is a natural product derived from plants such as willow bark and meadowsweet, and its medicinal properties of pain relief and fever reduction have been utilized for centuries (Vane 1971). Aspirin, or acetylsalicylic acid, is a synthetic drug made from salicylic acid. Aspirin irreversibly binds to the COX enzymes and inhibits the formation of all prostanoids (Flower 2003; KuKanich et al. 2012). While aspirin is effective in reducing fever, pain and inflammation, there are significant adverse effects of treatment with aspirin that are well-recognized in humans and animals, in particular gastrointestinal irritation and ulceration. Furthermore, irreversible inhibition of platelet TXA by aspirin leads to reduced aggregation that lasts up to 7–10 days (the life span of the affected platelets). This anti-thrombotic property can be useful in clinical conditions where reducing blood clotting is called for, but should also be recognized as a potentially significant unwanted side effect of aspirin administration.

Cyclo-oxygenase inhibiting non-steroidal anti-inflammatory drugs (COX inhibiting NSAIDs) decrease inflammation through inhibition of COX enzymes and subsequent inhibition of prostaglanoid production (Curry et al. 2005; KuKanich et al. 2012). This class includes aspirin, as described above, as well as other non-selective COX inhibitors (i.e. drugs that inhibit both COX 1 and COX 2 enzymes) such as ketoprofen and indomethacin. In addition, drugs have been developed that preferentially inhibit COX-2, such as carprofen, meloxicam, deracoxib, firocoxib and robenacoxib.

The two cyclo-oxygenase isoenzymes, COX-1 and COX-2, were isolated in the 1980s and shortly thereafter it was discovered that COX-2 is induced in response to tissue injury and is associated with inflammation and pain (Vane 1971; KuKanich et al. 2012). Drug development then concentrated on molecules that preferentially inhibited this enzyme in the hope of sparing the so-called 'house-keeping' prostaglandins produced by COX-1. The coxib class of drugs, or selective COX-2 inhibitors, were first marketed in human medicine in 1999. In humans, COX-2 selective products such as rofecoxib (Vioxx® Merck & Co., Inc. Kenilworth, NJ USA) and celecoxib (Celebrex®Pfizer Inc. New York, NY USA) did show improved GI tolerability; however, in some cases, the FDA reviewed evidence leading the agency to conclude that their use was related to significant cardiovascular side effects and thus, all but one product have been removed from the US market (Harirforoosh et al. 2013). The underlying cause for these adverse cardiovascular events may be attributed to inhibition of COX-2 synthesis of PGI_2 (prostacyclin). PGI_2 is a potent vasodilator and has anti-thrombotic properties (an endogenous antagonist of TXA), thus decreased production of PGI_2 by coxib-inhibiting NSAIDs may lead to increased thrombosis and vasoconstriction, two methods of potentiating cardiovascular disease (Harirforoosh et al. 2013). The cardiovascular adverse events associated with COX-2 selective NSAIDs in humans have not been observed in dogs taking COX-2 selective NSAIDs. However, severe gastrointestinal, renal and hepatic adverse events have been reported in dogs taking these products (Lascelles et al. 2005; KuKanich et al. 2012; Monteiro-Steagall et al. 2013).

Both COX-1 and COX-2 activity are important in maintaining gastrointestinal integrity and renal haemodynamics in dogs, primarily through the actions of PGE_2 and PGI_2 (Wilson et al. 2004; KuKanich et al. 2012). COX-2 is expressed in the canine kidney and involved in regulation of vessel tone and salt and water balance via synthesis of PGE_2 and PGI_2. In the stomach and intestinal tract, COX-1 is the primary mediator of gastro-protective prostanoid (PGE_2 and PGI_2) production in the healthy animal. COX-2 is up-regulated in areas of gastrointestinal irritation and it is important in promoting the healing of gastrointestinal ulcerations (KuKanich et al. 2012). This suggests that administration of a selective COX-2 inhibitor drug in the face of gastrointestinal ulceration, such as due to stress or administration of corticosteroids or a non-selective cyclo-oxygenase-inhibiting NSAID such as aspirin, may reduce healing and potentiate ulceration and perforation (Lascelles et al. 2005). Another potential mechanism for gastrointestinal injury secondary to cyclo-oxygenase inhibiting NSAID administration is the increased production of inflammatory leukotrienes (Curry et al. 2005). Inhibition of the COX pathways may result in increased AA that must be metabolized by the lipo-oxygenase enzyme (LOX) pathway.

The four FDA approved COX inhibitor NSAIDs for use in dogs, unless contra-indicated, are considered to be effective treatments for the pain associated with OA. However, these COX-inhibiting NSAIDs, as a class, carry the potential for adverse effects including gastrointestinal ulceration and perforation and renal insufficiency (Lascelles et al. 2005; Monteiro-Steagall et al. 2013). While COX-2 selective and preferential NSAIDs are associated with fewer side effects compared to aspirin and older, non-selective COX inhibitor NSAIDs, many dogs do not tolerate these drugs, and alternative pharmacologic pain relief is indicated. Currently, no other class of pharmaceuticals is approved by the FDA for the treatment of pain and inflammation associated with OA in dogs. Thus, it is evident that an FDA approved product that demonstrates targeted pain relief with improved tolerability is needed.

THE PIPRANT CLASS: PRA

After the identification of prostanoid receptors in the 1990s, significant research ensued into methods of targeting each receptor with synthetic agonists and antagonists (Woodward et al. 2011). In October 2013, the World Health Organization defined a newly recognized class of drugs that act as PRAs as the piprant class (World Health Organization, 2013).

EP4 PRAs and Anti-Inflammatory Effects: Experimental Models

Prostaglandin E_2 (PGE_2) is a key mediator of swelling, redness and pain, the classic signs of inflammation, with pain resulting from PGE_2-mediated sensitization of sensory neurons and swelling and redness resulting from PGE_2-mediated vasodilation and increased vascular permeability (Ricciotti & FitzGerald 2011). PGE_2 exerts its effects via four receptors, EP1, EP2, EP3 and EP4 (Woodward et al. 2011). The EP4 receptor is the primary mediator of the PGE_2-elicited sensitization of sensory neurons and PGE_2-elicited inflammation (Southall & Vasko 2001; McCoy et al. 2002; Lin et al. 2006; Nakao et al. 2007; Clark et al. 2008; Chen et al. 2010; Boyd et al. 2011). Grapiprant (AT-001) is a new analgesic and anti-inflammatory drug in the piprant class that functions as a selective EP4 PRA (Nakao et al. 2007). The following is a review of the literature and studies that demonstrate the anti-inflammatory effects of EP4 PRAs and of grapiprant in particular.

The use of receptor knockout mice has been helpful in understanding the roles of the specific EP receptors in inflammation. Collagen antibody-induced arthritis (CAIA) in mice is a model for the human inflammatory disorder rheumatoid arthritis (RA). The individual PGE_2receptors were evaluated by inducing CAIA in mice which were genetically modified to knock out the EP1, -2, -3, or -4 receptors and measuring the clinical, histopathological and cellular markers of disease (McCoy et al. 2002). When mice with one of these four receptors knocked out were evaluated for signs of pain and inflammation, the EP4 receptor knock-out mice, but not the EP1, EP2 or EP3 receptor knock-out mice, had decreased incidence and severity of disease, decreased histopathological deterioration associated with arthritis and decreased levels of inflammatory markers, implicating EP4 as a key mediator of inflammation. In a mouse model of acute inflammation, EP1, 2, 3 or 4 receptor knock-out mice were subjected to UV irradiation of the skin. EP4 and EP2 knock-out mice, but not EP1 or EP3 knock-out mice, had significantly decreased ear swelling compared to control mice. The reduction in swelling was also seen when the wild-type mice were treated with an EP4 PRA (Kabashima et al. 2007).

The anti-inflammatory effects of EP4 receptor antagonism have also been investigated in animal models of inflammation. In a study by Clark et al. (2008), joint inflammation (as measured by paw swelling) was created using an adjuvant-induced arthritis (AIA) model in rats. Rats treated with an EP4 PRA (MF498), but not an EP1 or an EP3 PRA, demonstrated reduced paw swelling. The reduction in swelling was similar to that seen in mice treated with a cyclo-oxygenase-2 (COX-2) inhibitor. In a study by Murase et al. (2008), the selective EP4 PRA, CJ-042,794, caused decreased paw swelling in a complete Freund's adjuvant model of chronic inflammatory pain in rats. The reductions in paw swelling in the CJ-042,794 treated rats were again similar to those seen with rofecoxib (a COX-2 inhibitor) treated rats. Using a complete Freund's adjuvant administration as a rodent model for pain and inflammation, treatment with an EP4 PRA, identified as 1a, also demonstrated reduced swelling of the paw (Boyd et al. 2011). In a series of experiments reported by Chen et al. (2010), an EP4 PRA, ER-819762, suppressed inflammatory cytokine production, suppressed disease and slowed disease progression in collagen and GPI-induced arthritis in mice. These data support the anti-inflammatory role of EP4 receptor antagonism in rodents. Indeed, these results demonstrated that EP4 PRAs can reduce inflammation as effectively as COX-2 inhibitors.

Several studies have been conducted examining the anti-inflammatory and analgesic effects of grapiprant (AT-001, referred to as CJ-023,423 in the publications) in rats (Nakao et al. 2007). Studies using rat models have demonstrated grapiprant's ability to reduce acute and chronic pain and inflammation (Nakao et al. 2007; RaQualia 2007a,b). The anti-inflammatory effect of grapiprant on paw swelling, inflammatory biomarkers in the serum and synovial inflammation was examined in the tarsal joint in AIA in rats (RaQualia 2007b). Grapiprant exhibited dose-dependent and significant anti-inflammatory effects on all parameters tested. The efficacy of grapiprant on paw swelling was comparable to those of rofecoxib and piroxicam (COX-inhibiting drugs). In another study, the anti-inflammatory activity of grapiprant on rat carrageenan-induced foot swelling was investigated (RaQualia 2007a). Grapiprant inhibited foot swelling in a dose-dependent manner compared to rats treated with placebo control. Nakao et al. (2007) investigated three different models of pain in rats: mechanical hyperalgesia, thermal hyperalgesia and weight bearing deficit. Oral administration of CJ-023,423 significantly reduced hyperalgesia in rodents in all three models, including significantly reversing complete Freund's adjuvant-induced chronic inflammatory pain.

Not only is the EP4 receptor prominently involved in inflammation and pain, but importantly this receptor may mediate central sensitization and play a role in chronic pain. Lin et al. (2006) reported that in rodents, the EP4 receptor is expressed by sensory neurons, and the level of EP4 receptors increased following peripheral inflammation. Administration of an EP4 PRA decreased pain and hypersensitivity in rodents.

EP4 PRA in Veterinary Medicine: Targeted Pain Management

The EP4 receptor in mice, humans and dogs has been cloned and characterized. The canine EP4 receptor has approximately 90% homology to the human receptor (Castleberry et al. 2001). Grapiprant is a PRA that selectively blocks the EP4 receptor in rodents, humans, and dogs (RaQualia 2007c). Grapiprant has undergone experimental and pilot studies in laboratory and client-owned dogs. A multi-site, masked, placebo-controlled, randomized field trial for the control of pain and inflammation associated with OA in dogs was recently completed and was submitted to and accepted by the FDA in support of regulatory approval (www.aratana.com). The results of these studies in client-owned dogs demonstrate that this drug provides control of the pain associated with OA. Studies are currently underway investigating the use of grapiprant in cats, and at this time data are not yet available.

As part of development of grapiprant for FDA approval for dogs with OA, a safety study in healthy Beagles investigated the effects of daily orally administered doses up to 50 mg kg^{-1} day^{-1} oral suspension (equivalent to approximately 30.5 mg kg^{-1} day^{-1} of the tablet formulation) for nine consecutive months (Rausch-Derra et al. 2015a,b). There were no drug-related effects on liver enzyme values, BUN/creatinine, or platelet function. Mild and reversible dose- and time-dependent decreases in total protein, albumin and calcium were seen. Clinical signs were also dose dependent and restricted to mild gastrointestinal signs including soft stool, occasional stool with mucus or blood, and sporadic vomiting. There were no histopathological changes to any tissues, including the stomach, kidneys or liver except in one dog in the 50 mg kg^{-1} group had mild mucosal regeneration of the ileum seen on histopathology.

The relative lack of toxic effects with grapiprant compared to those that have been reported in dogs treated with COX-inhibiting NSAIDs is not surprising. Grapiprant is a targeted approach to pain management – it selectively blocks the EP4 receptor, does not interfere with the production of prostanoids, and therefore does not affect the other PG receptor pathways that are affected in animals treated with COX inhibitor NSAIDs.

CONCLUSION

PGE_2 is a key mediator of pain and inflammation and has its effect through binding to the EP4 receptor. Grapiprant directly and specifically blocks the EP4 receptor, and therefore blocks PGE_2-elicited pain and inflammation. An EP4 PRA, such as grapiprant, which has been demonstrated to provide relief from arthritic pain in canine clinical patients, acts without affecting the synthesis and widespread activity of PGE_2 and other prostanoids.

Safety studies in laboratory dogs have demonstrated an excellent safety profile, and a wide safety margin, and this has been confirmed in two large field effectiveness studies in dogs with OA (Rausch-Derra et al. 2015a,b). The relative lack of toxic effects with grapiprant compared to those that have been reported in dogs treated with COX-inhibiting NSAIDs is consistent with grapiprant's unique mechanism of action, although until FDA review and approval, claims of safety and effectiveness cannot be made. Grapiprant may offer a more targeted, and potentially better tolerated, method of pain management in dogs with OA.

ACKNOWLEDGEMENT

We would like to acknowledge the scientists at RaQualia who pioneered basic research and development of EP4 PRAs.

CONFLICTS OF INTEREST

At the time of writing, all authors were employees of Aratana Therapeutics, Inc., Kansas City, KS, USA At the time of publication, KK Shaw will be a full time employee of Animal Surgical Clinic of Seattle; Seattle, WA, USA and a paid consultant for Aratana Therapeutics, Inc.

REFERENCES

1. Appelboom T. (2002) Arthropathy in art and the history of pain management – through centuries to cyclooxygenase-2 inhibitors.Rheumatology 41, 28–34.
2. Boyd M.J., Berthelette C., Chiasson J.F., Clark P., Colucci J., Denis D. et al. (2011) A novel series of potent and selective EP4 receptor ligands: facile modulation of agonism and antagonism. Bioorganic & Medicinal Chemistry Letters 21, 484–487.
3. Castleberry T.A., Lu B., Smock S.L. & Owen T.A. (2001) Molecular cloning and functional characterization of the canine prostaglandin E_2 receptor EP4 subtype. Prostaglandins & Other Lipid Mediators 65, 167–187.
4. Chen Q., Muramoto K., Masaaki N., Ding Y., Yang H., Mackey M. et al. (2010) A novel antagonist of the prostaglandin E(2) EP(4) receptor inhibits Th1 differentiation and Th17 expansion and is orally active in arthritis models. British Journal of Pharmacology160, 292–310.
5. Clark P., Rowland S. E., Denis D., Mathieu M. C., Stocco R., Poirier H. et al. (2008) MF498 [N-{[4-(5,9-Diethoxy-6-oxo-6,8-dihydro-7H-pyrrolo[3,4-g] quinolin-7-yl)-3-m ethylbenzyl]sulfonyl}-2-(2-methoxyphenyl)acetamide], a selective E prostanoid receptor 4 antagonist, relieves joint inflammation and pain in rodent models of rheumatoid and osteoarthritis. The Journal of Pharmacology and Experimental Therapeutics 325, 425–434.

6. Curry S.L., Cogar S.M. & Cook J.L. (2005) Nonsteroidal anti-inflammatory drugs: a review. Journal of the American Animal Hospital Association 41, 298–309.
7. Flower R. (2003) What are all the things that aspirin does? BMJ 327, 572–573.
8. Harirforoosh S., Asghar W. & Jamali F. (2013) Adverse effects of nonsteroidal anti-inflammatory drug: an update of gastrointestinal, cardiovascular and renal complications. Journal of Pharmacy and Pharmaceutical Sciences 16, 821–847.
9. Kabashima K., Nagamachi M., Honda T., Nishigori C., Miyachi Y., Tokura Y., Narumiya S. (2007) Prostaglandin E2 is required for ultraviolet B-induced skin inflammation via EP2 and EP4 receptors. Laboratory Investigation 87, 49–55.
10. Kawabata A. (2011) Prostaglandin E2 and pain–an update. Biological and Pharmaceutical Bulletin 34, 1170–1173.
11. KuKanich B., Bidgood T. & Knesl O. (2012) Clinical pharmacology of nonsteroidal ant-inflammatory drugs in dogs. Veterinary Anaesthesia and Analgesia 39, 69–90.
12. Lascelles B.D.X., Blikslager A.T., Fox S.M. & Reece D. (2005) Gastrointestinal tract perforation in dogs treated with a selective cyclooxygenase-2 inhibitor: 29 cases (2002–2003). Journal of the American Veterinary Medical Association 227, 1112–1117.
13. Lin C. R., Amaya F., Barrett L., Wang H., Takada J., Samad T. A., Woolf C. J. (2006) Prostaglandin E2 receptor EP4 contributes to inflammatory pain hypersensitivity. Journal of Pharmacology and Experimental Therapeutics 319, 1096–1103.
14. McCoy J.M., Wicks J.R. & Audoly L.P. (2002) The role of prostaglandin E2 receptors in the pathogenesis of rheumatoid arthritis. The Journal of Clinical Investigation 110, 651–658.
15. Monteiro-Steagall B.P., Steagall P.V.M. & Lascelles B.D.X. (2013) Systematic review of nonsteroidal anti-inflammatory drug-induced adverse effects in dogs. Journal of Veterinary Internal Medicine 27, 1011–1019.
16. Murase A., Okumura T., Sakakibara A., Tonai-Kachi H., Nakao K., Takada J. (2008) Effect of prostanoid EP4 receptor antagonist, CJ-042,794, in rat models of pain and inflammation. European Journal of Pharmacology 580, 116–121.
17. Nakao K., Murase A., Ohshiro H., Okumura T., Taniguchi K., Murata Y. et al. (2007) CJ-023,423, a novel, potent and selective prostaglandin EP4 receptor antagonist with antihyperalgesic properties. Journal of Pharmacology and Experimental Therapeutics322, 686–694.
18. RaQualia (2007a) Determination of the Dose Response Relationship of CJ-023423 in the Rat Carrageenin-Induced Foot Edema Model. SR_DB1_CJ-023423_RAT_CFE_1_2007.
19. RaQualia (2007b) Investigation of the Inhibitory Effects of CJ-023423 on Inflammation and Bone Destruction in Adjuvant-Induced Arthritis Rats. SR_DB1_CJ-023423_AIA_1_2007.

20. RaQualia (2007c) Determination of the Binding Affinity of CJ-023423 for the Cloned Dog EP4 Receptor. SR_PPL_CJ-02423_dog_EP4BD_2007.

21. Rausch-Derra L., Rhodes L., Freshwater L. (2015a) Pharmacokinetic Comparison of Oral Tablet and Suspension Formulations of Grapiprant, a Novel Therapeutic for the Pain and Inflammation of Osteoarthritis in Dogs. Presented at AAVPT Biennial Symposium, Fort Collins, CO.

22. Rausch-Derra L., Huebner M. & Rhodes L. (2015b) Evaluation of the safety of long-term, daily oral administration of grapiprant, a novel drug for treatment of osteoarthritic pain and inflammation, in health dogs. American Journal of Veterinary Research 76,853–859.

23. Ricciotti E. & FitzGerald G.A. (2011) Prostaglandins and inflammation. Arteriosclerosis, Thrombosis, and Vascular Biology 31,986–1000.

24. Simmons D.L., Botting R.M. & Hla T. (2004) Cyclooxygenase isozymes: the biology of prostaglandin synthesis and inhibition.Pharmacological Reviews 56, 387–437.

25. Southall M.D. & Vasko M.R. (2001) Prostaglandin receptor subtypes, EP3C and EP4, mediate the prostaglandin E2-induced cAMP production and sensitization of sensory neurons. The Journal of Biological Chemistry 276, 16083–16091.

26. Stahn C., Lowenberg M., Hommes D.W. & Buttgereit F. (2007) Molecular mechanisms of glucocorticoid action and selective glucocorticoid receptor agonists. Molecular and Cellular Endocrinology 275, 71–78.

27. Vane J.R. (1971) Inhibition of prostaglandin synthesis as a mechanism of action for aspirin-like drugs. Nature: New Biology 231,232–235.

28. Wilson J.E., Chandrasekharan N.V., Westover K.D. et al. (2004) Determination of expression of cyclooxygenase-1 and -2 isozymes in canine tissues and their differential sensitivity to nonsteroidal anti-inflammatory drugs. American Journal of Veterinary Research65, 810–818.

29. Woodward D.F., Jones R.L. & Narumiya S. (2011) International Union of basic and clinical pharmacology. LXXXIII: classification of prostanoid receptors, updating 15 years of progress. Pharmacological Reviews 63, 471–538.

30. World Health Organization (2013) Pre-stems: Suffixes Used in the Selection of INN.

13

CHAPTER

CYTOGENOMICS OF FELINE CANCERS: ADVANCES AND OPPORTUNITIES

Rachael Thomas

Keywords: Cat, feline, genomics, chromosome, cytogenomics, cancer, comparative, fibrosarcoma, lymphoma, mammary carcinoma

INTRODUCTION

The domestic cat offers a diverse range of opportunities to contribute to the "One Health" concept, which capitalizes on the integration of complementary human and veterinary biomedical research efforts for synergistic gain. Cats continue to grow in popularity as family-owned pets and benefit from increasingly comprehensive medical surveillance [1]. It has been estimated that one in three U.S. households owns at least one cat, equating to a total U.S. cat population of approximately 74 million and a total annual expenditure of approximately $7.4 billion on veterinary services [2]. Cats exhibit approximately 200 genetic diseases that are considered analogous to human disorders, many of which are rarely encountered in any other widely studied species [3]. The cat has served as a particularly powerful model system for studying facets of neuroscience, reproduction and both heritable and infectious disease, and the field of feline oncology offers several novel angles to the comparative medicine arena. The ability to explore these attributes from a molecular standpoint has become possible only relatively recently through intensive efforts to characterize domestic cat genome organization in detail. The combination of data from complementary approaches now allows us to explore the cat genome directly in context with that of humans and other key players in

Citation: Rachael Thomas, Cytogenomics of Feline Cancers: Advances and Opportunities, doi:10.3390/vetsci2030246.

comparative biomedical research. In turn we may now begin to investigate in earnest the causes and consequences of genomic abnormalities associated with heritable and spontaneous disease in our feline companions.

GROSS KARYOTYPIC ORGANIZATION IN THE DOMESTIC CAT

The genome of the domestic cat (*Felis catus*, FCA) is organized into 18 pairs of autosomes and two sex chromosomes. Unlike in other mammals, where autosomes are numbered consecutively in descending order of size, standardized nomenclature in the cat takes into account both chromosome size and morphology. The karyotype comprises six autosomal subgroups termed A-F, with between two and four members in each. All but two autosomal pairs, cat chromosomes (FCA) F1 and F2, are biarmed, as are both sex chromosomes. There is substantial variation in chromosome size throughout the karyotype, from the largest (FCA A1, 240Mb) to the smallest (FCA E3, 43Mb) [4,5]. This marked diversity in size and morphology, broadly comparable to that of the human karyotype, means that chromosome identification in the cat is generally less challenging than in other key model species that exhibit more limited karyotypic variation. Gross similarity in the architecture of the human and domestic cat karyotypes has long been evident through direct comparison of their chromosome banding patterns [6,7]. These observations were reinforced by a series of molecular cytogenetic studies that indicated a remarkably limited degree of divergent evolution between the human and domestic cat genomes over the 92 million years since they shared a common ancestor, compared to the more extensive reshuffling evident in other model species [4,8,9,10,11]. The passage towards development of whole genome sequence assemblies for diverse mammals has since provided a far more comprehensive appreciation of conserved genome organization and potential mechanisms for karyotypic evolution.

GENERATION OF A REFERENCE CAT GENOME SEQUENCE ASSEMBLY

The potential role of the domestic cat in comparative biomedical research was boosted substantially by the generation of a light (~two-fold) coverage feline genome sequence assembly of "Cinnamon", a female Abyssinian, which captured ~65% of euchromatic sequence [12]. This formed part of a broader initiative funded by the National Human Genome Research Institute (NHGRI) to aid interpretation of the human genome sequence assembly, and to investigate patterns of sequence conservation, divergence and rearrangement between rodents, primates and other carnivores [13]. These studies showed that genome evolution in canine, ursine and murine lineages was driven strongly by interchromosomal translocation events, while intrachromosomal inversions were predominant in felids and also most primates [10,12]. A ~14x coverage whole genome assembly has recently become available for "Cinnamon", spanning 2.35 Gb, with sequence annotation for almost 22,000 putative protein-coding cat genes [4,5]. This resource affords a fascinating insight into the genomic factors that provide the unique phenotypic attributes of the domestic cat, and firmly equips the cat to contribute to, and benefit from, a "One Health" approach to biomedical research. Among the most rapid and exciting advances in feline molecular medicine are now being made in the area of oncology.

FUNDAMENTALS OF CANCER CYTOGENOMICS

It is well established that the onset of a malignant phenotype is associated with the accumulation of both random and non-random genomic abnormalities [14,15]. Molecular characterization of numerous diverse human cancers has identified vast numbers of recurrent somatic abnormalities, of which a proportion have been shown to correlate with discrete clinicopathologic criteria [16]. The ability to screen individual patients for these genomic markers has revolutionized diagnostic and prognostic capabilities, refining historically broad tumor classifications into clinically predictive subcategories and paving the way towards personalized disease management strategies. "Genomic profiling" also provides insight into the molecular pathogenesis of disease, identifying gene dosage imbalances associated with functional disruption of regulatory pathways, revealing key mechanistic processes underlying neoplastic transformation and progression and highlighting opportunities for targeted therapeutics.

Techniques for molecular cytogenomic evaluation of tumors fall broadly into two categories (see [17] for a detailed review). Direct techniques, such as fluorescence *in situ* hybridization (FISH) analysis, enable both structural and numerical assessment of small numbers of discrete genomic loci (typically < five) within individual cells. In contrast, indirect methods, such as comparative genomic hybridization (CGH) analysis, permit semi-quantitative measurement of mean DNA copy number within a tumor cell population at many thousands of defined intervals selected throughout the genome, but cannot detect balanced structural rearrangements. Since cancers typically exhibit a combination of both structural and numerical aberrations coupled with cell-to-cell heterogeneity, these highly complementary approaches are often used in tandem. Modified protocols allow their application to challenging specimens, such as those where the availability of clinical material is limited, or where the integrity of the sample is compromised, such as archived histologic specimens. This opens up a multitude of possibilities for retrospective studies of case materials for which detailed clinical histories are available.

The concepts of cancer cytogenomics are well established in human medicine, and enormous strides have been made in translating the same fundamental principles to domestic dog cancers. This has revealed remarkable conservation of discrete molecular alterations in human and canine counterparts of the same cancer (reviewed in [18,19]), providing strong evidence in support of a shared pathogenesis. Progress in the feline field is now gaining momentum, particularly in those areas in which the cat offers a novel perspective that has not been explored in other model species.

INJECTION-SITE SARCOMA

It is now 25 years since concerns were first raised over the increasing number of reports of malignant lesions arising at routine vaccination sites in cats [20]. The masses, predominantly fibrosarcomas, were observed most commonly in association with inflammatory reactions following the use of adjuvanted vaccines against rabies and feline leukemia virus. Vaccine-site sarcomas typically exhibit a rapid, aggressive clinical course and a bleak long-term prognosis. Treatment often involves radical surgical intervention due to the highly invasive nature of the disease, despite which localized post-surgical recurrence is common [21]. Since wide surgical margins markedly reduce the risk of tumor regrowth, there has been widespread encouragement for a transition away from traditional interscapular and femoral vaccination sites where adequate resection is highly challenging. The introduction of non-adjuvanted vaccines has also gone some way to limit the impact of vaccine-site sarcoma; however it remains a substantial clinical concern in feline medicine [22].

Interestingly, histopathologically similar tumors have also been described, infrequently, in dogs, ferrets and rabbits [23,24]. Furthermore, this phenomenon is not restricted to vaccination, since there are reports, albeit rare, of apparently related tumors manifesting in conjunction with injection of other fluids, in response to non-absorbable suture materials and even following microchipping procedures [21]. This has led to increased usage of the term "injection-site sarcoma" (ISS). Additionally, ISS shares many features with lesions occurring following ocular trauma in cats, and also with tumors arising in people in response to prolonged contact with foreign materials, such as artificial implants [22,25]. Taken in combination, these observations provide intriguing evidence for an association between persistent inflammation and malignant transformation. More than two decades after the first description of ISS, however, there remains no solid, detailed explanation for their underlying etiology, and they remain somewhat of an enigma [26,27].

Recognition of the etiology, incidence and impact of feline ISS has been challenged by difficulty in conclusive distinction between these sarcomas and those arising spontaneously without an apparent underlying injection-related origin. ISS typically are more locally invasive and prone to local recurrence than fibrosarcomas of spontaneous origin (non-ISS). Consequently, ISS generally warrant highly extensive surgical margins followed by regular and meticulous monitoring for recurrence, while non-ISS tumors may respond favorably to more conservative clinical management [27,28]. The ability to distinguish ISS from non-ISS at diagnosis therefore has far-reaching implications for patient, owner and clinician; however their extensive clinicopathologic similarity often confounds prompt and unequivocal identification. Distinction between these subtypes currently involves combinatorial consideration of multiple histopathologic features in context with clinical history and anatomical location, and often remains subjective and inconclusive. Currently there are no robust and broadly consistent diagnostic features for distinction between these subtypes. Advances in feline genomics now offer a potential molecular means to address this need and comprehend the factors that underlie the differences in their biological behavior.

Prior to the genomics era, conventional cytogenetic studies identified highly disrupted karyotypic organization in feline fibrosarcomas, with frequent hyperdiploidy and broad cell-to-cell heterogeneity [29,30,31,32]. A putative link has since been reported between amplification of feline satellite DNA sequences and the onset of genomic instability in fibrosarcomas, likely through disruption of normal centromere activity and the formation of aberrant marker chromosomes [33]. A subsequent study of five established ISS cell lines by classical enumeration of banded chromosome preparations also showed tremendously complex karyotypic reorganization, with a range of 19 to 155 chromosomes per cell, as compared to the normal 2n = 38 [34]. None of these studies, however, included detailed assessment of the composition of these aberrant chromosome structures.

Towards this goal, a microarray platform was developed to permit CGH-based identification of recurrent genomic DNA copy number aberrations (CNAs) in feline tumors [35]. This "aneuploidy array" comprised 210 large-insert clones representing loci anchored at ~15 Mb intervals throughout the initial 2x-coverage cat genome sequence assembly. Microarray-based profiling of 46 retrospective primary feline fibrosarcomas identified an extensive range of highly recurrent CNAs, consistent with the high level of genomic instability identified in earlier chromosome-based studies. Targeted FISH analysis of tumor chromosome preparations demonstrated broad heterogeneity in the patterns of structural and numerical aberrations evident both within and between cases. Remarkably, combined CGH and FISH analyses showed that a subset of genomic regions exhibited in excess of 30 copies within individual tumor cells, which were distributed across as many as ten different chromosome structures. Also of note, ISS cases showed non-random reorganization of FCA E1 in conjunction with copy number amplification of a discrete region on FCA E1p12 [35], consistent with the location of a nucleolar organizing region (NOR) [36]. Elevated argyrophilic nucleolar organizing region (AgNOR) scores, as defined by silver staining analysis, are common indicators of increased cellular proliferation, and have been associated with decreased overall survival for canine soft tissue sarcomas [37]. It is tempting to consider that this may reflect the inferior outcome that is typically associated with ISS. Statistical comparison of genomic profiles across the cohort identified two subchromosomal regions that showed significant differences in DNA copy number status in ISS *versus* non-ISS cases. While providing support for molecular discrimination, the limited resolution capabilities of the aneuploidy array confounded the ability to refine the boundaries of these regions and in turn to assess their gene content [35].

A higher-density second-generation cat CGH microarray platform has since been developed utilizing the 14x coverage cat genome sequence assembly, comprising ~110,000 oligonucleotide probes distributed at mean intervals of ~21kb. This provides a >300-fold increase in resolution over the aneuploidy array, bringing feline resources closely in line with those of other model systems for the first time. Evaluation of the same cohort of feline fibrosarcomas with this more comprehensive platform [38] identified homozygous deletions of the tumor-suppressor gene *PTEN* and recurrent amplifications of the *KIT*proto-oncogene. Elevated *KIT* protein expression has been reported as a persistent finding in both ISS and non-ISS tumors [39]; however it is not yet clear whether upregulation is a direct consequence of increased *KIT* gene dosage, nor whether this confers potential for utilizing targeted therapies directed towards this receptor tyrosine kinase. ISS and non-ISS tumors showed grossly comparable profiles of DNA copy number imbalance; however ISS cases exhibited elevated levels of global genomic disruption, consistent with their typically more aggressive behavior and poorer outcome. Among these lay a subset of discrete regions with promise as discriminatory markers [38]. With focus on the most clinicopathologically compelling genomic regions, in combination with assessment of transcriptional and translational status, there is great promise for a more detailed definition of the molecular pathogenesis of feline fibrosarcomas, and in turn, for refinement of diagnostic and therapeutic modalities for both subtypes. In a broader sense, genomic characterization of ISS also may aid elucidation of molecular mechanisms involved in the passage from chronic inflammation to neoplastic transformation, which continues to challenge human medicine.

LYMPHOMA

Lymphoma is the most common hematopoietic malignancy of cats and the third most common feline cancer overall, comprising approximately one third of all cancer diagnoses. Moreover, cats are considered to show the highest relative incidence of lymphoma among all species studied to date (reviewed in [40]), offering another promising angle for comprehending key facets of tumor biology. Historically, cytogenetic studies of feline lymphomas have focused heavily on established cell lines, primarily those developed from tumors associated with infection by feline leukemia virus, which often are nodal or mediastinal in origin. Common observations from these reports include hyperdiploidies resulting from low amplitude copy number increases of a variety of chromosomes, with no strongly recurrent features. These investigations have greatly expanded our understanding of the mechanisms by which clonal proviral integration into a host genome can initiate tumorigenesis and genomic instability through oncogenic activation [41,42]. With the diminished incidence of retrovirus-associated feline lymphoma since the 1980's, as a result of increased testing, vaccination and global vigilance, the focus has since shifted toward subtypes that offer opportunities for a more comparative approach.

Extensive volumes of clinically predictive cytogenomic data are accumulating for nodal lymphomas in human patients, and more recently also in dogs [43,44]. In contrast, gastrointestinal (GI) lymphoma, which represents the most common extranodal form in people and comprises more than 50% of all feline lymphomas, remains vastly understudied at the molecular level [45,46,47,48]. Given the high incidence of the disease in cats there is an opportunity for feline studies to pave the way forward for mutual benefit. In cats, the overall survival time for low-grade small-cell GI-lymphomas is generally four-fold greater than for high-grade large-cell tumors, following standard of care chemotherapy [45,49]. The relative frequency of these histologic subtypes in different anatomical locations varies widely in prior reports [40,45,50,51,52], in part due to the logistical challenges of performing diagnostic evaluation of GI lesions by surgical biopsy [40,53]. This invites assessment of a genomic approach for comprehensive DNA-based subclassification. Initial observations from microarray-based CGH analysis have indicated that feline GI-lymphoma exhibits a relatively subtle degree of genomic copy number instability, with no evidence for recurrent high-level amplifications or homozygous deletions. The majority of aberrations are shared by fewer than 30% of cases, and include defects involving key cancer-associated genes, such as elevated copy number of the *MYC* proto-oncogene and deletion of *PTEN*. Efforts to identify candidates for molecular distinction between histologic and immunophenotypic subtypes are now underway [54].

MAMMARY CARCINOMA

Mammary tumors represent the third most commonly diagnosed feline neoplasm, the vast majority of which (in contrast to dogs) are malignant, primarily simple carcinomas. Feline mammary carcinomas (FMCs) generally are highly aggressive, infiltrative and metastatic and show extensive heterogeneity in outcome that is not readily predicted at the time of diagnosis [55]. FMC shares extensive clinicopathologic, demographic and epidemiological similarity with human breast carcinoma (HBC), the most frequently diagnosed cancer in women [56]. While there is evidence for steroid hormone involvement in some FMCs, 80%–90% are estrogen- and progesterone-receptor negative [57,58,59]. FMC therefore offers a particularly powerful spontaneous model of the ~30% of "basal-like" late-stage HBCs that are highly aggressive and unresponsive to hormone-antagonist therapies, with a lack of targeted treatments and a poor prognosis.

Diagnostic and prognostic descriptions for FMC frequently are limited in detail since there is little evidence to associate specific histomorphologic subtypes with outcome. In HBC histologic grade, typically defined using the Elston and Ellis scoring system, is one of the most robust prognostic factors [60]. Although inconclusive in dogs, it has been shown recently, using this same grading system, that invasive FMC also shows a significant incremental association between histologic grade and outcome [61]. In both human and feline patients, intermediate grade tumors show the lowest concordance in routine diagnosis and the broadest heterogeneity in outcome [60,61], and thus the greatest need for improved subclassification.

Genome-wide surveys of HBC have identified discrete genomic signatures that define clinically predictive subtypes, leading to effective treatment strategies based on molecular pathogenesis [62]. Assessment of evidence for corresponding molecular subtypes in FMC may confer potential to extrapolate these advances rapidly to feline patients. To date, the search for prognostic factors for FMC from a molecular perspective has been targeted to individual candidate genes known to be associated with HBC. Of particular note, approximately 25% of HBCs exhibit upregulation of the *ERBB2* gene encoding the receptor tyrosine kinase HER2/neu, of which >90% exhibit DNA copy number amplification of this region [63]. This aberration, historically considered to be an indicator of poor prognosis, also confers susceptibility to Trastuzamab (Herceptin®), a monoclonal antibody targeted against the HER2/neu receptor. Published estimates of HER2-positive FMCs by immunohistochemistry show tremendous variation between studies, largely due to the use of diverse patient cohorts and contrasting analytical techniques [64]. Consequently the true frequency of HER2-positive FMC, and the relationship between protein expression and gene copy number, is yet to be determined.

At the genome-wide level, early conventional chromosome banding studies of FMC identified highly disrupted karyotypes, including recurrent deletions of FCA B2 and gains of FCA E3 [65,66]. These long predated the "genomics era", precluding detailed interpretation in terms of their significance in disease pathogenesis. Microarray-based molecular profiling of FMC is now yielding more substantial insight. Preliminary results with the second-generation CGH array have demonstrated moderate DNA copy number instability in FMC that is distributed broadly throughout the genome, with very few CNAs shared by more than 50% of cases surveyed [67]. Overall, higher-grade tumors exhibit an elevated incidence of genomic imbalance, suggesting that increased chromosome instability may itself represent an indicator of inferior outcome. Interestingly, copy number gain of *ERBB2* was >3-fold more common in high-grade *versus* intermediate-grade tumors. The incidence of *PTEN* deletion was also increased in high-grade tumors, correlating with an earlier study that showed inferior outcome in FMC cases with decreased PTEN protein expression [68]. Gain of *ERBB2* and deletion of *PTEN* are among the most recurrent genomic imbalances in HBC and are associated with concomitant disregulation of gene expression and anti-apoptotic activity, and in turn with inferior outcome [69]. Continued efforts should offer new insight into the degree to which the clinicopathologic similarities between HBC and FMC are recapitulated at the genomic level, highlighting disrupted pathways and potential therapeutic targets for FMC.

CONCLUSIONS

The domestic cat is becoming increasingly well placed to stimulate new advances in molecular medicine. The unique range and distribution of cancers diagnosed in our feline companions fills a series of critical niches that have confounded progress in human medicine. Included among this diverse spectrum are those with direct human counterparts that have remained understudied due to their rarity in people, while others offer a means to study discrete facets of tumor biology that are largely peculiar to the cat. We are now in a position to perform rapid and comprehensive interrogation of normal and aberrant feline genomes and to interpret our observations directly in terms of gene content and potential dysfunction. In turn we have the ability to extrapolate with relative ease between the genomes of different species in the search for conserved molecular features that suggest a common disease mechanism. Given the gross similarity in the structural organization and evolutionary history of the human and cat genomes, it is conceivable that an integrated cytogenomic approach may help to reveal as yet unrecognized mechanisms of tumor-associated chromosome instability.

The field of personalized medicine continues to make tremendous strides in the human field, and opportunities to integrate similar concepts into the veterinary arena are gradually becoming a reality. Cytogenomic techniques are continuing to evolve, with increases in resolution, sensitivity, flexibility, throughput and cost-effectiveness, coupled with the ability to combine related techniques into single platforms that allow synergistic acquisition of data from complementary approaches in a single experiment. In the human field, cancer cytogenomic discovery is gradually transitioning from chromosome- and microarray-based techniques toward the use of next generation sequencing approaches [17]. These strategies provide substantially increased resolution capabilities and have the advantage of permitting concomitant assessment of both structural and numerical aberrations in conjunction with detection of sequence mutations. At the present time, however, their integration into the veterinary arena is constrained by high costs and intensive computational needs, and limited access to dedicated reagents and analytical tools for non-human species. Ten years ago, the same limitations applied to the use of microarray-based technologies such as those described here. Given that the field of veterinary molecular oncology is now well established, and its comparative and translational value is continually being proven, one must hope that the delay in widespread introduction of next generation sequencing strategies for use in companion animal medicine will be less profound.

REFERENCES

1. Cannon, C. Cats, cancer and comparative oncology. *Vet. Sci.* 2015, *2*, 111–126.
2. American Veterinary Medical Association (AVMA). *U.S. Pet Ownership and Demographics Sourcebook*; AVMA: Schaumburg, IL, USA, 2012.
3. Online Mendelian Inheritance in Animals (OMIA). Faculty of Veterinary Science, University of Sydney. Available online: http://omia.angis.org.au (accessed on 28 May 2015).
4. Montague, M.J.; Li, G.; Gandolfi, B.; Khan, R.; Aken, B.L.; Searle, S.M.; Minx, P.; Hillier, L.W.; Koboldt, D.C.; Davis, B.W.; *et al.* Comparative analysis of the domestic cat genome reveals genetic signatures underlying feline biology and domestication. *Proc. Natl. Acad. Sci. USA* 2014, *111*, 17230–17235.
5. Tamazian, G.; Simonov, S.; Dobrynin, P.; Makunin, A.; Logachev, A.; Komissarov, A.; Shevchenko, A.; Brukhin, V.; Cherkasov, N.; Svitin, A.; *et al.* Annotated features of domestic cat-*Felis catus* genome. *Gigascience* 2014, *3*.
6. Nash, W.G.; O'Brien, S.J. Conserved regions of homologous G-banded chromosomes between orders in mammalian evolution: Carnivores and primates. *Proc. Natl. Acad. Sci. USA* 1982, *79*, 6631–6635.
7. Yang, F.; Graphodatsky, A.S.; O'Brien, P.C.; Colabella, A.; Solanky, N.; Squire, M.; Sargan, D.R.; Ferguson-Smith, M.A. Reciprocal chromosome painting illuminates the history of genome evolution of the domestic cat, dog and human. *Chromosome Res.* 2000, *8*, 393–404.
8. Rettenberger, G.; Klett, C.; Zechner, U.; Bruch, J.; Just, W.; Vogel, W.; Hameister, H. Zoo-FISH analysis: Cat and human karyotypes closely resemble the putative ancestral mammalian karyotype. *Chromosome Res.* 1995, *3*, 479–486.
9. Stanyon, R.; Yang, F.; Cavagna, P.; O'Brien, P.C.; Bagga, M.; Ferguson-Smith, M.A.; Wienberg, J. Reciprocal chromosome painting shows that genomic rearrangement between rat and mouse proceeds ten times faster than between humans and cats. *Cytogenet. Cell Genet.* 1999, *84*, 150–155.
10. O'Brien, S.J.; Johnson, W.; Driscoll, C.; Pontius, J.; Pecon-Slattery, J.; Menotti-Raymond, M. State of cat genomics.*Trends Genet.* 2008, *24*, 268–279.
11. Graphodatsky, A.S.; Trifonov, V.A.; Stanyon, R. The genome diversity and karyotype evolution of mammals. *Mol. Cytogenet.* 2011, *4*.
12. Pontius, J.U.; Mullikin, J.C.; Smith, D.R.; Lindblad-Toh, K.; Gnerre, S.; Clamp,

M.; Chang, J.; Stephens, R.; Neelam, B.; Volfovsky, N.; *et al.* Initial sequence and comparative analysis of the cat genome. *Genome Res.* 2007, *17*, 1675–1689.

13. Lindblad-Toh, K.; Garber, M.; Zuk, O.; Lin, M.F.; Parker, B.J.; Washietl, S.; Kheradpour, P.; Ernst, J.; Jordan, G.; Mauceli, E.; *et al.* A high-resolution map of human evolutionary constraint using 29 mammals. *Nature* 2011, *478*, 476–482.
14. Bernheim, A. Cytogenomics of cancers: From chromosome to sequence. *Mol. Oncol.* 2010, *4*, 309–322.
15. Sandberg, A.A.; Meloni-Ehrig, A.M. Cytogenetics and genetics of human cancer: Methods and accomplishments.*Cancer Genet. Cytogenet.* 2010, *203*, 102–126.
16. Mitelman, F.; Johansson, B.; Mertens, F. Mitelman Database of Chromosome Aberrations and Gene Fusions in Cancer. Available online: http://cgap.nci.nih.gov/chromosomes/mitelman (accessed on 31 May 2015).
17. Le Scouarnec, S.; Gribble, S.M. Characterising chromosome rearrangements: Recent technical advances in molecular cytogenetics. *Heredity (Edinb)* 2012, *108*, 75–85.
18. Breen, M. Comparative Cytogenetics. Available online: http://www.els.net (accessed on 22 July 2015).
19. Schiffman, J.D.; Breen, M. Comparative oncology: What dogs and other species can teach us about humans with cancer. *Phil. Trans. Roy. Soc. B-Biol. Sci.* 2015, *370*.
20. Hendrick, M.J.; Goldschmidt, M.H. Do injection site reactions induce fibrosarcomas in cats? *J. Amer. Vet. Med. Assoc.*1991. Avaiable online: http://europepmc.org/abstract/med/1748617 (accessed 28 August 2015).
21. Martano, M.; Morello, E.; Buracco, P. Feline injection-site sarcoma: Past, present and future perspectives. *Vet. J.* 2011,*188*, 136–141.
22. Woodward, K.N. Origins of injection-site sarcomas in cats: The possible role of chronic inflammation—A review.*ISRN Vet. Sci.* 2011, *2011*.
23. Munday, J.S.; Stedman, N.L.; Richey, L.J. Histology and immunohistochemistry of seven ferret vaccination-site fibrosarcomas. *Vet. Pathol.* 2003, *40*, 288–293.
24. Vascellari, M.; Melchiotti, E.; Bozza, M.A.; Mutinelli, F. Fibrosarcomas at presumed sites of injection in dogs: Characteristics and comparison with non-vaccination site fibrosarcomas and feline post-vaccinal fibrosarcomas. *J. Vet. Med. A-Physiol. Pathol. Clin. Med.* 2003, *50*, 286–291.
25. Moizhess, T.G. Carcinogenesis induced by foreign bodies. *Biochemistry (Mosc.)* 2008, *73*, 763–775.
26. Hendrick, M.J. Musings on feline injection site sarcomas. *Vet. J.* 2011, *188*, 130–131.
27. Ladlow, J. Injection site-associated sarcoma in the cat: Treatment recommendations and results to date. *J. Feline Med. Surg.* 2013, *15*, 409–418.
28. Dobson, J.M.; Demetriou, J.; Seguin, B. Chapters 20: Skin tumors and 22: Injection site sarcomas. In *Feline Soft Tissue and General Surgery*, 1st ed.; Langley-Hobbs,

S., Demetriou, J., Ladlow, J., Eds.; Saunders Elsevier: Philadelphia, PA, USA, 2013; pp. 209–242.

29. Kalat, M.; Mayr, B.; Schleger, W.; Wagner, B.; Reifinger, M. Chromosomal hyperdiploidy in a feline sarcoma. *Res. Vet. Sci.* 1991, *51*, 227–228.

30. Mayr, B.; Bockstahler, B.; Loupal, G.; Reifinger, M.; Schleger, W. Cytogenetic variation between four cases of feline fibrosarcoma. *Res. Vet. Sci.* 1996, *61*, 268–270.

31. Mayr, B.; Eschborn, U.; Kalat, M. Near triploidy in a feline fibrosarcoma. *Zentralbl. Veterinarmed. A* 1991, *38*, 617–620.

32. Mayr, B.; Hofstadler, E.; Schleger, W.; Reifinger, M.; Eisenmenger, E. Trisomy D1, marker F1: New cytogenetic findings in two cases of feline fibrosarcoma. *Zentralbl. Veterinarmed. A* 1994, *41*, 197–201.

33. Santos, S.; Chaves, R.; Adega, F.; Bastos, E.; Guedes-Pinto, H. Amplification of the major satellite DNA family (FA-SAT) in a cat fibrosarcoma might be related to chromosomal instability. *J. Hered.* 2006, *97*, 114–118.

34. von Erichsen, J.; Hecht, W.; Lohberg-Gruene, C.; Reinacher, M. Cell lines derived from feline fibrosarcoma display unstable chromosomal aneuploidy and additionally centrosome number aberrations. *Vet. Pathol.* 2012, *49*, 648–657.

35. Thomas, R.; Valli, V.E.; Ellis, P.; Bell, J.; Karlsson, E.K.; Cullen, J.; Lindblad-Toh, K.; Langford, C.F.; Breen, M. Microarray-based cytogenetic profiling reveals recurrent and subtype-associated genomic copy number aberrations in feline sarcomas. *Chromosome Res.* 2009, *17*, 987–1000.

36. Szczerbal, I.; Michalak, E. FISH-localization of the nucleolar organizer region on the feline E1p12 chromosome. *Anim. Genet.* 2003, *34*, 386–387.

37. Ettinger, S.N.; Scase, T.J.; Oberthaler, K.T.; Craft, D.M.; McKnight, J.A.; Leibman, N.F.; Charney, S.C.; Bergman, P.J. Association of argyrophilic nucleolar organizing regions, Ki-67, and proliferating cell nuclear antigen scores with histologic grade and survival in dogs with soft tissue sarcomas: 60 cases (1996–2002). *J. Am. Vet. Med. Assoc.* 2006, *228*, 1053–1062.

38. Thomas, R.; Pontius, J.; Borst, L.; Lamm, C.; Breen, M. Development Of A Genome-Anchored Microarray Platform for Identification of Clinically Predictive Somatic DNA Copy Number Aberrations in Feline Cancers. In Proceedings of the 7th International Conference on Advances in Canine and Feline Genomics and Inherited Diseases, Cambridge, MA, USA, 23–27 September 2013.

39. Smith, A.J.; Njaa, B.L.; Lamm, C.G. Immunohistochemical expression of c-KIT protein in feline soft tissue fibrosarcomas. *Vet. Pathol.* 2009, *46*, 934–939.

40. Moore, P.F.; Rodriguez-Bertos, A.; Kass, P.H. Feline gastrointestinal lymphoma: Mucosal architecture, immunophenotype, and molecular clonality. *Vet. Pathol.* 2011, *49*, 658–668.

41. Wu, F.Y.; Iijima, K.; Tsujimoto, H.; Tamura, Y.; Higurashi, M. Chromosomal translocations in two feline T-cell lymphomas. *Leuk. Res.* 1995, *19*, 857–860.

42. Fujino, Y.; Ma, Z.; Satoh, H.; Mizuno, T.; Hisasue, M.; Baba, K.; Masuda, K.;

Ohno, K.; Onishi, T.; Tsujimoto, H. Characterization of a newly established nonproducer lymphoma cell line for feline leukemia virus. *Vet. Immunol. Immunopathol.* 2004, *102*, 429–439.

43. Breen, M.; Modiano, J.F. Evolutionarily conserved cytogenetic changes in hematological malignancies of dogs and humans—Man and his best friend share more than companionship. *Chromosome Res.* 2008, *16*, 145–154.

44. Thomas, R.; Seiser, E.L.; Motsinger-Reif, A.; Borst, L.; Valli, V.E.; Kelley, K.; Suter, S.E.; Argyle, D.; Burgess, K.; Bell, J.;*et al.* Refining tumor-associated aneuploidy through "genomic recoding" of recurrent DNA copy number aberrations in 150 canine non-Hodgkin lymphomas. *Leuk. Lymphoma* 2011, *52*, 1321–1335.

45. Wilson, H.M. Feline alimentary lymphoma: Demystifying the enigma. *Top. Companion Anim. Med.* 2008, *23*, 177–184.

46. Vail, D.M. Chapter 324: Hematopoetic tumors. In *Textbook of Veterinary Internal Medicine*, 7th ed.; Ettinger, S.N., Feldman, E.C., Eds.; Saunders: Philadelphia, PA, USA, 2009; p. 2148.

47. Rissetto, K.; Villamil, J.A.; Selting, K.A.; Tyler, J.; Henry, C.J. Recent trends in feline intestinal neoplasia: An epidemiologic study of 1129 cases in the veterinary medical database from 1964 to 2004. *J. Am. Anim. Hosp. Assoc.*2011, *47*, 28–36.

48. Jasdanwala, S.; Pitchumoni, C. Epidemiological spectrum of gastrointestinal lymphoma. *Pract. Gastroenterol.* 2014, *38*, 8–28.

49. Moore, P.F.; Woo, J.C.; Vernau, W.; Kosten, S.; Graham, P.S. Characterization of feline T cell receptor gamma (TCRG) variable region genes for the molecular diagnosis of feline intestinal T cell lymphoma. *Vet. Immunol. Immunopathol.*2005, *106*, 167–178.

50. Waly, N.E.; Gruffydd-Jones, T.J.; Stokes, C.R.; Day, M.J. Immunohistochemical diagnosis of alimentary lymphomas and severe intestinal inflammation in cats. *J. Comp. Pathol.* 2005, *133*, 253–260.

51. Briscoe, K.A.; Krockenberger, M.; Beatty, J.A.; Crowley, A.; Dennis, M.M.; Canfield, P.J.; Dhand, N.; Lingard, A.E.; Barrs, V.R. Histopathological and immunohistochemical evaluation of 53 cases of feline lymphoplasmacytic enteritis and low-grade alimentary lymphoma. *J. Comp. Pathol.* 2011, *145*, 187–198.

52. Pohlman, L.M.; Higginbotham, M.L.; Welles, E.G.; Johnson, C.M. Immunophenotypic and histologic classification of 50 cases of feline gastrointestinal lymphoma. *Vet. Pathol.* 2009, *46*, 259–268.

53. Scott, K.D.; Zoran, D.L.; Mansell, J.; Norby, B.; Willard, M.D. Utility of endoscopic biopsies of the duodenum and ileum for diagnosis of inflammatory bowel disease and small cell lymphoma in cats. *J. Vet. Intern. Med.* 2011, *25*, 1253–1257.

54. Thomas, R.; *et al.* Genomic profiling of feline gastrointestinal lymphoma (To be submitted).

55. Hughes, K.; Dobson, J.M. Prognostic histopathological and molecular markers in feline mammary neoplasia. *Vet. J.*2012, *194*, 19–26.

56. Siegel, R.; Naishadham, D.; Jemal, A. Cancer statistics, 2013. *CA Cancer J. Clin.* 2013, *63*, 11–30.

57. Burrai, G.P.; Mohammed, S.I.; Miller, M.A.; Marras, V.; Pirino, S.; Addis, M.F.; Uzzau, S.; Antuofermo, E. Spontaneous feline mammary intraepithelial lesions as a model for human estrogen receptor- and progesterone receptor-negative breast lesions. *BMC Cancer* 2010, *10*.

58. Gimenez, F.; Hecht, S.; Craig, L.E.; Legendre, A.M. Early detection, aggressive therapy: Optimizing the management of feline mammary masses. *J. Feline Med. Surg.* 2010, *12*, 214–224.

59. Zappulli, V.; De Zan, G.; Cardazzo, B.; Bargelloni, L.; Castagnaro, M. Feline mammary tumours in comparative oncology. *J. Dairy Res.* 2005, *72*, 98–106.

60. Rakha, E.A.; Reis-Filho, J.S.; Baehner, F.; Dabbs, D.J.; Decker, T.; Eusebi, V.; Fox, S.B.; Ichihara, S.; Jacquemier, J.; Lakhani, S.R.; *et al.* Breast cancer prognostic classification in the molecular era: The role of histological grade. *Breast Cancer Res.* 2010, *12*, 207.

61. Seixas, F.; Palmeira, C.; Pires, M.A.; Bento, M.J.; Lopes, C. Grade is an independent prognostic factor for feline mammary carcinomas: A clinicopathological and survival analysis. *Vet. J.* 2011, *187*, 65–71.

62. Curtis, C.; Shah, S.P.; Chin, S.F.; Turashvili, G.; Rueda, O.M.; Dunning, M.J.; Speed, D.; Lynch, A.G.; Samarajiwa, S.; Yuan, Y.; *et al.* The genomic and transcriptomic architecture of 2000 breast tumours reveals novel subgroups. *Nature*2012, *486*, 346–352.

63. Kiyose, S.; Igarashi, H.; Nagura, K.; Kamo, T.; Kawane, K.; Mori, H.; Ozawa, T.; Maeda, M.; Konno, K.; Hoshino, H.; *et al.* Chromogenic *in situ* hybridization (CISH) to detect HER2 gene amplification in breast and gastric cancer: Comparison with immunohistochemistry (IHC) and fluorescence *in situ* hybridization (FISH). *Pathol. Int.* 2012, *62*, 728–734.

64. Rasotto, R.; Caliari, D.; Castagnaro, M.; Zanetti, R.; Zappulli, V. An immunohistochemical study of HER-2 expression in feline mammary tumours. *J. Comp. Pathol.* 2011, *144*, 170–179.

65. Mayr, B.; Jugl, M.; Brem, G.; Reifinger, M.; Loupal, G. Cytogenetic variation in six cases of feline mammary tumours.*Zentralbl. Veterinarmed. A* 1999, *46*, 367–377.

66. Mayr, B.; Ortner, W.; Reifinger, M.; Loupal, G. Loss of chromosome B2-material in three cases of feline mammary tumours. *Res. Vet. Sci* 1995, *59*, 61–63.

67. Thomas, R.; Seixas, F.; Borst, L.; Breen, M. Landscapes of Genomic Copy Number Aberrations in Feline Mammary Cancer. In Proceedings of the 8th International Conference on Advances in Canine and Feline Genomics and Inherited Diseases, Cambridge, UK; Available online: http://www.caninefelinegenomicsconference.org/ (accessed on 22–26 June 2015).

68. Ressel, L.; Millanta, F.; Caleri, E.; Innocenti, V.M.; Poli, A. Reduced pten protein expression and its prognostic implications in canine and feline mammary tumors. *Vet. Pathol.* 2009, *46*, 860–868.

69. Curtis, C.; Lynch, A.G.; Dunning, M.J.; Spiteri, I.; Marioni, J.C.; Hadfield, J.; Chin, S.F.; Brenton, J.D.; Tavare, S.; Caldas, C. The pitfalls of platform comparison: DNA copy number array technologies assessed. *BMC Genom.* 2009, *10*.

14
CHAPTER

ANIMAL MODELS OF ALLERGIC DISEASES

Domenico Santoro and Rosanna Marsella

Keywords: Atopic dermatitis, food allergy, asthma, dogs, humans, mice

INTRODUCTION

Several types of allergic diseases affect the skin in both humans and animals. One of the most common is atopic dermatitis (AD), also referred to as eczema in human medicine. Atopic disease is genetically inherited in all species and results from complex interactions between genetic and environmental factors. In a subset of patients, AD is linked to allergies. In people, the first manifestation of atopic disease is cutaneous and is frequently first triggered by food allergens. The disease is chronic and relapsing in nature with acute exacerbations frequently associated with allergen exposure. Many studies have shown evidence of various mutations affecting skin barrier function highlighting the fact that sensitization occurs first through defective skin. Due to the increased permeability of the skin, allergens are more readily absorbed and this increased exposure leads to the development of allergic sensitization. As the disease progresses, sensitizations may develop against a variety of environmental allergens and not just foods. Some patients appear to progress from the cutaneous phase to respiratory signs such as asthma as part of the "atopic march", although debate still exists in human medicine regarding the existence of this phenomenon. Atopic disease has become very common in industrialized countries possibly due to changes in lifestyle and diet and much effort has been devoted to identifying the causes and mechanisms

Citation: Domenico Santoro and Rosanna Marsella, Animal Models of Allergic Diseases, doi:10.3390/vetsci1030192.

to either prevent or minimize this epidemic of allergies. For this reason many animal models have been studied for both environmental and food allergies. Many similarities, yet some differences exist in the manifestation of AD across species. Some of these differences can be leveraged to improve our understanding regarding the mechanisms involved in the pathogenesis of this complex disease and, in the future, to improve our understanding on why some individuals have multiple manifestations of atopic disease and some only have one clinical sign. In this review, we will discuss the various models by focusing on the primary manifestation of allergy that they were attempting to reproduce and study.

ATOPIC DERMATITIS: COMPARATIVE OBSERVATIONS

With this term in veterinary medicine, we refer to a recurrent chronic pruritic dermatitis with a characteristic distribution and most often associated with allergen specific IgE against environmental allergens [1]. People also suffer from AD. The term eczema is frequently used interchangeably with AD in human medicine while it has been abandoned in veterinary medicine. Eczema has become quite common in children in westernized countries and it is estimated to affect approximately 40% of preschool children in the USA and the UK [2,3]. This increase has a major impact both medically and financially and it has been referred to as an epidemic of allergies.

The clinical distribution of AD is very similar between children and dogs. Lesions are erythematous, pruritic and prone to be secondarily infected with *Staphylococcus spp.* Areas that are typically affected are folds and flexural surfaces such as the antebrachial area, axillary, and groin area. The perioral and periocular regions, hands and feet are also commonly involved.

In both species, AD is frequently *but not always* linked to an allergic sensitization. There is indeed a subset of patients in both humans and dogs in which the disease is not linked to allergies. This form of AD is called "intrinsic" or "not allergic" to differentiate it from the more classic "extrinsic" or "allergic" form of the disease in which allergen specific IgE are detectable [4,5,6]. Approximately 10% of people with AD are affected by the "intrinsic" form. Although the intrinsic form has been considered by some as a step toward the development of extrinsic form, it is becoming increasingly clear that it may actually represent a different subtype [5]. No difference in severity of disease is typically observed between the two subsets of patients although different frequency in distribution of lesions has been described [7]. The intrinsic form tends to develop in older patients and filaggrin mutations are not a characteristic of this form [8]. Studies investigating skin barrier function in patients diagnosed with intrinsic AD have shown that normal function and sensory reactivity to external stimuli is retained in these individuals, which is different from patients with the extrinsic form [9]. Immunologically, lower expression of T helper (Th)2 cytokines such as Interleukin (IL)-4, 5, and 13 are found in affected individuals. The same distinction has been proposed in the dog and the term atopic-like dermatitis" has been proposed for individuals in which no detectable IgE can be found. Multiple immune dysregulations have been reported in AD. It is generally accepted that AD may in part be due to defective immune tolerance [10]. Regulatory mechanisms are necessary to maintain peripheral tolerance by the immune system [11]. Regulatory T cells (Tregs) are a diverse subset of T cells capable of dampening inflammatory cell responses [12,13]. Several studies have shown that Tregs are dysfunctional in atopic patients [5,14] leading to aberrant immune response after allergen exposure. Other immune dysregulations described in allergic skin diseases have highlighted the role of basophils [15] and mast cells [16]. Interestingly, no increased skin mast cells' releasability [17] and no increased circulating levels of histamine have been reported in human AD patients [18]. Additionally, the usefulness of antihistamines H1 receptor blockers is limited [12]. More interest now exists in the role of H4 receptors and other mast cell products such as tryptase [19,20]. In particular, the histamine H4 receptor has been demonstrated to mediate inflammation and Th2-dependent inflammation and is a potential target for future therapies [21,22,23,24].

In dogs with AD, studies examining number of mast cells and the histamine release between normal and atopic dogs showed no differences or even a lower mast cell density in lesional and non-lesional atopic skin compared to healthy control skin [25]. In addition, studies evaluating serum histamine concentrations revealed that levels are similar [26] or lower [27] in dogs with AD compared to healthy controls, thus the role of histamine is still under debate. Interestingly, the few studies evaluating the effect of antihistamines, including H4 blockers, have failed to report a beneficial effect [28,29]. In a subset of human patients with AD, genetically inherited skin barrier defects are demonstrable and further skin barrier impairment occurs once sensitization develops and inflammation is triggered [30]. Thus, skin barrier impairment can be both primary and secondary and it plays some role in all patients at some point during the course of the disease. One of the most documented genetically inherited mutations is in the filaggrin gene. Filaggrin is very important for proper keratinization (the process of differentiation of cutaneous epithelial cells). Mutations in the filaggrin gene have been extensively studied and reported in people with AD to the point that null mutations in this gene, leading to a decrease expression of filaggrin, are considered one of the strongest risk factors for the development of the disease [31,32]. It is important to note that not all patients with AD have filaggrin mutations and that some patients with them do not necessarily develop the disease, highlighting the fact that the development of AD is multifactorial resulting from a complex interaction between genetics and environmental conditions. As primary skin barrier defect may not be present in all patients with AD, it is important to point out that AD may actually represent a clinical syndrome that could result from different mechanisms.

Recent research in dogs has highlighted that skin barrier impairment may be one of the mechanisms of allergic sensitization also in this species [33,34] when allergens come in contact with a more permeable and disrupted skin which results in a Th2 polarization and production of allergen specific IgE. Although it is not clear yet whether the skin barrier defect is primary in dogs, it is clear that the skin barrier function is impaired [35,36] in atopic dogs and it plays a role in the aggravation of the disease.

Interestingly, in people, AD is typically the first step in a progression of events called "atopic march" which starts in the skin and progresses in many, but not all cases, into respiratory signs (rhinitis and later on asthma) [37]. As mentioned above, it is important to point out that although this progression is noted in individual patients, debate exists on the evidence of this phenomenon. Some publications have questioned the existence of an actual atopic march [38,39] while more recent studies have provided renewed support of an actual temporal pattern of progression from eczema to allergic rhinitis and asthma and a correlation between early eczema and childhood asthma [40,41,42].

In dogs, atopic disease typically only manifests in the skin, without progression to respiratory signs in the vast majority of cases. On the contrary, in other domestic animals, such as cats and horses, the atopic disease can manifest as both dermatitis and respiratory disease. It is currently unclear why allergies have different forms of manifestations in various species and why some species are prone to skin manifestations while others are prone to respiratory disease. Allergic diseases have very complex pathogenesis and many genes have been considered as possible candidates to explain development of allergies. It is very likely that many different pathways can lead to the development of allergies and that even within one species allergies should be considered more like a syndrome rather than one disease. It is interesting to note that even within the canine species, different gene mutations may play a role in various breeds and various geographical areas [43]. As the recent literature has emphasized the role of increased penetration of allergens as one of the mechanisms to explain increased risk for sensitization, it is possible that different aberrations in the skin *versus* the respiratory epithelium may be one of the reasons for the various clinical manifestations of allergic disease in different species. The similarities and yet differences across species may actually constitute a key to understanding what determines the progression of the disease and hopefully allow early identification of the individuals that are at increased risk for the development of asthma.

Histologically and immunologically the similarity of AD between dogs and people is striking, making dogs the closest naturally occurring animal model to study this disease in people [44]. Atopy patch test reactions in dogs mimic naturally occurring lesions and are very similar to what is reported in human medicine [45]. AD type lesions may be experimentally induced in mice, but this species does not spontaneously develop the disease and the experimental models only reproduce limited aspects of the disease [46] and recent literature has questioned the value of mouse models [47] as mice appear to only reproduce a very simplistic approach to allergies as a Th2 mediated disease and fail to reproduce more complex aspects of the human condition [48]. Dogs, on the other hand, are genetically closer to people, they are spontaneously affected by AD, and they also share the same environment with their owners constituting a precious and better tool to fully understand this complex disease in people.

Dog Models of Atopic Dermatitis

A few canine models of AD have been identified and validated. One model is composed by a colony of high IgE producing atopic Beagles [49]. These dogs have skin barrier defects demonstrated by ultrastructural studies showing an abnormally organized lipid lamellae and retained lamellar bodies [50]. These changes are similar to what reported in human atopic patients in which disorganized intercellular lipids, decreased ceramides and defects of extrusion of lamellar bodies have been described [51,52].

The abnormalities in the skin barrier do not only affect lipids but also epidermal proteins. Filaggrin has also been studied in dogs, in particular in the atopic beagle colony mentioned above, and an irregular, patchy staining for filaggrin was found in immunohistochemical and immunofluorescence studies [53,54]. In addition, in histochemical studies, morphological differences have been identified when comparing the keratohyalin granules (granules where the filaggrin and its precursor are stored before complete keratinization) in the atopic beagles with age matched healthy controls. In people, the decreased expression of filaggrin is not always linked to genetic mutations, but it can also be caused by increased degradation of the protein. More specifically, two enzymes—caspase-14 and calpain-1—are responsible for the degradation of filaggrin into amino acids fundamental for proper miniaturization of the skin (natural moisturizing factors) [55]. A decreased expression of caspase-14 has been found in both people [56,57] and in the atopic Beagle [58] colony showing the relevance and the similarities between the canine model and the atopic condition in human patients.

In this Beagle model, the skin barrier defects are not only ultrastructural but also functional as demonstrated by an increased transepidermal water loss (TEWL) compared to age matched healthy controls [36]. Measurement of this parameter is a non-invasive approach to test skin permeability. Atopic people have increased TEWL when compared to healthy controls and skin barrier dysfunction correlates with disease activity [59]. It is believed that younger skin is more susceptible to sensitizations and interestingly puppies from this atopic colony have higher TEWL than adults of the same colony and age matched healthy Beagles kept in the same living conditions [36]. These findings seem to emphasize the existence of a window of opportunity of allergic sensitization. This leads to the fascinating hypothesis that maybe the development of AD could be prevented or at last minimized if skin barrier repair is enacted at a young age, before sensitization sets in. Indeed, pilot studies in infants showed a decrease sensitization in children at high risk for the atopic disease due to genetic predisposition in which emollients and occlusive therapy was started in the first few months of life [60,61]. Preventative studies are difficult to accomplish in people or in pet dogs with naturally occurring disease due to the variable environmental conditions which tend to make design and interpretation of studies quite challenging. That is where animal models can provide useful information that can benefit multiple species. One example of that is the proactive use of probiotics with the intention of preventing or at least lessening the severity of disease in highly predisposed individuals. One of the ideas behind this strategy is that allergies are partly due to improved hygiene conditions leading to less opportunity to have bacterial and parasitic exposure which helps to modulate the immune response toward a more protective cell mediated response. The exact mechanisms of probiotics in allergies are still under investigation and are more complex than the direct modulation of the immune response. With the development of methodologies targeting the 16S rRNA, knowledge of the importance of the microbiome in healthy and disease states is rapidly growing. It is becoming evident that loss of biodiversity can predispose to the development of allergies while high biodiversity can have a protective effect [62,63,64,65,66]. Oral assumption of probiotics can modulate gut microbiota [67] and this can be an additional mechanism by which probiotic can affect the immune response

[68], although this mechanism has not be confirmed in recent clinical trials in infants. In one study, skin and gut microbiome was investigated after oral administration of *Lactobacillus rahmnosus GG* (LGG) but no significant changes were detected when compared to the control group [69]. When studies on probiotic have been done in people, the results of clinical efficacy have been mixed [70] probably because it was not possible to control for genetic differences, variable diets and environmental conditions. In animal models, this can be done and even studies with a relatively low number of subjects can produce useful information. Using the colony of atopic Beagles, it was possible to breed the same parents twice, producing two litters, one used as control and the other one as probiotic litter. Puppies were raised under the same housing and dietary conditions, they were all exposed to house dust mites using the exact same doses and protocols and the only difference was the administration of LGG, which is a probiotic for both dogs and people. The results showed that prenatal and postnatal (for the first 6 months of life) exposure to LGG had a protective effect in decreasing the severity of sensitization [71]. Even more interestingly, the protective effect was long lasting and carried out for at least 3 years after the discontinuation of the LGG [72]. The probiotic litter continued to show significantly lower severity of clinical signs and was associated with increased regulatory cytokines such as transforming growth factor (TGF)-β. In the canine study, no investigation on the effects of LGG on skin or gut microbiome was done. This is an area that should be investigated further as preliminary studies on skin microbiome in allergic and normal dogs have shown that atopic dogs have less biodiversity and increased colonization by Staphylococcus compared to the healthy controls [73]. The preventative effects of this study echoed more recent metanalyses in human medicine that support a prophylactic role for probiotics, but not the therapeutic role once the disease has already been established [74].

A model for AD in dogs has also been described in Maltese-Beagles. In this model, pruritus and dermatitis can be elicited after epicutaneous application of house dust mites [75]. Lesions are consistent with naturally occurring AD lesions [76,77] making it a suitable model to test new therapies. No skin barrier defect has been described in this model compared to a control population. Ceramide reductions have been described as an effect of allergen exposure and development of inflammation [78]. Another well described but older model of AD and asthma was the one of Basenji-Greyhound dogs. While dogs typically do not develop asthma as progression of their skin disease, in this model both manifestations (skin and respiratory) of atopic disease were described [79] making them an appealing model to study the human condition [80,81]. No recent publications have been reported on this model.

Mouse Models of Atopic Dermatitis

Many different mouse models of AD have been described over time. The Nishiki-nezumi Cinnamon/Nagoya (NC/Nga) was the first AD-like murine model that spontaneously develops AD-like dermatitis only if raised under air-uncontrolled conventional conditions [82,83,84]. This model has been useful to test new treatments [85] although the fact that the NC/Nga mice exposure to only conventional environments is not enough to induce human AD-like clinical symptoms questions the relevance of such model to the human condition.

Other mouse models have been described by epicutaneous stimulation with certain environmental allergens [86]. SKH-1 hairless mice have been shown to be easily sensitized epicutaneously with allergens due to skin barrier impairment and reported to be helpful to test strategies such as probiotics [87]. Mice with a null mutation in the filaggrin gene develop flaky tails and that has been used as model for AD although this model may only represent one subset of AD [88,89].

FOOD ALLERGY

Food allergy is also becoming quite common in people. In people, food allergy is defined as "a pattern of immune reactivity to the ingestion of natural food components resulting in IgE mediated [reaction], which by nature routinely results in tolerance". In non-allergic individuals, the normal immune response to dietary protein is associated with a natural tolerance; on the contrary, in allergic patients, an excessive complex immune response against food proteins may occur. Several immune responses including an immediate and a delayed hypersensitivity have been associated with food allergy explaining the highly variable time of reaction after the ingestion of an allergen. Food allergy is extremely important in people due to the high variability of the clinical signs associated with it; the spectrum of clinical signs can range from mildly irritating to life-threatening conditions [90].

Food allergy is a substantial and evolving public health issue [91,92] with an increasing prevalence in the last decades [93] due to environmental changes [94]. In the USA, up to 8% of children and 4% of adults have food allergy [92]. Of major concern is the fact that, while previous generations of children would typically outgrow food allergies (particularly if not peanuts related), the new generations appear less able to outgrow food allergy. It is proposed that environmental factors have significant effect on this phenomenon and that "westernization" plays a role [95]. The most serious allergic response to food allergy is anaphylaxis [96,97]. More than 3 million Americans are allergic to peanuts and this is the leading cause of death by anaphylaxis [98]. In children, the most common foods able to trigger an immunological response include, but are not limited to, cow's milk, hen's egg, peanut, soybeans, wheat, fish, and tree nuts. Whereas, in adults, the most common food allergies are due to ingestion of peanuts, tree nuts, fish, and shellfish [99,100,101]. In people, most commonly food allergy started in the first 3 years of life; however, several studies have shown that most allergies that begin early in life (e.g., milk, egg, soy, and wheat) are generally outgrown. On the contrary, allergies to peanut, tree nuts, fish and shellfish tend to persist for life [102,103].

To better determine the immunological mechanisms and in order to develop safe therapeutic options for children and adults affected by food allergy, the use of animal models is fundamental. To date, animal models have been identified with some success in small animals (mice, rats, and guinea pigs) as well as in large animals (dogs, pigs, and sheep). Those species have been fundamental to assess routes of administration to induce sensitization and to better identify the gastrointestinal allergic response. However, each model has benefits and limitations.

Rodent Models of Food Allergy

Examples of murine model include strains like the BALB/c, DBA/2, C3H/HeJ, BDF-1, A/J, and the C57/Bl6. Of those, the most studied have been the C3H/HeJ and the BALB/c able to produce IgE and IgG1 anaphylactic antibodies [104,105]. The former has been used to investigate potential immunotherapeutic approaches to treat food allergy through intragastric administration of peanut and milk proteins [106,107]. The BALB/c mice have instead been used to evaluate the potential to predict the allergenicity of a novel protein for people through intraperitoneal administration of several proteins including ovalbumin, peanut agglutinin, and bovine serum albumin [108]. Due to the artificial sensitization methods it is unclear how well representative mouse models are for the natural disease in people and their usefulness in predicting efficacy of therapies [109].

Rats have also been used as an animal model for food allergy. The most commonly used strain is the brown Norway able to produce allergen specific IgE after oral sensitization and able to predict the allergenicity of novel proteins [110,111]. Other strains like Wistar, Hooded Lister, and Piebald Virol Glaxo have been studied, but not commonly used due to the inability to detect quantifiable levels of antigen specific IgE [112].

An alternative to mice and rats is the guinea pig. Indeed, these rodents are able to display fatal anaphylaxis after sensitization to cow's milk proteins. However, due to the technical difficulties (e.g., inability to directly quantify IgE production) and for the limited tools to study their immune system, guinea pigs have been abandoned as an animal model for food allergy [113].

Dog Models of Food Allergy

Dogs have been recently identified as a spontaneous model for food allergy in people. In fact, as in people, up to 8%–15% of the canine population is spontaneously affected by food allergy and it manifests more commonly during puppyhood [114]. Like in people, dogs may present with skin and gastrointestinal clinical signs, although these latter involves up to 10%–15% of the affected patients [113,115]. Contrary to the rodent models, dogs and people share the same food allergens: beef, dairy, wheat, lamb, egg, chicken, soy, oats, and pork [116]. In addition, they share similar gut anatomy and physiology, as well as nutritional requirements. On dogs, it is easier performing repeated endoscopic analysis, high IgE dogs are easy to identify, and the large size of immune organs along with larger blood volume facilitate certain analyses [104]. To date, three canine models have been well validated [117,118,119]. All the models include mixed breed atopic dogs. Two models are constituted by the same colony of inbred, high IgE producing, atopic spaniel/basenji dogs [117,118], whereas the other one is constituted by a colony of Maltese/Beagles atopic dogs [104,120]. The first generation of the spaniel/basenji model was developed by subcutaneous injection of wheat, cow's milk and beef extract showing signs of vomiting, diarrhea, or more rarely constipation [118]. The second generation was instead sensitized by subcutaneous injection of peanut, walnut, Brazil nut, wealth or barley developing vomiting and lethargy after oral challenge [117]. On the contrary, the Maltese/Beagle colony spontaneously developed food allergy (pruritus, diarrhea, and/or vomiting) to cow's milk, dairy products, corn, and soy without any experimental sensitization [104]. In all three models, the investigators were able to show clinical response to oral challenge between 1 h and 12 h, a higher production of total and allergen-specific serum IgE, and positive intradermal test [104,117,118]. Using the canine model for food allergy, the investigators proposed the hypothesis that in genetically predisposed children an early infection may stimulate the immune system to respond to "bystander" antigens more aggressively than healthy individuals. In the affected patients, the inflamed gut becomes more permeable to food allergens (proteins) leading to their exposure to the local immune system inducing sensitization of otherwise innocuous food proteins [105].

A recently described model for peanut allergy has been reported in atopic Beagles [121]. In this model, dogs were sensitized after epicutaneous application of a peanut paste and developed macular, popular dermatitis after oral challenge. No systemic effects were detected after oral challenge making it a safe model to test therapies. An IgE mediated response was detected on intradermal test and skin biopsies. This model could be useful to test new allergy vaccines to treat peanut allergy in children. The epicutaneous sensitization is very relevant to what is believed to occur in young atopic children where the perioral region is frequently one of the first affected areas, most likely due to increased penetration of food allergens through an impaired skin barrier [122].

Other Large Animal Models for Food Allergy

Another large animal model proposed for food allergy is constituted by neonatal pigs. This model, although very similar to the canine model, is much less commonly used due to several limitations. The major benefits of this model over the others include the strong similarity in anatomy and physiology of the gastrointestinal tract and the development of mucosal immunity between pigs and people [105]. Neonatal piglets have been used as an animal model for sensitization to cow's milk, soy, and peanuts. Sensitized piglets show a very similar immunological response occurring in sensitized children [105]. The induction of food sensitization in piglets involves the use of intraperitoneal injections (peanut extract) in the presence of cholera toxin as adjuvant and later on repeated oral challenges with sensitizing food allergen [105,123]. After challenge the pigs show clinical signs including vomiting, lethargy, diarrhea, bleeding, weight loss, and respiratory distress [123]. Finally, like in dogs, the clinical signs are associated with an increase in allergen-specific IgE and IgG, and a positive passive cutaneous anaphylaxis showing the involvement of IgE as cause of the allergic symptoms [105].

The last large animal model proposed for food allergy in people involves the use of sheep. Like dogs and pigs, also sheep are very similar in size and physiology to people. Sheep have been successfully used as model for peanut allergy [111]. Similarly to other animal models, sheep were sensitized by multiple subcutaneous injections of crude peanut extract and ovalbumin. As outcome the investigators were able to show the presence of Ara h 1- and Ara h 2-specific serum IgE in 100% and 80%, respectively, of the sensitized sheep and a positive intradermal test in 80% of the high-IgE producing sheep [111].

ASTHMA

Asthma in people is defined as "a [multiphenotypic] chronic inflammatory disorder of the airways associated with airway hyper-responsiveness [leading] to recurrent episodes of wheezing, breathlessness, chest tightness, coughing, [and] airflow obstruction often reversible with or without treatment" [124,125,126]. Asthma affects more than 10% of the North American population with the age of onset, pathophysiology, and response to treatment extremely variable [127,128]. In addition, a correlation between chronic obstructive pulmonary disease (COPD) has also been proven in patients with asthma [129].

Due to the high heterogeneity and the ethical problems in analyzing the pathomechanism of asthma in children, many disease models have been developed (mathematical modelling system as well as *in vitro* and *in vivo* models) [130]. The mathematical model has been used to describe patterns of flow limitations in the airways [131], whereas understanding of cell signaling, cellular responses under Th2 conditions, and wound repair have been facilitated by the use of primary or immortalized cell lines [132,133,134]. Although these two model systems have been largely used and are fundamental to unravelling the physical and immunological processes at a cellular and molecular level, their major limitation is the impossibility to evaluate such processes in a dynamic immunological milieu present in the asthmatic patient [130]. For this reason, the only model system able to reproduce the asthma in people is the animal (*in vivo*) model. In the past 100 years, the use of animal models have largely contributed to the identification of important immunological alterations in the lungs of asthmatic patients (e.g., the importance of Th2 phenotype in the progression and perpetuation of an inflammatory response in allergic asthma) as well as the development, safety, and efficacy of new drugs (e.g., montelukast, integrin antibodies, and tryptase inhibitors) [130].

Contrarily to AD and food allergy, an appropriate animal model for human asthma is lacking. Indeed, to date, a laboratory animal that spontaneously develops a disease with characteristics present in asthma has not been identified [135]. However, different species have diseases with some similarities to the human disease; cats spontaneously develop a bronchial disease similar to chronic asthma, horses are affected by a neutrophilic-dominated airway disease more close to COPD than asthma, sheep and dogs are naturally susceptible to allergen sensitization [135].

Mouse models have also been developed and use for identification of immunological alterations leading to pulmonary inflammation in asthmatic people; however, this model is not ideal for testing of new drugs due to the significant anatomic and immunological differences between mice and people [135,136]. Like mice, rats have also been largely used as animal model due to the abundance of reagents available, the ease handling and sensitization protocols, as well as the low maintenance expense. However, one advantage over mice is their larger size which determines an increase in sampling volume and possibility of testing compared with mice [135]. In addition, rats are able to develop an early- and a late-phase response as well as airway hyperresponsiveness to non-specific bronchoconstricting agents present in people but not in mice [135,137]. Although extremely useful to investigate the acute allergic reaction in asthma, the murine models have been largely criticized for their ability to easily develop tolerance following allergen sensitization limiting the use of such models for the investigation of chronic allergic response in asthmatic patients [135].

Contrary to the murine models, pet cats are spontaneously affected by a syndrome similar to human asthma [138]. In the past 10 years, such similarities have led to the development of two feline asthma models for preclinical studies [139,140,141]. Like in people, in cats asthma is extremely common and triggered by aeroallergens and the clinical manifestations include cough, wheeze and episodic expiratory respiratory distress [138]. In addition, cats with asthma have important features of asthma in people including recurrent and variable symptoms of chronic airway disease, airflow restriction, bronchial hyperresponsiveness, and airway inflammation [142]. However, contrarily to people in which airway hyperresponsiveness is triggered by drugs, pollutants, occupational factors, exercise, emotional stress, infections, and allergens; in cats the predominant triggers seem to be aeroallergens [138].

Like the feline models, the canine model has been identified as a better model due to the natural predisposition of dogs to develop allergic disease after exposure to allergens clinically relevant for people. However, naturally-occurring asthma is very uncommon in allergic dogs [143]. In fact, the most common clinical manifestations of allergy in dogs include dermatitis, otitis, and conjunctivitis [144]. However, many naturally or actively sensitized dogs to *Ascasis suum* larvae or ragweed have been used as canine model for asthma [134]. Although an increase in eosinophils have been identified in the airways of allergic dogs, this does not seem to be associated with an increase in responsiveness of the airways probably due to the significant anatomical difference of dogs with the other species; proportionally larger airways and less prone to bronchoconstriction [145]. Nevertheless, anatomical and clinical differences are evident between dogs and people; such model has been largely used due to the unique ability of dogs to show persistent sensitization (prolonged airways hyperresponsiveness) up to 5 months post challenge with *A. suum* [146]. The main drawback for this model is that dogs are labor intense and expensive, but these difficulties are easily overridden by the usefulness of such model to identify pathomechanisms and long term pulmonary changes related to the asthmatic disease [134]. The canine model has also been used as animal model for COPD in people. Although, no as much research as in asthma has been involved using the canine model, three model systems have been identified in dogs: inhalation of cigarette smoke, exposure to SO_2 gas and intratracheal or aerosolization of proteolytic enzymes [125].

Finally, the last animal model system used for asthma is sheep. Like dogs, sheep are naturally sensitized to *A. suum* and house dust mite [135,147,148]; although an inter-individual variability to mount an allergic physiological response to the allergen is present among sheep [149]. Similar to dogs, after challenges sheep develop an early- and late-phase as well as airway hyperresponsiveness [135]. In term of drug response, cromolyn and corticosteroids are highly effective in sheep with an allergic airway response [147]. In addition, sheep are more similar in size and physiology to people, they are very docile, and fewer ethical constraints are taken [147,150]. For all the reasons abovementioned sheep represent a very useful model system for asthma in people; however, relevant differences between sheep and people may affect the use of such model for development and testing of new drugs. One example is the efficacy of platelet activating factors extremely useful to modulate the inflammatory response in the sheep model, but not at all effective in people [151]. As in dogs, the main difficulties to work with sheep are the expense and the labor intensity; however, like for the canine model, such difficulties are easily overridden by the advantages of such model. Some key advantages of using large animal models include their outbred nature, allowing studies that are more comparable to humans, the ability to conduct serial experiments within the same cohort of animals, and their relative longevity, allowing more relevant investigations into chronic disease as well as the long-term evaluation of specific therapies.

CONCLUSIONS

Animals and people share many important allergic diseases, and animals have proven to be the key to improve our understanding on the mechanisms involved across species for the mutual benefit of people and animals. Animals and people share the same environment and are inextricably linked. A comparative approach to medicine has improved our appreciation of similarities and differences of diseases that affect multiple species and how that can be leveraged to improve our knowledge of the mechanisms involved. It is hoped that by improving our understanding on how we are all connected, veterinarians and physicians can collaborate across species to improve the lives of all species and develop therapies than can benefit multiple species.

ACKNOWLEDGMENTS

The authors would like to acknowledge Ahrens for helping with the editing of the manuscript.

AUTHOR CONTRIBUTIONS

Domenico Santoro and Rosanna Marsella equally contributed to the writing, revisions and editing of the paper. They are both veterinary dermatologists with extensive experience in animal models of allergy.

REFERENCES

1. Olivry, T.; DeBoer, D.J.; Griffin, C.E.; Halliwell, R.E.; Hill, P.B.; Hillier, A.; Marsella, R.; Sousa, C.A. The ACVD task force on canine atopic dermatitis: Forewords and lexicon. *Vet. Immunol. Immunopathol.* 2001, *81*, 143–146.
2. Thestrup-Pedersen, K. Atopic eczema. What has caused the epidemic in industrialised countries and can early intervention modify the natural history of atopic eczema? *J. Cosmet. Dermatol.* 2003, *2*, 202–210.
3. Giannetti, A.; Girolomoni, G. Skin diseases with high public health impact. Atopic dermatitis. *Eur. J. Dermatol.* 2007,*17*, 566.

4. Wüthrich, B.; Schmid-Grendelmeier, P. The atopic eczema/dermatitis syndrome. Epidemiology, natural course, and immunology of the IgE-associated ("extrinsic") and the nonallergic ("intrinsic") AEDS. *J. Investig. Allergol. Clin. Immunol.* 2003, *13*, 1–5.

5. Roguedas-Contios, A.M.; Misery, L. What is intrinsic atopic dermatitis? *Clin. Rev. Allergy Immunol.* 2011, *41*, 233–236.

6. Fujimura, M. The study of canine atopic dermatitis involving the isolation of dogs. *Pol. J. Vet. Sci.* 2011, *14*, 273–277.

7. Kulthanan, K.; Boochangkool, K.; Tuchinda, P.; Chularojanamontri, L. Clinical features of the extrinsic and intrinsic types of adult-onset atopic dermatitis. *Asia Pac. Allergy.* 2011, *1*, 80–86.

8. Tokura, Y. Extrinsic and intrinsic types of atopic dermatitis. *J. Dermatol. Sci.* 2010, *58*, 1–7.

9. Mori, T.; Ishida, K.; Mukumoto, S.; Yamada, Y.; Imokawa, G.; Kabashima, K.; Kobayashi, M.; Bito, T.; Nakamura, M.; Ogasawara, K.; *et al.* Comparison of skin barrier function and sensory nerve electric current perception threshold between IgE-high extrinsic and IgE-normal intrinsic types of atopic dermatitis. *Br. J. Dermatol.* 2010, *162*, 83–90.

10. Stelmaszczyk-Emmel, A.; Zawadzka-Krajewska, A.; Szypowska, A.; Kulus, M.; Demkow, U. Frequency and activation of CD4+CD25 FoxP3+ regulatory T cells in peripheral blood from children with atopic allergy. *Int. Arch. Allergy Immunol.* 2013, *162*, 16–24.

11. Rouse, B.T. Regulatory T cells in health and disease. *J. Intern. Med.* 2007, *262*, 78–95.

12. Bilate, A.M.; Lafaille, J.J. Induced CD4+Foxp3+ regulatory T cells in immune tolerance. *Annu. Rev. Immunol.* 2012, *30*, 733–758.

13. Daniel, C.; von Boehmer, H. Extrathymic generation of regulatory T cells—Chances and challenges for prevention of autoimmune disease. *Adv. Immunol.* 2011, *112*, 177–213.

14. Samochocki, Z.; Alifier, M.; Bodera, P.; Jeziorkowska, R.; Rosiak, E.; Jurkiewicz, B.; Glińska, O.; Gliński, W.; Stankiewicz, W. T-regulatory cells in severe atopic dermatitis: Alterations related to cytokines and other lymphocyte subpopulations. *Arch. Dermatol. Res.* 2012, *304*, 795–801.

15. Falcone, F.H.; Knol, E.F.; Gibbs, B.F. The role of basophils in the pathogenesis of allergic disease. *Clin. Exp. Allergy*2011, *41*, 939–947.

16. Ohsawa, Y.; Hirasawa, N. The role of histamine H1 and H4 receptors in atopic dermatitis: From Basic Research to Clinical Study. *Allergol. Int.* 2014.

17. Wahlgren, C.F.; Hägermark, O.; Bergström, R. Patients' perception of itch induced by histamine, compound 48/80 and wool fibres in atopic dermatitis. *Acta. Derm. Venereol.* 1991, *71*, 488–494.

18. Amon, U.; Menz, U.; Wolff, H.H. Investigations on plasma levels of mast cell mediators in acute atopic dermatitis. *J. Dermatol. Sci.* 1994, *7*, 63–67.

19. Sher, L.G.; Chang, J.; Patel, I.B.; Balkrishnan, R.; Fleischer, A.B., Jr. Relieving the pruritus of atopic dermatitis: A meta-analysis. *Acta. Derm. Venereol.* 2012, *92*, 455–461.
20. Darsow, U.; Pfab, F.; Valet, M.; Tölle, T.R.; Ring, J. Itch and eczema. *Chem. Immunol. Allergy* 2012, *96*, 81–88.
21. Cowden, J.M.; Zhang, M.; Dunford, P.J.; Thurmond, R.L. The histamine H4 receptor mediates inflammation and pruritus in Th2-dependent dermal inflammation. *J. Invest. Dermatol.* 2010, *130*, 1023–1033.
22. Gutzmer, R.; Mommert, S.; Gschwandtner, M.; Zwingmann, K.; Stark, H.; Werfel, T. The histamine H_4 receptor is functionally expressed on T_H2 cells. *J. Allergy Clin. Immunol.* 2009, *123*, 619–625.
23. Kollmeier, A.; Francke, K.; Chen, B.; Dunford, P.J.; Greenspan, A.J.; Xia, Y.; Xu, X.L.; Zhou, B.; Thurmond, R.L. The histamine H4 receptor antagonist, JNJ 39758979, is effective in reducing histamine-induced pruritus in a randomized clinical study in healthy subjects. *J. Pharmacol. Exp. Ther.* 2014, *350*, 181–187.
24. Dunford, P.J.; Williams, K.N.; Desai, P.J.; Karlsson, L.; McQueen, D.; Thurmond, R.L. Histamine H_4 receptor antagonists are superior to traditional antihistamines in the attenuation of experimental pruritus. *J. Allergy Clin. Immunol.* 2007, *119*, 176–183.
25. Welle, M.M.; Olivry, T.; Grimm, S.; Suter, M. Mast cell density and subtypes in the skin of dogs with atopic dermatitis.*J. Comp. Pathol.* 1999, *120*, 187–197.
26. Nimmo-Wilkie, J.S.; Yager, J.A.; Eyre, P.; Parker, W.M. Morphometric analyses of the skin of dogs with atopic dermatitis and correlations with cutaneous and plasma histamine and total serum IgE. *Vet. Pathol.* 1990, *27*, 179–186.
27. Helton-Rhodes, K.; Kerdel, F.; Soter, N.A.; Chinnici, R. Investigation into the immunopathogenesis of canine atopy.*Semin. Vet. Med. Surg. (Small Anim.)* 1987, *2*, 199–201.
28. Bäumer, W.; Stahl, J.; Sander, K.; Petersen, L.J.; Paps, J.; Stark, H.; Kietzmann, M.; Olivry, T. Lack of preventing effect of systemically and topically administered histamine H_1 or H_4 receptor antagonists in a dog model of acute atopic dermatitis. *Exp. Dermatol.* 2011, *20*, 577–581.
29. Olivry, T.; Mueller, R.S. International Task Force on Canine Atopic Dermatitis. Evidence-based veterinary dermatology: A systematic review of the pharmacotherapy of canine atopic dermatitis. *Vet. Dermatol.* 2003, *14*, 121–146.
30. Agrawal, R.; Woodfolk, J.A. Skin barrier defects in atopic dermatitis. *Curr. Allergy Asthma Rep.* 2014, *14*.
31. Kawasaki, H.; Kubo, A.; Sasaki, T.; Amagai, M. Loss-of-function mutations within the filaggrin gene and atopic dermatitis. *Curr. Probl. Dermatol.* 2011, *41*, 35–46.
32. O'Regan, G.M.; Sandilands, A.; McLean, W.H.; Irvine, A.D. Filaggrin in atopic dermatitis. *J. Allergy Clin. Immunol.*2008, *122*, 689–693.
33. Olivry, T.; Wofford, J.; Paps, J.S.; Dunston, S.M. Stratum corneum removal

facilitates experimental sensitization to mite allergens in atopic dogs. *Vet. Dermatol.* 2011, *22*, 188–196.

34. Marsella, R.; Olivry, T.; Carlotti, D.N.; International Task Force on Canine Atopic Dermatitis. Current evidence of skin barrier dysfunction in human and canine atopic dermatitis. *Vet. Dermatol.* 2011, *22*, 239–248.
35. Yoon, J.S.; Nishifuji, K.; Sasaki, A.; Ide, K.; Ishikawa, J.; Yoshihara, T.; Iwasaki, T. Alteration of stratum corneum ceramide profiles in spontaneous canine model of atopic dermatitis. *Exp. Dermatol.* 2011, *20*, 732–736.
36. Hightower, K.; Marsella, R.; Flynn-Lurie, A. Effects of age and allergen exposure on transepidermal water loss in a house dust mite-sensitized beagle model of atopic dermatitis. *Vet. Dermatol.* 2010, *21*, 88–95.
37. Shaker, M. New insights into the allergic march. *Curr. Opin. Pediatr.* 2014, *26*, 516–520.
38. Williams, H.; Flohr, C. How epidemiology has challenged 3 prevailing concepts about atopic dermatitis. *J. Allergy Clin. Immunol.* 2006, *118*, 209–213.
39. Curtiss, F.R. Atopic march to a dead end or does the theory really have legs? *J. Manag. Care Pharm.* 2007, *13*, 810–811.
40. Ker, J.; Hartert, T.V. The atopic march: What's the evidence? *Ann. Allergy Asthma Immunol.* 2009, *103*, 282–289.
41. Spergel, J.M. From atopic dermatitis to asthma: The atopic march. *Ann. Allergy Asthma Immunol.* 2010, *105*, 99–106.
42. Saunes, M.; Øien, T.; Dotterud, C.K.; Romundstad, P.R.; Storrø, O.; Holmen, T.L.; Johnsen, R. Early eczema and the risk of childhood asthma: A prospective, population-based study. *BMC Pediatr.* 2012, *12*.
43. Wood, S.H.; Ollier, W.E.; Nuttall, T.; McEwan, N.A.; Carter, S.D. Despite identifying some shared gene associations with human atopic dermatitis the use of multiple dog breeds from various locations limits detection of gene associations in canine atopic dermatitis. *Vet. Immunol. Immunopathol.* 2010, *138*, 193–197.
44. Marsella, R.; Girolomoni, G. Canine models of atopic dermatitis: A useful tool with untapped potential. *J. Invest. Dermatol.* 2009, *129*, 2351–2357.
45. Olivry, T.; Deangelo, K.B.; Dunston, S.M.; Clarke, K.B.; McCall, C.A. Patch testing of experimentally sensitized beagle dogs: Development of a model for skin lesions of atopic dermatitis. *Vet. Dermatol.* 2006, *17*, 95–102.
46. Amagai, Y.; Matsuda, H.; Tanaka, A. Abnormalities in itch sensation and skin barrier function in atopic NC/Tnd mice.*Biol. Pharm. Bull.* 2013, *36*, 1248–1252.
47. Takeda, K.; Gelfand, E.W. Mouse models of allergic diseases. *Curr. Opin. Immunol.* 2009, *21*, 660–665.
48. Graham, M.T.; Nadeau, K.C. Lessons learned from mice and man: Mimicking human allergy through mouse models.*Clin. Immunol.* 2014, *155*, 1–16.
49. Marsella, R.; Olivry, T.; Nicklin, C.; Lopez, J. Pilot investigation of a model for canine atopic dermatitis: Environmental house dust mite challenge of high-IgE-

producing beagles, mite hypersensitive dogs with atopic dermatitis and normal dogs. *Vet. Dermatol.* 2006, *17*, 24–35.

50. Marsella, R.; Samuelson, D.; Doerr, K. Transmission electron microscopy studies in an experimental model of canine atopic dermatitis. *Vet. Dermatol.* 2010, *21*, 81–88.
51. Fartasch, M.; Bassukas, I.D.; Diepgen, T.L. Disturbed extruding mechanism of lamellar bodies in dry non-eczematous skin of atopics. *Br. J. Dermatol.* 1992, *127*, 221–227.
52. Fartasch, M.; Diepgen, T.L. The barrier function in atopic dry skin. Disturbance of membrane-coating granule exocytosis and formation of epidermal lipids? *Acta. Derm. Venereol. Suppl. (Stockh.)* 1992, *176*, 26–31.
53. Marsella, R.; Samuelson, D.; Harrington, L. Immunohistochemical evaluation of filaggrin polyclonal antibody in atopic and normal beagles. *Vet. Dermatol.* 2009, *20*, 547–554.
54. Santoro, D.; Marsella, R.; Ahrens, K.; Graves, T.K.; Bunick, D. Altered mRNA and protein expression of filaggrin in the skin of a canine animal model for atopic dermatitis. *Vet. Dermatol.* 2013, *24*, 329–336.
55. Eckhart, L.; Tschachler, E. Cuts by caspase-14 control the proteolysis of filaggrin. *J. Invest. Dermatol.* 2011, *131*, 2173–2175.
56. Hvid, M.; Johansen, C.; Deleuran, B.; Kemp, K.; Deleuran, M.; Vestergaard, C. Regulation of caspase 14 expression in keratinocytes by inflammatory cytokines—A possible link between reduced skin barrier function and inflammation?*Exp. Dermatol.* 2011, *20*, 633–636.
57. Yamamoto, M.; Kamata, Y.; Iida, T.; Fukushima, H.; Nomura, J.; Saito, M.; Tajima, M.; Okubo, Y.; Momoi, T.; Tsuboi, R.; *et al.* Quantification of activated and total caspase-14 with newly developed ELISA systems in normal and atopic skin. *J. Dermatol. Sci.* 2011, *61*, 110–117.
58. Papastavros, V.; Marsella, R.; Cronin, M.; Ahrens, K.; Kim, H.J.; Santoro, D. Investigation of caspase-14 expression in canine atopic dermatitis. *Vet. Dermatol.* 2014, *25*, 155.
59. Addor, F.A.; Takaoka, R.; Rivitti, E.A.; Aoki, V. Atopic dermatitis: Correlation between non-damaged skin barrier function and disease activity. *Int. J. Dermatol.* 2012, *51*, 672–676.
60. Simpson, E.L.; Berry, T.M.; Brown, P.A.; Hanifin, J.M. A pilot study of emollient therapy for the primary prevention of atopic dermatitis. *J. Am. Acad. Dermatol.* 2010, *63*, 587–593.
61. Williams, H.C.; Chalmers, J.R.; Simpson, E.L. Prevention of atopic dermatitis. *F1000 Med. Rep.* 2012, *4*.
62. Haahtela, T.; Holgate, S.; Pawankar, R.; Akdis, C.A.; Benjaponpitak, S.; Caraballo, L.; Demain, J.; Portnoy, J.; von Hertzen, L.; WAO Special Committee on Climate Change and Biodiversity. The biodiversity hypothesis and allergic disease: World allergy organization position statement. *World Allergy Organ. J.* 2013, *6*.

63. Hanski, I.; von Hertzen, L.; Fyhrquist, N.; Koskinen, K.; Torppa, K.; Laatikainen, T.; Karisola, P.; Auvinen, P.; Paulin, L.; Mäkelä, M.J.; *et al.* Environmental biodiversity, human microbiota, and allergy are interrelated. *Proc. Natl. Acad. Sci. USA* 2012, *109*, 8334–8339.

64. Legatzki, A.; Rösler, B.; von Mutius, E. Microbiome diversity and asthma and allergy risk. *Curr. Allergy Asthma Rep.*2014, *14*.

65. Sjögren, Y.M.; Jenmalm, M.C.; Böttcher, M.F.; Björkstén, B.; Sverremark-Ekström, E. Altered early infant gut microbiota in children developing allergy up to 5 years of age. *Clin. Exp. Allergy* 2009, *39*, 518–526.

66. Sjögren, Y.M.; Tomicic, S.; Lundberg, A.; Böttcher, M.F.; Björkstén, B.; Sverremark-Ekström, E.; Jenmalm, M.C. Influence of early gut microbiota on the maturation of childhood mucosal and systemic immune responses. *Clin. Exp. Allergy* 2009, *39*, 1842–1851.

67. Kwok, L.Y.; Wang, L.; Zhang, J.; Guo, Z.; Zhang, H. A pilot study on the effect of Lactobacillus casei Zhang on intestinal microbiota parameters in Chinese subjects of different age. *Benef. Microbes.* 2014, *5*, 295–304.

68. Geuking, M.B.; Köller, Y.; Rupp, S.; McCoy, K.D. The interplay between the gut microbiota and the immune system.*Gut Microbes.* 2014, *5*, 411–418.

69. Nermes, M.; Kantele, J.M.; Atosuo, T.J.; Salminen, S.; Isolauri, E. Interaction of orally administered *Lactobacillus rhamnosus* GG with skin and gut microbiota and humoral immunity in infants with atopic dermatitis. *Clin. Exp. Allergy.* 2011, *41*, 370–377.

70. Ismail, I.H.; Licciardi, P.V.; Tang, M.L. Probiotic effects in allergic disease. *J. Paediatr. Child. Health.* 2013, *49*, 709–715.

71. Marsella, R. Evaluation of *Lactobacillus rhamnosus* strain GG for the prevention of atopic dermatitis in dogs. *Am. J. Vet. Res.* 2009, *70*, 735–740.

72. Marsella, R.; Santoro, D.; Ahrens, K. Early exposure to probiotics in a canine model of atopic dermatitis has long-term clinical and immunological effects. *Vet. Immunol. Immunopathol.* 2012, *146*, 185–189.

73. Rodrigues Hoffmann, A.; Patterson, A.P.; Diesel, A.; Lawhon, S.D.; Ly, H.J.; Elkins Stephenson, C.; Mansell, J.; Steiner, J.M.; Dowd, S.E.; Olivry, T.; *et al.* The skin microbiome in healthy and allergic dogs. *PLOS ONE* 2014, *9*.

74. Panduru, M.; Panduru, N.M.; Sălăvăstru, C.M.; Tiplica, G.S. Probiotics and primary prevention of atopic dermatitis: A meta-analysis of randomized controlled studies. *J. Eur. Acad. Dermatol. Venereol.* 2014.

75. Pucheu-Haston, C.M.; Jackson, H.A.; Olivry, T.; Dunston, S.M.; Hammerberg, B. Epicutaneous sensitization with Dermatophagoides farinae induces generalized allergic dermatitis and elevated mite-specific immunoglobulin E levels in a canine model of atopic dermatitis. *Clin. Exp. Allergy* 2008, *38*, 667–679.

76. Olivry, T.; Dean, G.A.; Tompkins, M.B.; Dow, J.L.; Moore, P.F. Toward a canine model of atopic dermatitis: Amplification of cytokine-gene transcripts in the skin of atopic dogs. *Exp. Dermatol.* 1999, *8*, 204–211.

77. Pucheu-Haston, C.M.; Shuster, D.; Olivry, T.; Brianceau, P.; Lockwood, P.; McClanahan, T.; de Waal Malefyt, R.; Mattson, J.D.; Hammerberg, B. A canine model of cutaneous late-phase reactions: Prednisolone inhibition of cellular and cytokine responses. *Immunology* 2006, *117*, 177–187.
78. Stahl, J.; Paps, J.; Bäumer, W.; Olivry, T. Dermatophagoides farinae house dust mite allergen challenges reduce stratum corneum ceramides in an experimental dog model of acute atopic dermatitis. *Vet. Dermatol.* 2012, *23*.
79. Butler, J.M.; Peters, J.E.; Hirshman, C.A.; White, C.R., Jr.; Margolin, L.B.; Hanifin, J.M. Pruritic dermatitis in asthmatic basenji-greyhound dogs: A model for human atopic dermatitis. *J. Am. Acad. Dermatol.* 1983, *8*, 33–38.
80. Peters, J.E.; Hirshman, C.A.; Malley, A. The Basenji-Greyhound dog model of asthma: Leukocyte histamine release, serum IgE, and airway response to inhaled antigen. *J. Immunol.* 1982, *129*, 1245–1249.
81. Hirshman, C.A.; Downes, H.; Leon, D.A.; Peters, J.E. Basenji-greyhound dog model of asthma: Pulmonary responses after beta-adrenergic blockade. *J. Appl. Physiol. Respir. Environ. Exerc. Physiol.* 1981, *51*, 1423–1427.
82. Shiohara, T.; Hayakawa, J.; Mizukawa, Y. Animal models for atopic dermatitis: Are they relevant to human disease? *J. Dermatol. Sci.* 2004, *36*, 1–9.
83. Suto, H.; Matsuda, H.; Mitsuishi, K.; Hira, K.; Uchida, T.; Unno, T.; Ogawa, H.; Ra, C. NC/Nga mice: A mouse model for atopic dermatitis. *Int. Arch. Allergy Immunol.* 1999, *120*, S70–S75.
84. Matsuda, H.; Watanabe, N.; Geba, G.P.; Sperl, J.; Tsudzuki, M.; Hiroi, J.; Matsumoto, M.; Ushio, H.; Saito, S.; Askenase, P.W.; *et al.* Development of atopic dermatitis-like skin lesion with IgE hyperproduction in NC/Nga mice. *Int. Immunol.*1997, *9*, 461–466.
85. Yang, F.; Tanaka, M.; Wataya-Kaneda, M.; Yang, L.; Nakamura, A.; Matsumoto, S.; Attia, M.; Murota, H.; Katayama, I. Topical application of rapamycin ointment ameliorates Dermatophagoides farina body extract-induced atopic dermatitis in NC/Nga mice. *Exp. Dermatol.* 2014.
86. Kim, J.Y.; Jeong, M.S.; Park, M.K.; Lee, M.K.; Seo, S.J. Time-dependent progression from the acute to chronic phases in atopic dermatitis induced by epicutaneous allergen stimulation in NC/Nga mice. *Exp. Dermatol.* 2014, *23*, 53–57.
87. Kim, H.J.; Kim, Y.J.; Kang, M.J.; Seo, J.H.; Kim, H.Y.; Jeong, S.K.; Lee, S.H.; Kim, J.M.; Hong, S.J. A novel mouse model of atopic dermatitis with epicutaneous allergen sensitization and the effect of *Lactobacillus rhamnosus*. *Exp. Dermatol.*2012, *21*, 672–675.
88. Vercelli, D. Of flaky tails and itchy skin. *Nat. Genet.* 2009, *41*, 512–513.
89. Presland, R.B.; Boggess, D.; Lewis, S.P.; Hull, C.; Fleckman, P.; Sundberg, J.P. Loss of normal profilaggrin and filaggrin in flaky tail (*ft/ft*) mice: An animal model for the filaggrin-deficient skin disease ichthyosis vulgaris. *J. Invest. Dermatol.* 2000, *115*, 1072–1081.

90. NIAID-Sponsored Expert Panel; Boyce, J.A.; Assa'ad, A.; Burks, A.W.; Jones, S.M.; Sampson, H.A.; Wood, R.A.; Plaut, M.; Cooper, S.F.; Fenton, M.J.; *et al.* Guidelines for the diagnosis and management of food allergy in the United States: Report of the NIAID-sponsored expert panel. *J. Allergy Clin. Immunol.* 2010, *126*, S1–S58.

91. Prescott, S.; Allen, K.J. Food allergy: Riding the second wave of the allergy epidemic. *Pediatr. Allergy Immunol.* 2011,*22*, 155–160.

92. Amin, A.J.; Davis, C.M. Changes in prevalence and characteristics of IgE-mediated food allergies in children referred to a tertiary care center in 2003 and 2008. *Allergy Asthma Proc.* 2012, *33*, 95–101.

93. Gupta, R.S.; Springston, E.E.; Warrier, M.R.; Smith, B.; Kumar, R.; Pongracic, J.; Holl, J.L. The prevalence, severity, and distribution of childhood food allergy in the United States. *Pediatrics* 2011, *128*, e9–e17.

94. Pałgan, K.; Bartuzi, Z. Gene and environmental interactions of food allergy. *Postepy. Hig. Med. Dosw. (Online)* 2012, *66*, 385–391.

95. Chiang, W.C.; Pons, L.; Kidon, M.I.; Liew, W.K.; Goh, A.; Wesley Burks, A. Serological and clinical characteristics of children with peanut sensitization in an Asian community. *Pediatr. Allergy Immunol.* 2010, *21*, e429–e438.

96. Levy, M.B.; Goldberg, M.R.; Nachshon, L.; Tabachnik, E.; Katz, Y. Lessons from cases of mortality due to food allergy in Israel: Cow's milk protein should be considered a potentially fatal allergen. *Isr. Med. Assoc. J.* 2012, *14*, 29–33.

97. Vetander, M.; Helander, D.; Flodström, C.; Ostblom, E.; Alfvén, T.; Ly, D.H.; Hedlin, G.; Lilja, G.; Nilsson, C.; Wickman, M. Anaphylaxis and reactions to foods in children—A population-based case study of emergency department visits. *Clin. Exp. Allergy* 2012, *42*, 568–577.

98. De Leon, M.P.; Rolland, J.M.; O'Hehir, R.E. The peanut allergy epidemic: Allergen molecular characterisation and prospects for specific therapy. *Expert Rev. Mol. Med.* 2007, *9*, 1–18.

99. Hefle, S.; Nordlee, J.A.; Taylor, S.L. Allergenic foods. *Crit. Rev. Food Sci. Nutr.* 1996, *36*, S69–S89.

100. Sicherer, S.H.; Sampson, H.A. Food allergy. *J. Allergy Clin. Immunol.* 2010, *125*, S116–S125.

101. Wang, J.; Sampson, H.A. Food allergy. *J. Clin. Invest.* 2011, *121*, 827–835.

102. Helm, R.M.; Ermel, R.W.; Frick, O.L. Nonmurine animal models of food allergy. *Environ. Health Perspect.* 2003, *111*, 239–244.

103. Maloney, J.M.; Rudengren, M.; Ahlstedt, S.; Bock, S.A.; Sampson, H.A. The use of serum-specific IgE measurements for the diagnosis of peanut, tree nut, and seed allergy. *J. Allergy Clin. Immunol.* 2008, *122*, 145–151.

104. Helm, R.M.; Burks, Q.W. Animal models of food allergy. *Curr. Opin. Allergy Clin. Immunol.* 2002, *2*, 541–546.

105. Helm, R.M. Food allergy animal models: An overview. *Ann. N. Y. Acad. Sci.* 2002, *964*, 139–150.

106. Srivastava, K.D.; Kattan, J.D.; Zou, Z.M.; Li, J.H.; Zhang, L.; Wallenstein, S.; Goldfarb, J.; Sampson, H.A.; Li, X.M. The Chinese herbal medicine formula FAHF-2 completely blocks anaphylactic reactions in a murine model of peanut allergy. *J. Allergy Clin. Immunol.* 2005, *115*, 171–178.
107. Li, X.M.; Schofield, B.H.; Huang, C.K.; Kleiner, G.I.; Sampson, H.A. A murine model of IgE-mediated cow's milk hypersensitivity. *J. Allergy Clin. Immunol.* 1999, *103*, 206–214.
108. Dearman, R.J.; Stone, S.; Caddick, H.T.; Basketter, D.A.; Kimber, I. Evaluation of protein allergenic potential in mice: Dose-response analyses. *Clin. Exp. Allergy.* 2003, *33*, 1586–1594.
109. Gonipeta, B.; Kim, E.; Gangur, V. Mouse models of food allergy: How well do they simulate the human disorder? *Crit. Rev. Food Sci. Nutr.* 2013.
110. Van Gramberg, J.L.; de Veer, M.J.; O'Hehir, R.E.; Meeusen, E.N.T.; Bischof, R.J. Induction of allergic responses to peanut allergen in sheep. *PLOS ONE* 2012, *7*.
111. Ladics, G.S.; Knippels, L.M.; Penninks, A.H.; Bannon, G.A.; Goodman, R.E.; Herouet-Guicheney, C. Review of animal models designed to predict the potential allergenicity of novel proteins in genetically modified crops. *Regul. Toxicol. Pharmacol.* 2010, *56*, 212–224.
112. Knippels, L.M.; Penninks, A.H.; van Meeteren, M; Houben, G.F. Humoral and cellular immune responses in different rat strains on oral exposure to ovalbumin. *Food Chem. Toxicol.* 1999, *37*, 881–888.
113. Van Gramberg, J.L.; de Veer, M.J.; O'Hehir, R.E.; Meeusen, E.N.; Bischof, R.J. Use of animal models to investigate major allergens associated with food allergy. *J. Allergy (Cairo)* 2013.
114. Favrot, C.; Steffan, J.; Seewald, W.; Picco, F. A prospective study on the clinical features of chronic canine atopic dermatitis and its diagnosis. *Vet. Dermatol.* 2010, *21*, 23–31.
115. Carlotti, D.N.; Remy, I.; Prost, C. Food allergy in dogs and cats: A review and report of 43 cases. *Vet. Dermatol.* 1990, *1*, 55–62.
116. Verlinden, A.; Hesta, M.; Millet, S.; Janssens, G.P. Food allergy in dogs and cats: A review. *Crit. Rev. Food Sci. Nutr.*2006, *46*, 259–273.
117. Jackson, H.A.; Jackson, M.W.; Coblentz, L.; Hammerberg, B. Evaluation of the clinical and allergen specific serum immunoglobulin E responses to oral challenge with cornstarch, corn, soy and a soy hydrolysate diet in dogs with spontaneous food allergy. *Vet. Dermatol.* 2003, *14*, 181–187.
118. Teuber, S.S.; del Val, G.; Morigasaki, S.; Jung, H.R.; Eisele, P.H.; Frick, O.L.; Buchanan, B.B. The atopic dog as a model of peanut and tree nut food allergy. *J. Allergy Clin. Immunol.* 2002, *110*, 921–927.
119. Buchanan, B.B.; Frick, O.L. The dog as a model for food allergy. *Ann. N. Y. Acad. Sci.* 2002, *964*, 173–183.
120. Kennis, R.A. Use of atopic dogs to investigate adverse reactions to food. *J. Am. Vet. Med. Assoc.* 2002, *221*, 638–640.

121. Marsella, R.; Ahrens, K. Experimental model of peanut allergy in dogs after epicutaneous sensitization. *Br. J. Dermatol.*2014, *170*, E4.

122. Matsumoto, K.; Saito, H. Epicutaneous immunity and onset of allergic diseases—Per-"eczema"tous sensitization drives the allergy march. *Allergol. Int.* 2013, *62*, 291–296.

123. McClain, S.; Bannon, G.A. Animal models of food allergy: Opportunities and barriers. *Curr. Allergy Asthma Rep.* 2006,*6*, 141–144.

124. Global Strategy for Asthma Management and Prevention. Available online: http://erj.ersjournals.com/content/31/1/143.full.pdf+html (accessed on 10 October 2014).

125. Chapman, R.W. Canine models for asthma and COPD. *Pulm. Pharmacol. Ther.* 2008, *21*, 731–742.

126. Cabana, M.D.; Kunselman, S.J.; Nyenhuis, S.M.; Wechsler, M.E. Researching asthma across the ages: Insights from the National Heart, Lung, and Blood Institute's Asthma Network. *J. Allergy Clin. Immunol.* 2014, *133*, 27–33.

127. Masoli, M.; Fabian, D.; Holt, S.; Beasley, R. The global burden of asthma: Executive summary of the GINA Dissemination Committee Report. *Allergy* 2004, *59*, 469–478.

128. Subbarao, P.; Mandhane, P.J.; Sears, M.R. Asthma: Epidemiology, etiology and risk factors. *CMAJ* 2009, *181*, E181–E190.

129. Gershon, A.; Guan, J.; Victor, J.C.; Wang, C.; To, T. The course of asthma activity: A population study. *J. Allergy Clin. Immunol.* 2012, *129*, 679–686.

130. Zosky, G.R.; Sly, P.D. Animal models of asthma. *Clin. Exp. Allergy* 2007, *37*, 973–988.

131. Bates, J.H.T. Stochastic-model of the pulmonary airway tree and its implications for bronchial responsiveness. *J. Appl. Physiol.* 1993, *75*, 2493–2499.

132. Barnes, P.J. Corticosteroid effects on cell signalling. *Eur. Respir. J.* 2006, *27*, 413–426.

133. Eriksson, U.; Egermann, U.; Bihl, M.P.; Gambazzi, F.; Tamm, M.; Holt, P.G.; Bingisser, R.M. Human bronchial epithelium controls TH2 responses by TH1-induced, nitric oxide-mediated STAT5 dephosphorylation: Implications for the pathogenesis of asthma. *J. Immunol.* 2005, *175*, 2715–2720.

134. Howat, W.J.; Holgate, S.T.; Lackie, P.M. TGF-β isoform release and activation during *in vitro* bronchial epithelial wound repair. *Am. J. Physiol.* 2002, *282*, L115–L123.

135. Szelenyi, I. Animal models of bronchial asthma. *Inflamm. Res.* 2000, *49*, 639–654.

136. Taube, C.; Dakhama, A.; Gelfand, E.W. Insights into the pathogenesis of asthma utilizing murine models. *Int. Arch. Allergy Immunol.* 2004, *135*, 173–186.

137. Turner, D.J.; Myron, P.; Powell, W.S.; Martin, J.G. The role of endogenous corticosterone in the late-phase response to allergen challenge in the brown

Norway rat. *Am. J. Respir. Crit. Care Med.* 1996, *153*, 545–550.

138. Reinero, C.; DeClue, A.; Rabinowitz, P. Asthma in humans and cats: Is there a common sensitivity to aeroallergens in shared environments? *Environ. Res.* 2009, *109*, 634–640.
139. Kirschvink, N.; Leemans, J.; Delvaux, F.; Snaps, F.; Clercx, C.; Gustin, P. Non-invasive assessment of airway responsiveness in healthy and allergen sensitized cats by use of barometric whole body plethysmography. *Vet. J.* 2007,*173*, 343–352.
140. Norris Reinero, C.; Decile, K.; Berghaus, R.; Williams, K.; Leutenegger, C.; Walby, W.; Schelegle, E.; Hyde, D.; Gershwin, L. An experimental model of allergic asthma in cats sensitized to house dust mite or Bermuda grass allergen. *Int. Arch. Allergy Immunol.* 2004, *135*, 117–131.
141. Padrid, P.; Snook, S.; Finucane, T. Persistent airway hyperresponsiveness and histologic alterations after chronic antigen challenge in cats. *Am. J. Resp. Crit. Care Med.* 1995, *151*, 184–193.
142. Expert Panel Report 3: Guidelines for the Diagnosis and Management of Asthma. Available online: http://www.nhlbi.nih.gov/health-pro/guidelines/current/asthma-guidelines/full-report (accessed on 20 October 2014).
143. Haliwell, R.E.W.; Schwartzmann, R.M. Atopic diseases in the dog. *Vet. Rec.* 1971, *89*, 209–214.
144. De Weck, A.L.; Mayer, P.; Stumper, B.; Schiessel, B.; Pickat, L. Dog allergy, a model for allergy genetics. *Int. Arch. Allergy Immunol.* 1997, *113*, 55–57.
145. Collie, D.D.; DeBoer, D.J.; Muggenburg, B.A.; Bice, D.E. Evaluation of association of blood and bronchoalveolar eosinophil number and serum total immunoglobulin. *Am. J. Vet. Res.* 1997, *58*, 34–39.
146. Redman, T.K.; Rudolph, K.; Barr, E.B.; Bowan, L.E.; Muggenburg, B.A.; Bice, D.E. Pulmonary immunity to ragweed in a beagle dog model of allergic asthma. *Exp. Lung Res.* 2001, *27*, 433–451.
147. Meeusen, E.N.; Snibson, K.J.; .Hirst, S.J.; Bischof, R.J. Sheep as a model species for the study and treatment of human asthma and other respiratory diseases. *Drug Discov. Today* 2009, *6*, 101–106.
148. Bischof, R.J.; Snibson, K.; Shaw, R.; Meeusen, E.N. Induction of allergic inflammation in the lungs of sensitized sheep after local challenge with house dust mite. *Clin. Exp. Allergy* 2003, *33*, 367–375.
149. Abraham, W.M. Pharmacology of allergen-induced early and late airway responses and antigen-induced airway hyperresponsiveness in allergic sheep. *Pulm. Pharmacol.* 1989, *2*, 33–40.
150. Scheerlinck, J.P.; Snibson, K.J.; Bowles, V.M.; Sutton, P. Biomedical applications of sheep models: From asthma to vaccines. *Trends Biotechnol.* 2008, *26*, 259–266.
151. Gomez, F.P.; Rodriguez-Roisin, R. Platelet-activating factor antagonists—Current status in asthma. *BioDrugs* 2000, *14*, 21–30.

15
CHAPTER

FROM "ONE HEALTH" TO "ONE COMMUNICATION": THE CONTRIBUTION OF COMMUNICATION IN VETERINARY MEDICINE TO PUBLIC HEALTH

Micaela Cipolla, Luigi Bonizzi and Alfonso Zecconi

Keywords: Communication, One Health, public health, antimicrobial resistance, food safety, food-producing animals, risk communication, companion animal practice

INTRODUCTION

Health Communication is a discipline only recently developed, and it is "The study of how health information is generated and disseminated and how that information affects individuals, community groups, institutions and public policy" [1].

The aim of health communication is to inform and influence people's behaviour and attitude in order to improve health [2,3,4]. This is possible because it concerns all aspects of health, including, *i.e.*, research, clinical practice, public health, global health and policy making [5,6]. Different approaches are available to investigate all of the aspects, *i.e.*, health campaigns, risk communication and patient-provider communication.

An effective communication is essential to public health. It can be written and verbal, taking many forms and using various channels such as physicians and other health professionals, family, friends and mass media, Internet, advertisement. For its growing importance, the World Health Organization (WHO) includes health communication in its activities and provides several guides supporting communication strategies development for different situations, such as health emergencies and disease

Citation: Micaela Cipolla, Luigi Bonizzi and Alfonso Zecconi, From "One Health" to "One Communication": The Contribution of Communication in Veterinary Medicine to Public Health, doi:10.3390/vetsci2030135.

prevention [7,8,9,10,11,12,13]. Moreover, WHO considers communication expertise as essential to outbreak control as well as epidemiological training and laboratory analysis, and demonstrated a significant reduction of cases during an outbreak when applied a proactive communication [14,15]. Many other institutions, such as UNICEF, FAO, CDC, Johns Hopkins University and others agree that communication is a necessary tool for public health [16,17,18,19,20,21,22,23,24,25,26,27,28].

Any advice aiming to enhance health by changing people's behaviour is a communicative act. Health communication allows to identify contexts, channels, messages and factors having the potential to motivate individuals to use correctly health information. Therefore, health communication supports health professionals in their daily work, educates patients and helps policy makers; it has a powerful role in disease prevention and health promotion. It is part of health management, even in settings with limited resources, helping to use information and interacting with the community or other partners.

Due to its pivotal importance, health communication became part of the curriculum in several Medicine and Veterinary Medicine Schools worldwide, but usually health communication refers to human health and it is generally less considered in veterinary medicine. The intended outcome of this article is to describe this new aspect of veterinary medicine—the health communication—and its contribution to public health. With our paper we highlight the role of communication in the main branches of veterinary activity, to help veterinarians to find their role in the "One communication" perspective. Indeed, communication in veterinary medicine has the potential to contribute to public health and should be considered in a One Health perspective.

One Health

The One Health concept links human, animal and environmental health, it is "a worldwide strategy for expanding interdisciplinary collaborations and communications in all aspects of health care for humans, animals and the environment. The synergism achieved will advance health care for the 21st century and beyond by accelerating biomedical research discoveries, enhancing public health efficacy, expeditiously expanding the scientific knowledge base, and improving medical education and clinical care."[29]. This approach considers all global health threats to gain cross-disciplinary collaboration, especially between physicians and veterinarians. The result is a collaborative effort to enhance human and animal health between the health professions.

One Health has its origins in the 1800s, when Rudolf Virchow, the German physician who coined the term "zoonosis", highlighted the linkages between human and veterinary medicine [30]. In the following years, other physicians and veterinarians recognized the importance of good animal health for the public health. One of them, Calvin Schwabe, made important contributions to epidemiology, zoonoses, tropical health and public health. He coined the term "One medicine", emphasizing the close interdependence and similarities between human and veterinary medicine [31]. More recently, the Wildlife Conservation Society promoted a symposium to discuss the movements of diseases among human, domestic animal and wildlife populations. The symposium set twelve priorities—the Manhattan Principles—for an interdisciplinary strategy to combat diseases and maintain the ecosystem integrity. These principles considered, with human and animal health, also environment health [32].

The One Health approach has been endorsed by the main global health organizations, such as WHO, CDC, EFSA, OIE, FAO [33,34,35,36,37]. The collaborative effort between human and veterinary medicine should be applied not only at global level but also at local level, where it could be a new paradigm of health management [38]. This will result in a more effective and sustainable organization of public health, reducing the risk of zoonotic diseases such as rabies, H5N1 avian influenza, West Nile disease, TBC and diseases caused by E. coli STEC, *Staphylococcus aureus* MRSA, Nipah and Hendra viruses, Hantaviruses, Filovirus such as Ebola and Marburg viruses.

VETERINARY MEDICINE AND PUBLIC HEALTH

The purpose of veterinary medicine is to protect public health, through the promotion of animal health and food safety. To fulfil this objective, veterinary medicine has many arenas of activity in public health, including (Figure 1):

- Institutions (health authority, healthcare system)
- Food safety and nutrition
- Clinical practice
    - companion animals
    - food-producing animals
- Pharmacology and drugs
- Wildlife fauna
- Environment

In all these fields, communication has a key role and can contribute to public health by influencing people's behaviour and attitude.

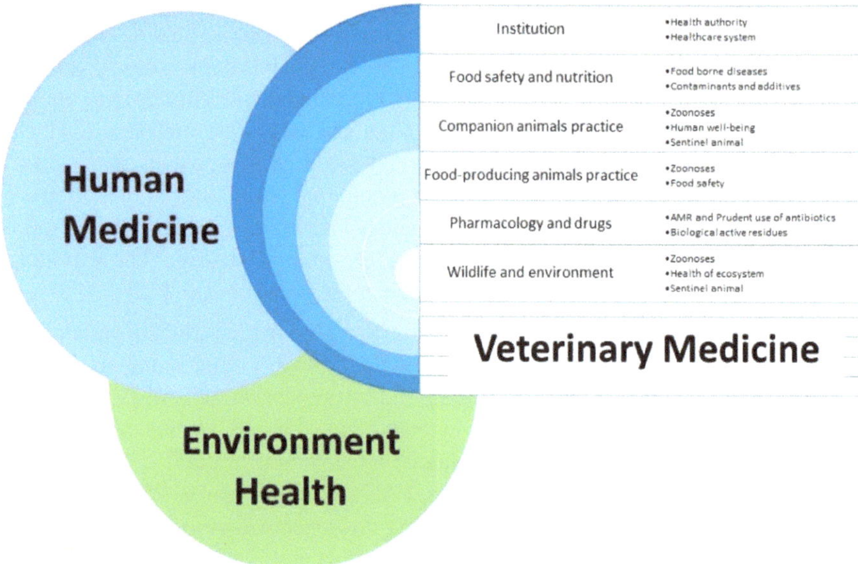

Figure 1: Potential contributes of veterinary medicine to public health in a One Health and One Communication perspective.

Institutions

Health care authorities and systems have the responsibility to manage health system, and communication is part of the management. Therefore, the role of communication is related to the institutional setting. We reported, as example, one European health system. In the Italian health system, communication for human and veterinary medicine is unique at the higher institutional level, because the Ministry of Health (Ministero della Salute) manages both. At lower regional and local institutional level, health authorities work separately on human and animal health, so the communication efforts often are uncoordinated. However, the institutional communication in veterinary medicine gives a high contribution to public health, because of the continuous overlapping between veterinary and human medicine in public health. This institutional activity includes, for example, health campaigns on zoonoses or food safety [39,40].

This organization of veterinary system has both pros and cons. The major benefit of the integration in the Ministry of Health is that the veterinary health system has a peculiar focus on health, and it is much less biased by production aspects, when compared to the systems under the Ministry of Agriculture. However, the focus on health, sometimes, put an excessive pressure on the production system, reducing its efficiency, by applying unnecessary barriers to the production process. At the local level, the system splits into the two components of human and veterinary medicine, and this disconnection gives to the veterinary medicine the opportunity to be more independent and effective in a given area, even if a coordination would be hopeful.

Moreover, the veterinary diseases surveillance networks have a key role in human surveillance and its utility would be increased through a better integration between the two systems, as happens through the joining of health service [41]. Likewise, a coordination also at the communicative level would produce more efficient efforts in enhancing public health. Also at policy and management levels, communication has a key role, as demonstrated by the example of Regional Veterinary Prevention Plan 2012–2014 (Piano Regionale della Prevenzione Veterinaria 2012–2014) of Regione Lombardia [42]. This was a new and powerful tool for public health, supporting veterinary health system at regional level, giving to all the operative units and officers an unique and coherent frame of reference [43]. Indeed, our research group developed a model (scorecard) to assess zoonoses and food safety issues. The scorecard supports daily practice setting priority in prevention and risk management, by assigning different scores to various risk and management aspects of each disease or food safety problem. Once this assignation has been done, the veterinary officers know the priority of each intervention and, also, if there is a lack of information about the specific disease. This model established a completely new approach to risk characterization in Italian public health authorities; it had to be understood and adopted by all the personnel involved in the regional veterinary system and, for this reason, communication was crucial. Both internal and external communication strategies were needed. All the members of the regional healthcare system were the audiences of internal communication: Regione Lombardia, local health authorities (Azienda Sanitaria Locale), regional diagnostic and surveillance laboratory (Istituto Zooprofilattico Sperimentale della Lombardia e dell'Emilia Romagna), research centers. At internal level, the aims of communication were to verify the outcomes of the plan application, to share information and to consolidate cooperation. External communication was addressed to stakeholders, with the aims to involve people, gather information and share results. All the initiatives, planned to inform and involve the target audience, were focused on objectives and results of the prevention plan application. However, the first communication need concerned the plan itself, and the understanding of the new risk characterization praxis. Indeed, the document was very articulated; it had many tables (the scorecards) and schemes for disease control plans, prevention protocols and risk characterization, each one concerning one of the veterinary areas. Indeed, in Italy the veterinary health system has three areas: A for animal health, B for food safety and C for herd management and animal welfare. One of the parameters considered for an effective communication of the plan was its graphic aspect. Due to the high amount and complexity of information delivered, we chose a simple and immediate graphic aspect, assigning a specific colour to each area. Every piece of information addressed to the animal health sector was green, to the food safety sector was red and to the herd management and animal welfare sector was yellow. Everything concerning the past or general topics was blue. This simple color code had a very useful function clarifying the whole document and making it more understandable. Moreover, this code made every local health authority having the same color for the same unit. All the veterinary officers recognized themselves in the color of their area, independently by the district of the local health authority. Therefore, the primary aim of the plan—to make uniform veterinary health system to improve public health—was achieved also with this simple communicative choice, and it was maintained also in the subsequent edition of the plan [44].]

Food Safety and Nutrition

Communication on food safety and nutrition frequently pertains to veterinary medicine, being related to food-borne disease, GMO, contaminants, additives and foods of animal origin.

Consumers receive much information about food, but often it is contradictory and conflicting. This includes alerts, recommendation on what is good for health and what could be dangerous, risks and benefits associate in the same food, food components to reduce, nutrients to increase, warning on different diets and eating styles. All this information provide a non-unique frame of reference, which is difficult to manage and to understand by consumers. Sometimes unfounded concerns may overlap reliable messages from health authorities, resulting in more confusion and uncertainty [45]; especially during an alert or an outbreak, this situation may lead to fear and distrust in the product involved. Examples are the recent European food scares on *E. coli* in vegetables, horsemeat scandal, blue mozzarella cheese, BSE and avian influenza.

The health and welfare of food-producing animals during breeding, transportation and slaughtering have consequences for human health and are responsibility of veterinarians. Therefore, due to the pivotal role of veterinary medicine in animal nutrition, animal health, food inspection and food safety, communication in this area is important for public health, contributing to consumers' protection from field to fork.

Communication about food is often risk communication. Accordingly with the Codex Alimentarius Commission (CAC), risk communication is "an interactive exchange of information and opinions concerning risk among risk assessors, risk managers, consumers and other interested parties [46]. Therefore, food risk communication enables informed decision-making to promote health, fosters the understanding of both the real and the perceived food risk, and shares knowledge between government officials, health professionals, academicians, food producers, stakeholders, journalists and public. Misleading messages can have serious consequences not only on public health but also on the entire food supply chain. Thanks to a proper communication, authorities, experts and other stakeholders can communicate more successfully, making the public reacting properly [47].

To meet these needs, many local and international organizations, such as EFSA and FAO, promoted food risk communication [48,49].

Clinical Practice

Companion Animals

Companion animals, due to their close relationship with people, are important in the prevention of zoonoses and in their management. Moreover, pets have a role as sentinel animal and could be used to protect human health. For example, they are useful in cancer prevention and treatment in humans, because often they share the same risk and carcinogen factors, have many of the same types of cancer and are treated almost with the same drugs as humans [50]. Communication on such topics can contribute significantly to public health [51].

However, the focus of veterinary medicine in public health is not limited to zoonoses, because the One Health concept involves all of the aspects of health, including mental health via the human-animal bond phenomenon [52]. This latter aspect gives to the veterinary medicine a further role in public health, through disciplines centred on human-animal bond such as pet therapy. Moreover, the One Health statement amplifies the role of companion animals clinical practice in maintaining and improving human health, because it concerns not only zoonoses but also the owner-pet relationship.

The importance of communication in clinical practice has been widely recognized, even if only recently in veterinary medicine, where effective communication increases client satisfaction and compliance [53,54,55,56,57,58,59,60]. Therefore, this skill has become part of the veterinary education programs in many countries, being as important as other clinical skills [54,61,62,63].

However, in many European countries communication is still poorly considered. This situation may lead to communication errors, failures in meeting client expectations and, eventually, to complaint or malpractice claim as has been observed in human medicine [64]. Recent studies showed that in one of these countries, the large majority of pet owners consider the own pet as family member and this also affected owner responses and attitudes towards the veterinarian [65]. These results confirm the role of communication in improving veterinary practice and promoting clients' comfort, satisfaction and well-being.

Food-Producing Animals

Communication has a key role also in food-producing animals practice, improving management and animal health, as demonstrated for example in dairy farms [66,67,68].

Communication strategies are essential in promoting dairy herd health and are required to support diseases control programs [69,70]. Indeed, how consultant delivers information affects ideas, beliefs and motivation of the farmer, thus his/her behaviour and actions. [71,72,73]. Therefore, the leading role of communication in dairy herds is due to its power in influencing how farmers apply consultants' advice and, thus, in improving animal health and food safety. It is crucial for public health in a "from field to fork" perspective, because farmer's actions and management directly influence the quality of meat, milk and milk products.

All these aspects improve also herd sustainability. An effective communication in food-producing area supports development and improves health and innovation, also in emerging countries.

However, communication in veterinary practice is poorly considered in many countries including Italy. In this country, recent studies showed that dairy farmers are not satisfied with their consultants' communication [74]. This gap in veterinarians' skill represent a problem because an effective farmer-veterinarian communication is essential to improve farm management, herd health, food safety and herd sustainability.

Pharmacology and Drugs

The activity of veterinarians related to pharmacology and drugs is often cross-disciplinary, covering companion and food producing animal practice, food security, and official drugs residue controls. However, the rising importance of prudent use of antibiotics makes this topic suitable to become a specific area under the One Health approach. Indeed, the concern on antimicrobial resistance (AMR) increased in recent years; it is considered a major public health threat, due to misuse of antibiotics in both human and animal therapy. Therefore, it is a cross-disciplinary issue, engaging veterinarians to reduce and monitor antimicrobial usage in livestock [75,76].

Many veterinary organisations promote the responsible and prudent use of antimicrobial agents in animals, such as The World Organisation for Animal Health (OIE) [77]. Moreover, OIE developed standards and guidelines for OIE Member Countries to address the risk of the emergence or spread of resistant bacteria that result from the use of antimicrobial agents in food producing animals [78].

The European Medicines Agency (EMA) implemented the European Surveillance of Veterinary Antimicrobial Consumption (ESVAC) project, to identify possible risk factors that could lead to the development and spread of antimicrobial resistance in animals. The aim was to develop a harmonised approach for the collection and reporting of data on the use of antimicrobial agents in animals from EU Member States. Thus, EMA published reports on sales of veterinary antimicrobial agents in EU/EEA countries [79]. The International Dairy Federation (FIL-IDF) published a Guide to Prudent Use of Antimicrobial Agents in Dairy Production [80] and also the Federation of Veterinarians of Europe (FVE) developed a document on AMR and prudent use of antibiotics in Veterinary Medicine [81]. A specific interest on this topic was shown by U.S. Food and Drug Administration (FDA) and the U.S. Centers for Disease Control and Prevention (CDC) [82,83]. The latter one funded the development of the Antimicrobial Resistance Learning Site (AMRLS), which is a suite of educational materials promoting the prudent use of antimicrobial agents in veterinary practice [84]. Despite the large interest of veterinary sector on AMR, the communication was poorly considered. However, communication in veterinary medicine can promote the prudent use of antimicrobials, being synergic with the initiatives in human medicine. To highlight the problem and to support a rational antimicrobial use, the European Union promoted the European Awareness Day, an health initiative marked annually on 18 November and coordinated by European Center for Diseases Prevention and Control (ECDC). For this event, ECDC provides campaign communication materials for the European national health authorities in order to develop a consistent communication campaign on the prudent use of antibiotics. National campaigns use several communication tools, such as leaflets, poster, videos, websites and social media, that are aimed to both prescribers and the general public. Many communication initiatives take place across Europe, to disseminate messages on risks related to the antibiotic misuse and explaining how to take antibiotics responsibly [85,86,87]. Similar campaigns are promoted also in the United States, Canada and Australia [88,89].

All these programs show the importance of communication in human medicine to contain AMR, but communication in veterinary medicine is equally indispensable to promote a rational use of antibiotics and enhance the collaboration of veterinary organisations with the public health sector to reduce the antimicrobial resistance.

Wildlife Fauna and Environment

The One Health concept considers also the health of ecosystem, being health of humans, animals and environment interrelated. Indeed, both animals and humans live in the same environment, sharing air, water and food. If there is a poor health for the environment, there is a poor health for people and animals. The environmental pollution is a health hazards but it is not the only threat, because the health of plants is indispensable for having food [90]. Through an effective and responsible management of the natural resources, the One Health approach protects human and animal health and ensures a safe food supply [36,37]. Veterinary medicine can contribute to the health of the ecosystem, because agricultural contamination may lead to contamination of foods of animal origin. Moreover, these foods can be used as sentinel for monitoring contamination in the environment. For example, pesticide contamination of honey can be related to the contamination source and could reflect the specific pollution of an environment [91]. The use of animal sentinel for health hazards is very helpful to detect and manage more quickly and efficiently shared health risks [92]. Also when considering toxic risk, as shown by the potentials of "One Toxicology", the protection of domestic and wild animals' health is relevant to protecting humans [93].

In recent years the emerging diseases gained a leading role in epidemics on a global scale, and zoonoses were dominant [94]. These diseases are currently the main and global threat for human health, and are related to both domestic and wildlife fauna. Therefore, the synergy between medicine and veterinary medicine is indispensable for the research, the surveillance, the control and the communication of global health challenges at the animal-human-ecosystem interface [95]. The result of this cooperation is well known in developing countries, where it already resulted in an improved health care for the local populations [96]. Also in this area of veterinary medicine, coordinated communication efforts make an important contribution to public health.

CONCLUSIONS

In almost all the areas of veterinary activity communication can contribute to human health. It takes many forms and employs several channels, and this variety of communication opportunities represent a challenge for veterinarians. For this reason, communication courses should be included in the curricula of Veterinary Medicine Schools, as it happened in some already in North America.

Veterinarians should improve their communication skills because human and animal health are interrelated, as is health communication in human and veterinary sectors. Both of them cover the same issue (zoonoses, food safety *etc.*) and use the same channels. For example, it is not possible to differentiate between food risk communication in human and veterinary areas, having the same target, using the same strategies and considering the same risks.

Despite the fact that health communication is a recent matter, it has a growing importance in human medicine but it is less considered in veterinary medicine. However, because of the role of veterinary medicine in public health, communication in veterinary area also has the potential to improve public health. Therefore, a One Health approach applies to communication as well, leading to the "One Communication" concept, which is the result of the synergy in communicative efforts both in human and in veterinary medicine. As One Health, One Communication is a strategy for expanding collaborations in health communication and it will enhance health care.

AUTHOR CONTRIBUTIONS

Micaela Cipolla conceived and designed the study, wrote the paper; Luigi Bonizzi designed the study, revised the paper; Alfonso Zecconi designed the study, revised the paper.

REFERENCES

1. Harvard School of Public Health. The Field of Health Communication. Available online: http://www.hsph.harvard.edu/health-communication/ (accessed on 17 May 2015).
2. Hornik, R.C. *Public Health Communication—Evidence for Behavior Change*; Routledge-Lawrence Erlbaum Associates: Mahwah, NJ, USA, 2002.
3. CDC. What is Health Communications? Available online: http://www.cdc.gov/healthcommunication/healthbasics/whatishc.html (accessed on 17 May 2015).
4. National Cancer Institute; Public Health Service; National Institutes of Health. *Making Health Communication Programs Work (Pink Book)*; U.S. Department of Health & Human Services: Washington, DC, USA, 2002.
5. Wickremasinghe, D. What makes for good health communication? In *Global Health Communication—Global Health Histories*; WHO: Geneve, Switzerland, 2013.
6. Rajiv, N.; Rimal, M.; Lapinski, K. Why health communication is important in public health. *Bull. WHO* 2009, *87*, 247–247.
7. WHO. Special theme issue: Public health communication. *Bull. WHO* 2009, *87*, 565–644.
8. *Afghanistan Report—Health Communication*; WHO: Geneve, Switzerland, 2003; p. 19.
9. Obregón, R.; Chitnis, K.; Morry, C.; Feek, W.; Bates, J.; Galway, M.; Ogden, E. Achieving polio eradication: A review of health communication evidence and lessons learned in India and Pakistan. *Bull. WHO* 2009, *87*, 624–630.

10. WHO. Create HPV vaccination communication strategies. Available online: http://www.who.int/immunization/hpv/communicate/en/ (accessed on 17 May 2015).

11. WHO. *HPV Vaccine Communication—Special Considerations for A Unique Vaccine*; WHO: Geneve, Switzerland, 2013.

12. Parks, W.; Lloyd, L. *Planning Social Mobilization and Communication for Dengue Fever Prevention and Control*; WHO: Geneve, Switzerland, 2004.

13. *Effective Media Communication During Public Health Emergencies*; WHO: Geneve, Switzerland, 2005.

14. WHO. *World Health Organization Outbreak Communication Planning Guide*; WHO: Geneve, Switzerland, 2008.

15. WHO. *Outbreak Communication Guidelines*; WHO: Geneve, Switzerland, 2005.

16. UNICEF. Communication for development. Available online: http://www.unicef.org/cbsc (accessed on 17 May 2015).

17. Waisbord, S.; Larson, H.J. Why Invest in Communication for Immunization? Evidence and Lessons Learned. A Joint Publication the Health Communication Partnership Based at Johns Hopkins Bloomberg School of Public Health/Center for Communication Programs (Baltimore) and the United Nations Children's Fund (New York). 2005. Available online: http://www.who.int/immunization/hpv/communicate/why_invest_in_communication_for_immunization_unicef_healthcommunicationspartnership_path_usaid.pdf (accessed on 10 July 2015).

18. O'Sullivan, G.A.; Yonkler, J.A.; Morgan, W.; Merritt, A.P. *A Field Guide to Designing a Health Communication Strategy*; Johns Hopkins Bloomberg School of Public Health/Center for Communication Programs: Baltimore, MD, USA, 2003.

19. United Nations Children's Fund Regional Office for South Asia. *Strategic Communication for Behaviour and Social Change in South Asia*; UNICEF: Kathmandu, Nepal, 2005.

20. Wittet, S. *Hepatitis B Vaccine Introduction—Lessons Learned in Advocacy,Communication and Training*; PATH: Seattle, WA, USA, 2001.

21. WHO; UNICEF; FAO. *Communication for Behavioural Impact—A Toolkit for Behavioural and Social Communication in Outbreak Response*; WHO: Geneve, Switzerland, 2012.

22. Feig, C. WHO: Communicating for health. In *Global Health Communication—Global Health Histories*; WHO: Geneve, Switzerland, 2013.

23. Zaman, F.; Underwood, C. *The Gender Guide for Health Communication Programmes*; Johns Hopkins Bloomberg School of Public Health, Center for Communication Programs: Baltimore, MD, USA, 2003.

24. U.S. Department of Health and Human Services Office of Disease Prevention and Health Promotion. *A Quick Guide to Health Literacy: Fact Sheets, Strategies, Resources*; U.S. Department of Health and Human Services, Office of Disease Prevention and Health Promotion: Washington, DC, USA, 2005.

25. Department for International Development. *Radio Broadcasting for Health—A*

Decision Makers Guide; Information and Communication for Development, UK Department for International Development: London, UK, 2004.

26. CDC. Gateway to Health Communication & Social Marketing Practice. Available online: http://www.cdc.gov/healthcommunication/about.html (accessed on 17 May 2015).
27. US Department of Health and Human Services. Health Communication, Health Literacy, and E-Health. Available online: http://www.health.gov/communication/Default.asp (accessed on 17 May 2015).
28. FAO; OIE. *Global Animal Health Communication Strategy to Support Prevention and Control of H5N1*; HPAI FAO/OIE International Animal Health Communicators' Roundtable in Support of the FAO/OIE Global Strategy for the Prevention and Control of HPAI: Rome, Italy; Paris, France, 2007.
29. One Health Initiative. About the One Health Initiative. Available online: http://www.onehealthinitiative.com/about.php (accessed on 17 May 2015).
30. CDC. History of One Health. Available online: http://www.cdc.gov/onehealth/people-events.html (accessed on 16 June 2015).
31. Schwabe, C. *Veterinary Medicine and Human Health*; Williams & Wilkins Co.: Baltimore, MD, USA, 1964.
32. The Manhattan Principles. Available online: http://www.cdc.gov/onehealth/pdf/manhattan/twelve_manhattan_principles.pdf (accessed on 16 June 2015).
33. CDC. One Health. Available online: http://www.cdc.gov/onehealth/ (accessed on 17 May 2015).
34. EFSA. *Programming Document 2015-2017*; EFSA: Parma, Italy, 2014.
35. OIE. One Health. Available online: http://www.oie.int/for-the-media/onehealth/oie-involvement/ (accessed on 17 May 2015).
36. FAO. *One Health: Food and Agriculture Organization of the United Nations Strategic Action Plan*; FAO: Rome, Italy, 2011.
37. FAO. FAO workshop leverages country case studies for stronger collaboration on One Health. Available online: http://www.fao.org/ag/againfo/programmes/en/empres/news_041013.html (accessed on 17 May 2015).
38. OIE. One Health at a Glance. Available online: http://www.oie.int/for-the-media/onehealth/ (accessed on 17 May 2015).
39. Ministero della Salute. Influenza Aviaria. Available online: http://www.salute.gov.it/portale/temi/p2_6.jsp?lingua=italiano&id=816&area=Malattie%20infettive&menu=altremalattie (accessed on 17 May 2015).
40. Ministero della Salute. Infezione da Virus West Nile. Available online: http://www.salute.gov.it/portale/temi/p2_6.jsp?lingua=italiano&id=1201&area=Malattie%20infettive&menu=altremalattie (accessed on 17 May 2015).
41. Zinsstag, J.; Schelling, E.; Bonfoh, B.; Fooks, A.R.; Kasymbekov, J.; Toews, D.W.; Tanner, M. Towards a One Health research and application tool box. *Vet. Ita.* 2009, *45*, 121–133.

42. Bonizzi, L.; Cipolla, M.; Grieco, V.; Grilli, G.; Lanfranchi, P.; Mortarino, M.; Zecconi, A. *Piano regionale della prevenzione veterinaria 2012-2014*; Regione Lombardia: Milano, Italy, 2011.

43. Scali, F.; Bonizzi, L.; Ferrero, F.; Frazzi, P.; Grilli, G.; Lanfranchi, P.; Mortarino, M.; Sala, V.; Taloni, D.; Zecconi, A. Risk prioritization as a tool to guide veterinary public health activities at regional level. *Vet.Ita.* 2014. in press.

44. Alfonso Zecconi, U.O.V.R. *Piano regionale integrato della sanità pubblica veterinaria 2015-2018*; Regione Lombardia DG Sanità: Milano, Italy, 2014.

45. EFSA. Risk Communication. Available online: http://www.efsa.europa.eu/en/efsawhat/riskcommunication.htm(accessed on 17 May 2015).

46. FAO; WHO. *Codex Alimentarius Commission Report of the Twenty-Second Session*; FAO: Rome, Italy, 1997.

47. EFSA. Risk communication: Making it clear, timely and relevant. Available online: http://www.efsa.europa.eu/en/press/news/120711e.htm (accessed on 17 May 2015).

48. FAO. *The Application of Risk Communication to Food Standards and Safety Matters*; FAO: Rome, Italy, 1998.

49. EFSA. *When Food is Cooking Up a Storm—Proven Recipes for Risk Communications*; EFSA: Parma, Italy, 2012.

50. Thamm, D.; Dow, S. How companion animals contribute to the fight against cancer in humans. *Vet. Ita.* 2009, *45*, 111–120.

51. Ministero della Salute. *Rabbia—conoscere per prevenire*; Istituto Zooprofilattico Sperimentale delle Venezie: Legnaro, Italy, 2010.

52. One Health Initiative. Mission Statement. Available online: http://www.onehealthinitiative.com/mission.php (accessed on 17 May 2015).

53. Grant, C.H.; Cissna, K.N.; Rosenfeld, L.B. Patients' perceptions of physicians communication and outcomes of the accrual to trial process. *Health Commun.* 2000, *12*, 23–39.

54. Shaw, J.R.; Adams, C.L.; Bonnett, B.N. What can veterinarians learn from studies of physician-patient communication about veterinarian-client-patient communication? *J. Am. Vet. Med. Assoc.* 2004, *224*, 676–684.

55. Kurtz, S.M. *Teaching and Learning Communication Skills in Medicine*, 2nd ed.; Radcliffe Publishing: Oxford, UK, 2005.

56. Kanji, N.; Coe, J.B.; Adams, C.L.; Shaw, J.R. Effect of veterinarian-client-patient interactions on client adherence to dentistry and surgery recommendations in companion-animal practice. *J. Am. Vet. Med. Assoc.* 2012, *240*, 427–436.

57. Chadderdon, L.M.; King, L.J.; Lloyd, J.W. The skills, knowledge, aptitudes, and attitudes of successful veterinarians: A summary of presentations to the NCVEI subgroup (Brook Lodge, Augusta, Michigan, December 4–6, 2000). *J. Vet. Med. Educ.* 2001, *28*, 28–30.

58. Coe, J.B.; Adams, C.L.; Bonnett, B.N. A focus group study of veterinarians'

and pet owners' perceptions of veterinarian-client communication in companion animal practice. *J. Am. Vet. Med. Assoc.* 2008, *233*, 1072–1080.

59. Shaw, J.R.; Bonnett, B.N.; Roter, D.L.; Adams, C.L.; Larson, S. Gender differences in veterinarian-client-patient communication in companion animal practice. *J. Am. Vet. Med. Assoc.* 2012, *241*, 81–88.
60. Shaw, J.R.; Adams, C.L.; Bonnett, B.N.; Larson, S.; Roter, D.L. Veterinarian satisfaction with companion animal visits.*J. Am. Vet. Med. Assoc.* 2012, *240*, 832–841.
61. Adams, C.L.; Kurtz, S.M. Building on existing models from human medical education to develop a communication curriculum in veterinary medicine. *J. Vet. Med. Educ.* 2006, *33*, 28–37.
62. Latham, C.E.; Morris, A. Effects of formal training in communication skills on the ability of veterinary students to communicate with clients. *Vet. Rec.* 2007, *160*, 181–186.
63. Martin, F.; Ruby, K.L.; Deking, T.M.; Taunton, A.E. Factors associated with client, staff, and student satisfaction regarding small animal euthanasia procedures at a veterinary teaching hospital. *J. Am. Vet. Med. Assoc.* 2004, *224*, 1774–1779.
64. Beckman, H.B.; Markakis, K.M.; Suchman, A.L.; Frankel, R.M. The doctor-patient relationship and malpractice. Lessons from plaintiff depositions. *Arch. Intern. Med.* 1994, *154*, 1365–1370.
65. Cipolla, M.; Bonizzi, L.; Zecconi, A. Attitude toward companion animals and breaking bad news: The role of caretakers' attitude and other factors on client-veterinarian communication. *Soc. Anim.* 2015. submitted.
66. Kleen, J.L.; Atkinson, O.; Noordhuizen, J.P. Communication in production animal medicine: Modelling a complex interaction with the example of dairy herd health medicine. *Ir. Vet. J.* 2011, *64*, 8.
67. Jansen, J.; Steuten, C.D.; Renes, R.J.; Aarts, N.; Lam, T.J. Debunking the myth of the hard-to-reach farmer: Effective communication on udder health. *J. Dairy Sci.* 2010, *93*, 1296–1306.
68. Jansen, J.; Lam, T.J. The role of communication in improving udder health. *Vet. Clin. North Am. Food Anim. Pract.* 2012,*28*, 363–379.
69. Jansen, J.; Renes, R.J.; Lam, T.J. Evaluation of two communication strategies to improve udder health management. *J. Dairy Sci.* 2010, *93*, 604–612.
70. Lievaart, J.J.; Noordhuizen, J.P.T.M.; Buckley, D.; Van Winden, S.C.L. The marketing of herd health and production management services on dutch dairy farms: Perceptions of dairy farmers and their veterinary surgeons. *Ir. Vet. J.* 2008,*61*, 668–676.
71. Jansen, J.; van den Borne, B.H.P.; Renes, R.J.; van Schaik, G.; Lam, T.J.G.M.; Leeuwis, C. Explaining mastitis incidence in dutch dairy farming: The influence of farmers' attitudes and behaviour. *Prev. Vet. Med.* 2009, *92*, 210–223.
72. Valeeva, N.I.; Lam, T.J.G.M.; Hogeveen, H. Motivation of dairy farmers to improve mastitis management. *J. Dairy Sci.*2007, *90*, 4466–4477.

73. Kristensen, E.; Jakobsen, E.B. Challenging the myth of the irrational dairy farmer; understanding decision-making related to herd health. *N. Z. Vet. J.* 2011, *59*, 1–7.
74. Cipolla, M.; Zecconi, A. Short communication: Study on veterinarian communication skills preferred and perceived by dairy farmers. *Res. Vet. Sci.* 2015, *99*, 60–62.
75. WHO. Antimicrobial Resistance. Available online: http://www.euro.who.int/en/health-topics/disease-prevention/antimicrobial-resistance (accessed on 17 May 2015).
76. WHO Regional Office for Europe. Tackling antibiotic resistance from a food safety perspective in europe. WHO Regional Office for Europe: Copenhagen, 2011.
77. OIE. Antimicrobial agents and antimicrobial resistance. Available online: http://www.oie.int/our-scientific-expertise/veterinary-products/antimicrobials/ (accessed on 17 May 2015).
78. OIE. Antimicrobial Resistance (AMR). Available online: http://www.oie.int/en/for-the-media/amr/ (accessed on 17 May 2015).
79. EMA. European surveillance of veterinary antimicrobial consumption (ESVAC). Available online: http://www.ema.europa.eu/ema/index.jsp?curl=pages/regulation/document_listing/document_listing_000302.jsp (accessed on 17 May 2015).
80. International Dairy Federation. *Guide to Prudent Use of Antimicrobial Agents in Dairy Production*; International Dairy Federation: Brussels, Belgium, 2013.
81. Federation of Veterinarians of Europe. *Antibiotic Resistance & Prudent Use of Antibiotics in Veterinary Medicine*; FVE: Brussels, Belgium, 2012.
82. FDA. Antimicrobial Resistance. Available online: http://www.fda.gov/AnimalVeterinary/SafetyHealth/AntimicrobialResistance/default.htm (accessed on 17 May 2015).
83. CDC. Antibiotic use in food-producing animals. Available online: http://www.cdc.gov/narms/animals.html (accessed on 17 May 2015).
84. College of Veterinary Medicine, Michigan State University; College of Veterinary Medicine, University of Minnesota. Antimicrobial resistance learning site. Available online: http://amrls.cvm.msu.edu/ (accessed on 17 May 2015).
85. ECDC. European antibiotics awareness day. Available online: http://ecdc.europa.eu/en/eaad/Pages/Home.aspx(accessed on 17 May 2015).
86. ECDC. Antimicrobial resistance. Available online: http://www.ecdc.europa.eu/en/healthtopics/antimicrobial_resistance/Pages/index.aspx (accessed on 17 May 2015).
87. AIFA. Campagne di comunicazione. Available online: http://www.agenziafarmaco.gov.it/it/content/campagne-di-comunicazione-0 (accessed on 17 May 2015).
88. CDC. Get smart about antibiotics week. Available online: http://www.cdc.gov/getsmart/campaign-materials/week/index.html (accessed on 17 May 2015).

89. NPS MedicineWise. Join the fight against antibiotic resistance. Available online: http://www.nps.org.au/about-us/what-we-do/campaigns-events/antibiotic-resistance-fighter (accessed on 17 May 2015).

90. Fletcher, J.; Franz, D.; LeClerc, E. Healthy plants: Necessary for a balanced One Health concept. *Vet. Ita.* 2009, *45*, 79–95.

91. Panseri, S.; Catalano, A.; Giorgi, A.; Arioli, F.; Procopio, A.; Britti, D.; Chiesa, L. Occurrence of pesticide residues in italian honey from different areas in relation to its potential contamination sources. *Food Control* 2014, *38*, 150–156. [CrossRef]

92. Rabinowitz, P.; Scotch, M.; Conti, L. Human and animal sentinels for shared health risks. *Vet. Ita.* 2009, *45*, 23–24.

93. Beasley, V. One Toxicology, ecosystem health and One Health. *Vet. Ita.* 2009, *45*, 97–110.

94. Gibbs, E.P.; Anderson, T.C. One World—One Health' and the global challenge of epidemic diseases of viral aetiology. *Vet. Ita.* 2009, *45*, 35–44.

95. FAO; OIE; WHO; UN System Influenza Coordination; UNICEF; The World Bank. *Contributing to One World, One Health—A Strategic Framework for Reducing Risks of Infectious Diseases at the Animal–Human–Ecosystems Interface*; FAO: Rome, Italy, 2008.

96. FAO. *FAO's Support to the One Health Regional Approach—Towards Integrated and Effective Animal Health—Food Safety Surveillance Capacity Development in Eastern Africa*; FAO: Rome, Italy, 2013.

16
CHAPTER

ENHANCING SURVIVAL OF TRANSPLANTED STEM CELLS IN THE WOUND BED

Alan Wells

Transplantation of stem cells to augment the intrinsic regenerative capacity is a potential therapy for non-healing wounds. However, such approaches have been less than successful, as the majority of introduced cells are lost within days due to cell death from the harsh wound environment that lacks nutrients and presents apoptosis inducing cytokines. A cellular engineering approach to enhanced survival could overcome this obstacle. Activation of the EGF receptor at the cell surface, but not from internalized receptors in the endosomes, promotes cell survival in the face of cellular starvation, death cytokine signaling and toxic agents. The signaling cascade involves tonic low-level activation of Erk MAPK and PI3K/Akt pathways. To achieve this mode of signaling the triggering ligand must be retained in or attached to the substratum or matrix. This can be accomplished by either tethering classical EGF receptor ligands to the substratum or activating the EGF receptor with cryptic ultralow affinity matrikines present in tenascin-C and laminin V. We have creating matrices with or without tethered EGF or tenascin-C. These were introduced into acute full thickness wounds in mice, internal soft tissue in mice (subfascial) and critical cortical bone defects in dogs. In all three instances wound healing and vascularization was significantly increased in the presence of EGF receptor ligand. Xenotransplanted stem cells were retained up to one month in immunocompetent mice, compared to less than a week without the tEGF or tenascin-C. The presence of these cells with the tenascin-C limited scarring in a hypertrophic scar model, even 6 months after wounding, when all the transplanted stem cells have been rejected. The extended survival of these transplanted stem cells allows them to educate the local wound environment and turn the healing towards

Citation: Alan Wells, Enhancing survival of transplanted stem cells in the wound bed, DOI: 10.4172/2157-7013.C1.035.

regeneration and away from non-functional scarring or failure to heal. This represents a new approach to cellular support for dysrepair.

BIOGRAPHY

Alan Wells is an Executive Vice-Chair and Thomas J Gill III Professor of the Departments of Pathology and Bioengineering. He holds an AB in Biochemistry from Brown University (1979), DMSc in Tumor Biology from the Karolinska Institute (1982) and MD from Brown University (1988). Following his studies, he has completed a Postdoctoral Fellowship in Tumor Biology at the University of California in San Francisco, California and a Residency in Laboratory Medicine at the University of California in San Diego, California. He has over 230 scholarly publications that have been cited over 15,000 times. These advances have been recognized by numerous grants, patents and invited keynote talks and professorships, as well as election to the American Society for Clinical Investigation and the American Association of University Pathologists (Pluto Club). He has consulted extensively to industry and has cofounded two companies.

17
CHAPTER

DOGS ON THE FRONT LINE OF CARE: TIMELY INFORMATION FOR FAMILY PHYSICIANS

Mariely Lima and Karine Silva

Recent years have witnessed a surge of interest in the relationship between dogs and human health with a concurrent emergence of new and exciting 'medical' roles for these animals. Not only studies show that owning a pet dog can have prophylactic and therapeutic value, but that incorporating these animals into clinical practice, can have a number of benefits for different types of patients. Dogs can also fill the role of assistants for people with disabilities, bringing important physical, psychological and social positive effects for their handlers, and even be trained to alert to seizures in epileptic patients and to changes in blood sugar levels in diabetics. In light of this, a significant "push" is currently being made by a number of researchers to integrate dogs into mainstream healthcare, notably through family medicine. Data, however, suggest that family physicians do not explicitly enquire their patients about dog ownership and feel uncomfortable to discuss the benefits of acquiring assistance or alert dog, and recommend dog-assisted interventions. In this communication, a timely and comprehensive update on the scientifically stronger evidence supporting the positive effects of dogs for human health will be provided. With it, one aims at calling for the attention of family care practitioners on the clinical potential of pet dogs, namely as motivators for adherence to treatment plans, and on the importance of ensuring their patients knowledge about the possibility of engaging in dog-assisted interventions and/or acquiring an assistance or alert dog.

Citation: Mariely Lima and Karine Silva, Dogs on the front line of care: Timely information for family physicians, DOI: 10.4172/2167-1079.C1.002.

BIOGRAPHY

Mariely Lima completed her degree in Speech Therapy and PhD in Biomedical Sciences. She is an invited Professor at two Universities in Portugal, where she lectures Post-Graduate and Master's courses and supervises academic research. She is a founding member of ÂNIMAS, a Portuguese association, accredited by the Assistance Dogs International, which implements dog-assisted interventions and educates assistance dogs. She has been responsible for a number of dog-assisted activities and therapy programs for individuals with different diagnoses. She has attended different conferences as an invited speaker and published a number of scientific papers in peer-reviewed journals with impact factor.

INDEX

G

H

I

L

M

N

O

P

R

S

T

V

W